CRC SERIES IN AGING

Editors-in-Chief

HANDBOOK OF BIOCHEMISTRY IN AGING
Editor
James Florini, Ph.D.
Department of Biology
Syracuse University
Syracuse, New York

HANDBOOK OF IMMUNOLOGY IN AGING
Editors
Marguerite M. B. Kay, M.D. and
Takashi Makinodan, Ph.D.
Geriatric Research Education and Clinical Center
V.A. Wadsworth Medical Center
Los Angeles, California

SENESCENCE IN PLANTS
Editor
Kenneth V. Thimann, Ph.D.
The Thimann Laboratories
University of California
Santa Cruz, California

HANDBOOK OF PHYSIOLOGY IN AGING
Editor
Edward J. Masoro, Ph.D.
Department of Physiology
University of Texas
Health Science Center
San Antonio, Texas

IMMUNOLOGICAL TECHNIQUES APPLIED TO AGING RESEARCH
Editors
William H. Adler, M.D. and
Albert A. Nordin, Ph.D.
Gerontology Research Center
National Institute on Aging
Baltimore City Hospitals
Baltimore, Maryland

CURRENT TRENDS IN MORPHOLOGICAL TECHNIQUES
Editor
John E. Johnson, Jr., Ph.D.
Gerontology Research Center
National Institute on Aging
Baltimore City Hospitals
Baltimore, Maryland

Additional topics to be covered in this series include Cell Biology of Aging, Microbiology of Aging, Pharmacology of Aging, Evolution and Genetics, Animal Models for Aging Research, Hormonal Regulatory Mechanisms, Detection of Altered Proteins, Insect Models, Lower Invertebrate Models, Testing the Theories of Aging, and Nutritional Approaches to Aging Research.

CRC Handbook of Immunology in Aging

Editors

Marguerite M. B. Kay, M.D.
Chief, Laboratory of Molecular and Clinical Immunology
Geriatric Research, Education, and Clinical Center
V. A. Wadsworth Medical Center and Department of Medicine
University of California
Los Angeles, California

Takashi Makinodan, Ph.D.
Director, Geriatric Research, Education, and Clinical Center
V. A. Wadsworth Medical Center
Los Angeles, California

CRC Series in Aging

Editors-in-Chief

Richard C. Adelman, Ph.D.
Executive Director
Institute on Aging
Temple University
Philadelphia, Pennsylvania

George S. Roth, Ph.D.
Research Chemist
Gerontology Research Center
National Institute on Aging
Baltimore City Hospitals
Baltimore, Maryland

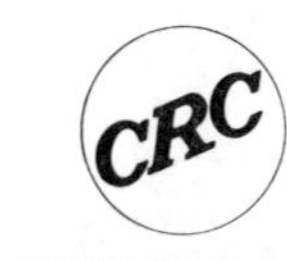

CRC Press, Inc.
Boca Raton, Florida

Library of Congress Cataloging in Publication Data

Main entry under title:

CRC handbook of immunology in aging.
(CRC series in aging)

Bibliography: p.
Includes index.
1. Aging—Immunological aspects—Handbooks, manuals, etc. I. Makinodan, T. II. Kay, Marguerite M. B. III. Chemical Rubber Company. IV. Series. [DNLM: 1. Aging. 2. Immunity—In old age. WT104 C1044]
QP86.C19 612'.67 80-24315
ISBN 0-8493-3144-7 AACR1

This book represents information obtained from authentic and highly regarded sources. Reprinted material is quoted with permission, and sources are indicated. A wide variety of references are listed. Every reasonable effort has been made to give reliable data and information, but the author and the publisher cannot assume responsibility for the validity of all materials or for the consequences of their use.

Direct all inquiries to CRC Press, Inc., 2000 N.W. 24th Street, Boca Raton, Florida 33431.

International Standard Book Number 0-8493-3144-7

Library of Congress Card Number 80-24315
Printed in the United States

FOREWORD

The purpose of this book on aging and immunology is to provide a reference for both investigators in the field and those entering it. Background information essential for understanding the immunobiology of aging is provided in the first six chapters (aging theories, genetics, behavior, homeostatic mechanisms, and development and aging of the immune system).

Areas of immunology which are crucial to understanding human health and disease (diet, immunity and infection, intrinsic and extrinsic immunosuppression, and experimental models for neoplasia) are covered in the next section. These aspects of immunobiology have often been overlooked in the past.

Critical reviews of methods for assessing both cellular and humoral immune function during the aging process are included to assist investigators in selecting techniques for aging studies. The applicability and limitations of these techniques are discussed.

We have included a section on maintenance of animals for aging studies (specific pathogen free [SPF] and germfree animal systems) because an adequate supply of well-characterized animals is an absolute requirement for aging research. Since the maintenance of animals throughout their life span is costly, animal colonies used for aging studies should be protected from infections. Thus, they should be established with pathogen free animals and maintained under barrier conditions. Differences between rodents reared under different environmental conditions are discussed in this section.

In summary, this volume is intended as a reference book for those actively engaged in aging research, those anticipating entering the field, and those who simply desire guidance in evaluating the rationale, strategies, and methodologies employed by investigators in the area of immunobiology of aging. It is our hope that the information contained in this volume will act as catalyst to current research and serve to initiate new interest and new research in the area of aging.

Marguerite M. B. Kay
Los Angeles, California
January 1980

EDITORS-IN-CHIEF

Dr. Richard C. Adelman is currently Executive Director of the Temple University Institute on Aging, Philadelphia, Pa., as well as Professor of Biochemistry in the Fels Research Institute of the Temple University College of Medicine. An active gerontologist for more than 10 years, he has achieved international prominence as a researcher, educator, and administrator. These accomplishments span a broad spectrum of activities ranging from the traditional disciplinary interests of the research biologist to the advocacy, implementation, and administration of multidisciplinary issues of public policy of concern to elderly people.

Dr. Adelman pursued his pre- and postdoctoral research training under the guidance of two prominent biochemists, each of whom is a member of the National Academy of Sciences: Dr. Sidney Weinhouse as Director of the Fels Research Institute, Temple University, and Dr. Bernard L. Horecker as Chairman of the Department of Molecular Biology, Albert Einstein College of Medicine, Bronx, N.Y. His accomplishments as a researcher can be expressed in at least the following ways. He is the author and/or editor of more than 70 publications, including original research papers in referred journals, review chapters, and books. His research efforts have been supported by grants from the National Institutes of Health for the past 10 years, at a current annual level of approximately $300,000. He continues to serve as an invited speaker at seminar programs, symposiums, and workshops all over the world. He is the recipient of the IntraScience Research Foundation Medalist Award, an annual research prize awarded by peer evaluation for major advances in newly emerging areas of the life sciences. He is the recipient of an Established Investigatorship of the American Heart Association.

As an educator, Dr. Adelman is also involved in a broad variety of activities. His role in research training consists of responsibility for pre- and postdoctoral students who are assigned specific projects in his laboratory. He teaches an Advanced Graduate Course on the Biology of Aging, lectures on biomedical aspects of aging to medical students, and is responsible for the biological component of the basic course in aging sponsored by the School of Social Administration. Training activities outside the University include membership in the Faculty of the National Institute on Aging summer course on the Biology of Aging; programs on the biology of aging for AAA's throughout Pennsylvania and Ohio; and the implementation and teaching of Biology of Aging for the Nonbiologist locally, for the Gerontology Society of America and other national organizations, as well as for the International Association of Gerontology.

Dr. Adelman has achieved leadership positions across equally broad areas. Responsibilities of this position include the integration of multidisciplinary programs in research, consultation and education, and health service, as well as advocacy for the University on all matters dealing with aging. He coordinates a city-wide consortium of researchers from Temple University, the Wistar Institute, the Medical College of Pennsylvania, Drexel University, and the Philadelphia Geriatric Center, conducting collaborative research projects, training programs, and symposiums. He was a past President of the Philadelphia Biochemists Club. He serves on the editorial boards of the *Journal of Gerontology, Mechanisms of Ageing and Development, Experimental Aging Research*, and *Gerontological Abstracts.* He was a member of the Biomedical Research Panel of the National Advisory Council of the National Institute on Aging. He chairs a subcommittee of the National Academy of Sciences Committee on Animal Models for Aging Research. As an active Fellow of the Gerontological Society of America, he is a past Chairman of the Biological Sciences section; a past Chairman of the Society Public Policy Committee for which he prepared Congressional testimony and represented the Society on the Leadership Council of the Coalition of National Aging Organizations; and is Secretary-Treasurer of the North American Executive

Committee of the International Association of Gerontology. Finally, as the highest testimony of his leadership capabilities, he continues to serve on National Advisory Committee which impact on diverse key issues dealing with the elderly. These include a 4-year appointment as a member of the NIH Study Section on Pathobiological Chemistry; the Executive Committee of the Health Resources Administration Project on publication of the recent edition of *Working with Older People — A Guide to Practice;* a recent appointment as reviewer of AOA applications fo Career Preparation Programs in Gerontology; and a 4-year appointment on the Veterans Administration Long-Term Care Advisor Council responsible for evaluating their program on Geriatric Research, Education, and Clinical Centers (GRECC).

Dr. George S. Roth is a Research Chemist at the Gerontology Research Center of the National Institute on Aging, Baltimore, Md. Dr. Roth received his B.S. in Biology from Villanova University in 1968 and his Ph.D. in Microbiology from Temple University School of Medicine in 1971. He received postdoctoral training in Biochemistry at the Fels Research Institute in Philadelphia, Pa. Since coming to NIA in 1972, Dr. Roth has also been affiliated with the Graduate Schools of Georgetown University and George Washington University, Washington, D.C.

He is an officer of the Gerontological Society of America, a co-editor of the CRC series, *Methods of Aging Research,* an associate editor of *Neurobiology of Aging,* and a referee for numerous other journals. Dr. Roth has published extensively in the area of hormone action and aging and has lectured throughout the world on this subject.

THE EDITORS

Dr. Marguerite M. B. Kay is Chief of the Laboratory of Molecular and Clinical Immunology, Geriatric Research, Education, and Clinical Center, V.A. Wadsworth Medical Center, and the Department of Medicine, University of California, Los Angeles.

Dr. Kay received her A.B. in Zoology from the University of California, Berkeley, in 1970, and her M.D. from the University of California, San Francisco, in 1974. After six months as a Staff Fellow, National Institute of Child Health and Human Development, Dr. Kay was appointed Chief of the High Resolution Membrane Laboratory and Coordinator, Human Immunoepidemiology Program, Gerontology Research Center, National Institute on Aging, Baltimore, Md., from 1975 to 1977.

Dr. Kay has published more than 50 scientific papers and has been on the Editorial Board of *Mechanisms of Ageing and Development* since 1979. She has been an invited speaker and chairman at numerous international and national meetings and organized national symposia on aging. Her current research interests are in immune aging. T-cell differentiation, physiological autoantibodies and molecular aging, and membrane biology.

Dr. Takashi Makinodan entered the University of Michigan in 1949 and completed his graduate training in 1953 when he received his doctoral degree in zoology and biochemistry. He then became an Associate Biologist at the Biology Division of the Oak Ridge National Laboratory, a position he held until 1957, when he was promoted to Biologist and Head of the Immunology Group at Oak Ridge. In 1972, he was appointed Chief of the Laboratory of Cellular and Comparative Physiology at the Gerontology Research Center, NIA, NIH, Bethesda, Md., a position he held until 1976. Dr. Makinodan then became Director of the Geriatric Research, Education, and Clinical Center at the V.A. Wadsworth Medical Center in Los Angeles, a position he currently holds.

Throughout his career, Dr. Makinodan has been involved in teaching and training. At Oak Ridge National Laboratory, Dr. Makinodan was a lecturer at the University of Tennessee, Oak Ridge Biomedical Graduate School. In 1968, he became a professor of that school, and was also the director of an NICHD-sponsored Training Program in Research on Aging at the University of Tennessee. When at the Gerontology Research Center in Baltimore, Dr. Makinodan was a lecturer at Johns Hopkins University in Advanced Seminars in Immunology. Presently, Dr. Makinodan is a lecturer at the USC School of Gerontology, presenting courses on the biology of aging, and is a Professor of Medicine in Residence at the Department of Medicine, UCLA. He currently supervises and trains graduate and undergraduate biochemistry students.

Dr. Makinodan has had an impressive research career in the biology of aging. His accomplishments include demonstrating the nature and magnitude of the decline in immune response with age. He has published over 150 full-length papers since 1950.

He is a member of the editorial board of many peer-reviewed professional journals; a member of the NIH Study Section, Immunological Sciences; a member of the Steering Committee on Animal Models for Research in Aging, Chairman of the Subcommittee on Mice, National Research Council; and Science Council Member of the Intra-Science Research Foundation. In addition, he is a consultant to several institutes, including the Radiation Effects Research Foundation, Hiroshima, Japan.

ADVISORY BOARD

CONTRIBUTORS

Robert C. Allen, Ph.D.
Professor and Chairman
Department of Laboratory Animal Medicine
Medical University of South Carolina
Charleston, South Carolina

Robin E. Callard, Ph.D.
ICRF Human Tumor Immunology Group
University College Hospital Medical School
London, England

Conrad H. Casavant, Ph.D.
Assistant Director
Immunology Laboratory
Assistant Clinical Professor of Laboratory Medicine
University of California, San Francisco
San Francisco, California

Neal K. Clapp, D.V.M., Ph.D.
Experimental Pathologist
Biology Division
Oak Ridge National Laboratory
Oak Ridge, Tennessee

Nicola Fabris, M.D.
Professor of Immunology
Medical Faculty
University of Pavia
Director Immunology Center
I.N.R.C.A. Research Department
Ancona, Italy

H. Hugh Fudenberg, M.D.
Professor and Chairman
Department of Basic and Clinical Immunology and Microbiology
Professor of Medicine
Medical University of South Carolina
Charleston, South Carolina

Jeffrey E. Galpin, M.D.
Chief, Postgraduate Training in Medicine
Assistant Professor of Medicine, UCLA
Veterans Administration
Department of Infectious Diseases
V.A. Wadsworth Medical Center
Los Angeles, California

Justine S. Garvey, Ph.D.
Professor of Immunochemistry
Syracuse University
Biological Research Laboratories
Syracuse, New York

Chou C. Hong, D.V.M., Ph.D.
Associate Professor and Vice Chairman
Department of Laboratory Animal Medicine
Medical University of South Carolina
Charleston, South Carolina

Julian R. Pleasants, Ph.D.
Associate Professor of Microbiology
University of Notre Dame
Notre Dame, Indiana

Diana M. Popp, B.S., M.T.
Research Associate
Biology Division
Oak Ridge National Laboratory
Oak Ridge, Tennessee

Raymond A. Popp, Ph.D.
Senior Research Biologist
Biology Division
Oak Ridge National Laboratory
Oak Ridge, Tennessee

David V. Safranski, M.S.
Research Instructor
Department of Foods and Nutrition
Purdue University
West Lafayette, Indiana

Richard L. Sprott, Ph.D.
Health Scientist Administrator
Division of Research Resources
National Institutes of Health
Bethesda, Maryland

Daniel P. Stites, M.D.
Director, Immunology Laboratory
Associate Professor of Laboratory Medicine and Medicine
University of California, San Francisco
San Francisco, California

Bernard L. Strehler, Ph.D.
Professor of Biology
Molecular Biology Division
University of Southern California
University Park
Los Angeles, California

Marvin L. Tyan, M.D.
Professor of Medicine
Department of Medicine
UCLA School of Medicine and Medical
and Research Services
V.A. Wadsworth Medical Center
Los Angeles, California

Ronald Ross Watson, Ph.D.
Associate Professor of Nutrition and
Immunology
Department of Foods and Nutrition
Purdue University
West Lafayette, Indiana

DEDICATION

To: This book is dedicated with respect and affection to my mentor, Dr. Fred Wilt, Professor of Zoology, University of California, Berkeley.

For: my Students . . .

Marguerite M. B. Kay
Los Angeles, California
January 1980

TABLE OF CONTENTS

General Topics

AGING THEORIES AND IMMUNOLOGICAL SENESCENCE: PERSPECTS AND PROSPECTS*

Bernard L. Strehler

INTRODUCTION

Among the almost universal properties of highly evolved forms of life is the process of aging, a process which colors nearly all human activities and attitudes. Interest in the causes of aging is as old as recorded human history and together with love, death, and curiosity about the future and the nature of selfness is the focus of much of humanity's great literary, artistic, musical, and philosophical creativity. It seems likely that the basic causes of the aging process in humans will be understood within the next decades and that this knowledge will give man at least some measure of control over the rate of the process and thereby add healthful years to the human life span. Individuals may differ about the personal or social desirability of such effects of scientific inquiry, but it is almost as inevitable as sin that, like it or not, future generations will be faced with the additional problems and potentialities that an increase in healthy life span will confer on them. This insight into the future implies an obligation on present societies to anticipate these new problems and to devise solutions for them.

Any rational discussion of a complex biological phenomenon makes at least an operational definition of the underlying process desirable, so as to have a common conceptual base for research and to avoid needless confusion or mindless controversy. It should be remembered, though, that a definition of a phenomenon only partially understood is just an arbitrary assignment of qualities to such an entity or process, and that the usefulness of a definition is only as good as is its consistency with existing experimental observations and common sense. Nevertheless, it is desirable to pose a working definition before theories of aging, particularly as they impinge on the mechanisms of immune failure during aging, are discussed.

Definition

Aging may conveniently be defined as that set of deteriorative processes which (a) occurs primarily after reproductive maturity is reached[1-3] and (b) which processes have the following four properties in common:

Universality — These processes occur in all members of a species.

Intrinsicality — Built into the genetic makeup of a species and can at best only be modified by environmental influences.

Progressiveness — Occur gradually with the passage of time, rather than as discrete events such as specific disease episodes. Aging is thus a *process* rather than an *event*. (For these purposes, a process is defined as the cumulative effect of many separate molecular-cellular events.)

Deleteriousness — Aging processes *reduce* the functional capacity of an aging system to withstand challenges from the environment or from within the system; they also eventually cause the system to succumb to even a minor challenge to its existence.

General Postulates on the Origins of Aging

Weismann[4] and more recently others have postulated that aging, per se, serves an evolutionary function. This thesis is difficult to defend because no one has yet pro-

* Work supported in part by NASA grant NSF7367 and by gifts from Mrs. B. Hubbard, Mrs. J. Barnett, and the Glenn Foundation.

posed a mechanism through which a limited life span has an evolutionary benefit, except perhaps in very special cases where it improves the chances of reproduction or survival of a species. Examples which fall into this category are the sudden senescence of salmon and the regular regression (every 4 days) of the individual hydra-like bodies in colonial coelenterates such as *Campanularia flexuosa.* These species seem to be the exception to the rule for the simple reason that the evolutionary trend among land animals (vertebrates) is selection for ever increasing longevity. Mutation and sexual reproduction (and the recombination of genetic materials it permits) provide quite adequate means for evolutionary progress and it has therefore been concluded that the Weismannian thesis is in fact a circular argument, a view emphasized by Comfort[5] in his excellent monograph.

In this writer's opinion, the key to the nearly universal presence of the aging process in higher animals lies in a suggestion by an English physician, Bidder.[6] Bidder proposed that aging is a harmful side effect of the fact that land animals, at least, have a species-specific optimum size. A mouse the size of an elephant would be a most fragile giant and an elephant the size of a mouse would be at best awkward and be unable to survive in a cat-ridden environment. Therefore, the very simple idea that a fixed body size has as a (pleiotropic) side effect a limited lifetime is both logical and consistent with observation. A detailed analysis of pleiotropy and the genetics of aging was presented some years ago by Williams.[7]

Second, the usual mechanism that limits body size is the arresting of growth, usually through the arrest of mitosis of key body cells as maturity is reached. In some cases, such as in the nervous system, cell division is arrested for still another pleiotropic reason — namely, that a continually growing brain would have grave deficits in memory retention, certainly a key function of the organ called the brain.[8] Experimental proof that long-term memory retention is better in adult animals than in growing ones was provided by Campbell.[9]

Given the above two concepts, one would expect that the primary, possibly even exclusive, sites of age-dependent declines in function are to be found in *post-mitotic cell types.* That this is consistent with observation is documented in Reference 10.

A fourth generalization is that although aging occurs in many different cell types, it is likely that very similar processes, if not identical ones, underly this deterioration in different cells and species and that no single system is more likely to fail than others. The reason, as Williams[7] pointed out, is that evolutionary forces tend to select against any dominant source of age-related failure. Thus, animals without major inheritable diseases are not unlike O. W. Holmes' "Wonderful One-Hoss Shay"!

The fifth generalization is that longevity among primates has evolved at an unprecedented rate. During the last 2 to 5 million years there has been at least a doubling of maximum life span potential, compared to that our prehominid ancestors possessed. This remarkably high rate of evolution of longevity has been variously interpreted,[11,12] but one newly suggested possibility is that the social structures of the prehominid tribes led to the polygamous dominance of one or a very few males with respect to fathering of the next generation.[13] One effect of such polygamous practices is to *greatly accelerate the rate at which even slight selective advantages of new genes or gene combinations can become predominant in the gene pool of a species.* Thus, the still present, though socially disapproved inclination of male humans to engage in polygamy, albeit secretly or successively, perhaps reflects specific evolved social qualities which were a major factor in man's rapid rise to preminence and dominance on this globe. Straightforward population genetics analyses indicate that, in the presence of polygamous practices, the rate of evolution of longevity (and of intelligence) may be increased by factors of 50 to 100 over what would be anticipated if random, monogamous reproduction were the rule.[13]

The hypothesis set forth by Sacher,[11] and subsequently by Cutler[12] in greater detail, holds that modern man differs from prehominid ancestors of a few million years ago by only a few dozen to a few hundred adaptive genes. But polygamy may well have provided a means through which many thousands of longevity and intelligence-conferring genetic changes (mutations) could have become incorporated in relatively brief evolutionary time spans.

The above paragraphs set forth the main theses upon which the following analysis of specific theories of aging is based.

CATEGORIZATION OF AGING THEORIES

In the interest of clarity, the various theories of aging are subdivided here into three major groupings, each of which will be described separately. These categories are (a) cellular-molecular theories, (b) systemic deterioration theories, and (c) focal "death clock" theories.

Cellular-Molecular Theories of Aging

Cellular-molecular theories of aging may be further subdivided into two different categories, *depletional* theories and *accumulational* theories. The first of these is based on the concept that during aging important components necessary for life are lost or eroded with use and is derivative of the Pearl-Rubner hypothesis.[14,15] The second, the accumulation theories postulate the accretion, during aging, of various kinds of substances which interfere with cell function.

Depletional Theories

Among the most important of the depletional theories of aging are those that have to do with the loss of genetic information due to genetic instability. This concept was first set forth by Henshaw et al.[16] about 1947 and was restated in various forms, particularly by Curtis,[17,18] during the 1960s. The essence of this theory is that aging is due to the accumulation of damage to DNA (i.e., either a depletion of or change in the structure of the genetic material). The primary argument against a simple mutational hypothesis is the fact that the amount of mutagen (e.g., radiation) required to shorten the life span of an animal appreciably is much greater — by a factor of 12 to 20 — than that required to double the dose of measurable mutations as detected through chromosomal abnormalities. Specifically, the dose of radiation that is required to produce an entire lifetime's dose of chromosomal aberrations in liver cells of mice is about 65 R equivalents; this dose actually enhances the life span of at least some experimental species, including the laboratory mouse. A variant of this theory, however, does appear to be valid. Namely, it has been shown that the apparent dose of redundant copies of rDNA sequences, absolutely essential to optimal cell function, decrease substantially during aging[19,20] (see Figure 1).

A second depletional theory is related to the concept that the translational ability of cells is modified during development and subsequent aging and that this "modulation" in codon usage is a primary cause of ultimate senescence. Simply stated, the idea embraced in the quote "Codon Restriction Theory of Aging"[21] is that the messages produced by specific cells use particular combinations of codons and that the cell must be able to translate every codon in a message in order to form the completed product — a relatively obvious conclusion. Evidence relating the codon restriction theory to aging has been presented elsewhere,[1,3] as it demonstrates that during the aging of cotyledons, at least, there is a loss of ability completely to amino-acylate certain tRNA species. Table 1 shows the substantial restriction of codon usages in specific messages.

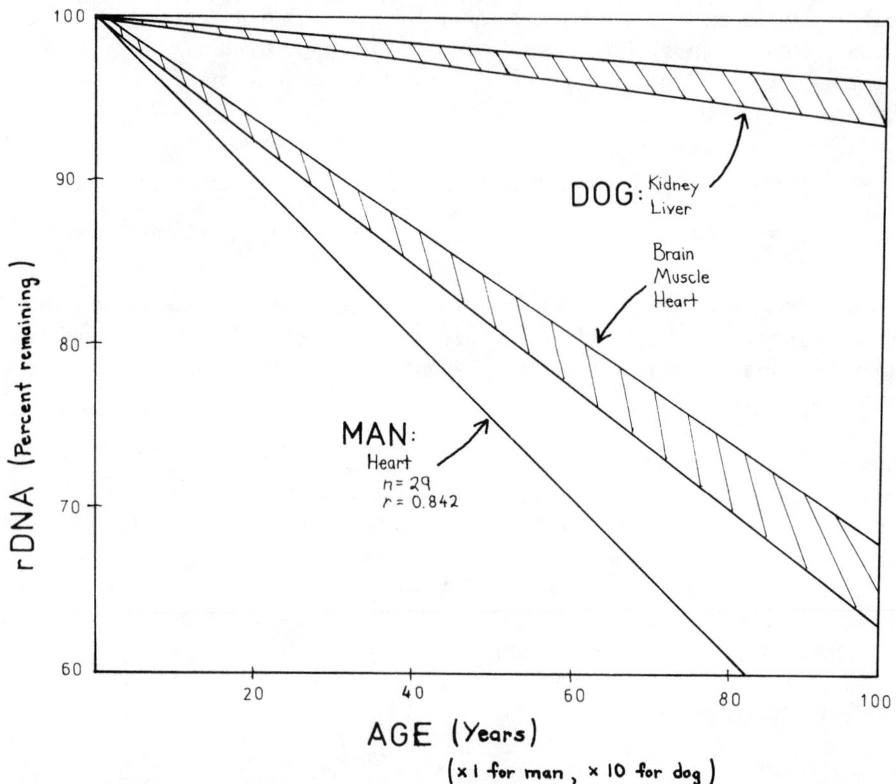

FIGURE 1.. Evidence for loss of rDNA genes in human myocardium during aging. The values of tritium counts for each of the three samples run concurrently in separate experiments (including one young, one old, and one middle-aged specimen) were averaged and the values obtained were normalized to 100% at the average age of the three samples. The regression line was calculated from a least squares fit, assuming linear regression. The regression was highly significant. The actual percent hybridization was about 0.08% at age 40.[20]

Note that similar cells from different species have similar codon usages, but that messages from dissimilar cells from the same species differ in their codon usages.[22-26]

A third theory is that of "mitotic exhaustion", a depletion of the reserve capacity of cells to undergo mitosis. This theory is quite consistent with the in vitro observations of Hayflick[27,28] who noted that only a limited number of divisions is possible in cell culture. It was also shown that the number of divisions that can take place under culture conditions is a direct function of the life span of the source tissue.[29] Although this is an attractive hypothesis and the observations on the number of divisions which fibroblasts are capable of undergoing under culture conditions is slightly dependent on the age of the donor,[30] one major objection to the theory is that the culture conditions may not be appropriate to the continued division potential of cells. Of particular interest in this regard is the recent discovery of Doldavsky et al.[31] that the division potential of endothelial cells derived from the vascular system are capable of indefinite numbers of replications in the presence of an appropriate growth factor. However, when this growth factor is omitted they have the Hayflick-type limitation in division potential.

Table 1
CODON USAGE IN VARIOUS EUKARYOTIC mRNA MESSAGES

			RA[a]	RB[b]	HB[c]	RPGH[d]	HCS[e]	OVA[f]	VLCM[g]	IM[h]	INS[i]
UUU	= 1	= PH1	—	3	5	6	2	11	2	1	1
UUC	= 2	= PH2	8	5	3	6(1)	8	9	4(1)	2	2
UUA	= 3	= LU1	—	—	—	1	—	3	1(1)	—	—
UUG	= 4	= LU2	1	—	—	2	—	4	—	2	1
CUU	= 5	= LU3	—	—	—	1	—	8	1(1)	—	2
CUC	= 6	= LU4	2	2	3	6(2)	7	6	6(2)	1	3
CUA	= 7	= LU5	—	—	—	—	3	1	2(2)	1	—
CUG	= 8	= LU6	14	16	14	15(4)	11	10	3	—	8
AUU	= 9	= IL1	—	1	—	3	2	6	2	2	1
AUC	= 10	= IL2	3	—	—	5	5	16	1(1)	2	1
AUA	= 11	= IL3	—	—	—	—	—	3	3	1	—
AUG	= 12	= MEU	1	2	2	6(1)	5	17	2(2)	1	—
GUU	= 13	= VA1	—	4	2	—	—	9	4	—	1
GUC	= 14	= VA2	—	2	3	2	1	7	2	3	2
GUA	= 15	= VA3	—	—	—	—	—	5	—	2	—
GUG	= 16	= VA4	10	12	13	2	4	10	1(1)	2	5
UCU	= 17	= SR1	3	3	—	0(1)	2	10	3(1)	1	—
UCC	= 18	= SR2	4	3	3?	3	5	5	2(1)	6	2
UCA	= 19	= SR3	—	—	—	2	1	7	5	4	—
UCG	= 20	= SR4	—	—	—	2	4	1	—	—	—
CCU	= 21	= PR1	1	3	5	1(1)	—	6	2	1	2
CCC	= 22	= PR2	5	—	—	5(1)	2	1	—	4	2
CCA	= 23	= PR3	—	1	2	1	1	7	2	5	1
CCG	= 24	= PR4	1	—	—	—	1	—	—	—	2
ACU	= 25	= TH1	2	2	3	1(1)	1	4	8(1)	5	—
ACC	= 26	= TH2	10	2	3	7(1)	5	4	4(1)	10	2
ACA	= 27	= TH3	—	—	1	—	3	7	4(3)	3	1
ACG	= 28	= TH4	—	—	—	—	2	—	—	2	—
GCU	= 29	= AL1	1	7	7?	7(3)	—	10	7	2	3
GCC	= 30	= AL2	10	6	7	8	2	9	4	3	3
GCA	= 31	= AL3	—	1	1	1(1)	1	16	4	2	1
GCG	= 32	= AL4	2	1	—	2	0	—	—	—	—
UAU	= 33	= TY1	2	1	2	4	4	3	2	2	—
UAC	= 34	= TY2	1	2	1	3	4	7	2(2)	5	3
UAA	= 35	= STP	1	—	1	—	—	1	—	—	—
UAG	= 36	= STP	—	—	—	1	1	—	—	—	—
CAU	= 37	= HS1	1	4	2	—	2	4	2	1	—
CAC	= 38	= HS2	10	5	7	3	2	3	—(1)	2	2
CAA	= 39	= GN1	—	—	—	1(1)	2	8	1	2	3
CAG	= 40	= GN2	1	4	3	12(1)	7	7	3	2	5
AAU	= 41	= AN1	1	4	1	2	1	10	—(1)	3	—
AAC	= 42	= AN2	3	4	5	3	6	7	3	8	3
AAA	= 43	= LY1	2	3	3	3	1	11	1	6	1
AAG	= 44	= LY2	10	9	8	8	8	9	1	10	2
GAU	= 45	= AS1	—	1	4	1	1	6	4	3	2
GAC	= 46	= AS2	7	3	3	9(1)	13	6	2(1)	2	1
GAA	= 47	= GL1	3	4	2	4	5	18	2	1	2
GAG	= 48	= GL2	4	6	6	10(1)	8	15	1	1	7
UGU	= 49	= CY1	—	1	2	2	1	5	2(2)	1	2
UGC	= 50	= CY2	1	—	—	2(1)	3	1	1	1	4
UGA	= 51	= STP	—	1	—	—	—	—	—	—	1
UGG	= 52	= TRP	1	2	2	1(2)	1	3	4(2)	1	1
CGU	= 53	= AR1	1	—	—	2	—	—	—	—	4
CGC	= 54	= AR2	—	—	—	6	4	2	1	—	—
CGA	= 55	= AR3	—	—	—	1	—	—	1	1	—
CGG	= 56	= AR4	1	—	—	1	2	—	—	2	1
AGU	= 57	= SR5	1	4	2	1	1	6	3(2)	1	—

Table 1 (continnued)
CODON USAGE IN VARIOUS EUKARYOTIC mRNA MESSAGES

	RA[a]	RB[b]	HB[c]	RPGH[d]	HCS[e]	OVA[f]	VLCM[g]	IM[h]	INS[i]
AGC = 58 = SR6	3	—	—	6(1)	4	9	2	5	1
AGA = 59 = AR5	—	—	—	1	—	10	1(3)	—	—
AGG = 60 = AR6	1	3	3	1	3	3	—	1	—
GGU = 61 = GY1	1	4	4	1(1)	—	3	6(1)	1	3
GGC = 62 = GY2	8	6	8	3	4	8	1(1)	2	2
GGA = 63 = GY3	—	—	—	1	—	6	3(1)	1	1
GGG = 64 = GY4	—	1	1	3	3	2	2	—	2

[a] RA = Rabbit α chain.
[b] RB = Rabbit β chain.
[c] HB = Human β chain.
[d] RPGH = Rat pregrowth hormone (parenthentical numbers not in final product).
[e] HCS = Human chorioallantoic somatotropin.
[f] OVA = Chick ovalbumin.
[g] VLCM = Variable light chain mouse (numbers in parentheses are present in part of constant chain coding region).
[h] IM = Mouse immunoglobulin.
[i] INS = Rat insulin.

A fourth general "depletional" hypothesis which has not been subjected to any extensive experimental study is the gradual hydrolysis of nonreplenishing components in cells. Because the DNA, RNA, proteins, polysaccharides, and fats cells contain are all synthesized through the removal of water from between precursor molecules (a process that requires the expenditure of energy), nearly all, if not all, biological molecules are inherently unstable in an aqueous environment (i.e., within cells.) Therefore, it is to be expected that hydrolysis including depurination, chain scission, etc., of DNA will occur in all biomacromolecules at some rate during aging, particularly in nondividing cells whose DNA is not replenished. The degree to which this interferes with function is not known, but it is interesting that Makinodan et al.[32] have demonstrated that there is an *increased* capacity of denatured DNA in brain tissue sections to act as a template for RNA polymerase, an observation which is consistent with the concept that hydrolysis-fragmentation of DNA may be important in aging.

A fifth possiblity is the stereo-isomerization of amino acids in long-lived proteins from the l to the d form. This process has been documented in tooth- and eye-lens proteins by Bada et al.[33] of the Scripps Institute, although evidence on this is still essentially lacking as to whether the rates of racemizaton are sufficiently high to contribute to the decrease in function which is observed in post-mitotic tissues.

A sixth possibility suggested by the work of Robinson[34] is the deamidination of the amino acids asparagine and glutamine, particularly in proteins that are not subject to rapid turnover. Robinson used model systems and showed that the half-life of the amide linkage at the terminus of the R group of these two amino acids is sufficiently short that major changes in nonreplenishing enzymes and structural proteins may well occur during aging.

Related to this concept is the depletion of active enzymes as the result of reduced rate of turnover in important proteins. This hypothesis is consistent with the observations of the Gershons[35,36] since confirmed by others[37,38] that the specific activity (i.e., the number of catalytic events per second per unit enzyme) decreases with age, at least in the case of some enzymes.

Denaturation is a final possibility to be listed here. This is the potential denaturation of protein catalysts in post-mitotic cells through thermal accidents and otherwise. No substantial evidence is available either to contradict or support this hypothesis.[39]

Accumulational Theories

This group of theories suggests that there is an accumulation of ineffectual biological materials in cells as they age.

The most well-documented example of such an accumulation is the gradual accretion of so-called age pigments in post-mitotic cells such as heart, brain, etc.[40-43] It is of particular interest that the amount of such waste products (also known as lipofuscin) may be sufficient to occupy up to 75% of the intracellular volume of large neurons in the brain.[44] Moreover, Mann and Yates[45] have shown that the amount of ribosomal RNA which is present in such cells decreases in rough proportion to the accumulation of age pigments.

A second major category is the accumulation of errors, particularly errors in the translational apparatus as first suggested by Medvedev[46] and later more concisely stated by Orgel et al.[47] The essential concept is that if certain kinds of errors should occur in the transcriptional or translational apparatus of a cell, a delayed effect of certain such errors will be a self-reinforcing accumulation of further errors. Although some evidence has been presented[48] which is consistent with this theory, Orgel has presented evidence that there is a low probability that it applies in real systems. Moreover, Popp et al.[49] have shown that misrepresentation errors do *not* increase during age as measured in β-hemoglobin chains derived from individuals of different ages.

Cell surface changes are among the most important of changes that occur during aging. These are changes in cell surfaces, e.g., in the numbers and kinds of mitotic repressor substances, in the receptor proteins for various hormones, and in phagocytic recognition sites. For example, it has recently been shown[50] that the amount of certain mitogens which are capable of binding to the membranes of clonally aged cells increases with age and this is consistent with the concept that mitotic inhibitors become irreversibly bound to cells, even cells which are slowly undergoing mitosis. The responsivity of the endocrine system is also decreased with time, particularly as shown by Adelman in the response of the intact aging-rodent pancreatic β-cells to a glucose challenge.[51,52] Kay[53] has demonstrated the interesting fact that, in aged erythrocytes, antigens are exposed which react with circulating auto-antibodies to these substances — thus leading to selective phagocytosis of "old" red cells.

A fourth category of accumulation theories is that of accumulation of viruses of various types. It is known that certain diseases (such as Kuru which previously was endemic to certain parts of New Guinea[54]) lead to an early deterioration — at age 30 to 40 — of infected individuals. Similar so-called slow viruses may also well be present in other groups of humans, but take a longer time to express themselves. For example, Alzheimer's disease, so-called presenile dementia, may be a reflection of a similar kind of viral effect. There is evidence for the accumulation of viral particles in various species including Drosophila as is shown by Miquel.[55]

One of the most popular accumulation theories of aging has to do with the accumulation of cross-linkages in collagen.[56-59] Cross-linkages, of course, are involved in the formation of age pigments, but at least some collagen cross-linkages are probably in a different category in that they are part of the process of maturation of collagen. However, some kinds of collagen, such as those which are constituents of the basement membranes and of glomeruli may be very important (should they become cross-linked) in impeding the flow of waste products between parenchymal cells and the vasculature.

Systemic Theories of Aging

In contrast to the above "accumulational" and "depletional" theories, some workers have suggested that aging occurs because of ineffectual communication between different kinds of cells in different parts of the body. The systems in which such secondary effects of changes at the cell-molecular level are probably particularly important include the endocrine system, the neural system (including the brain), and the immunological system; all of which are involved in the transmission of information from one portion of an organism to another.

There is certainly good evidence that endocrine decline occurs with aging particularly, as shown in Figure 2, with respect to the beginning of so-called adult-onset diabetes as measured through glucose tolerance tests. Neural functions and particularly neural-endocrine functions mediated through the hypothalamic-pituitary axis are also of importance, particularly those that occur during menopause.

Of crucial importance is the aging of the immune system. This functional decline appears to be the key to the gradual decrease in the body's ability to coordinate its defenses against exogenous agents such as viruses, including oncogenic viruses and pathogenic bacteria as well as transformed (neoplastic) cells. Evidence for immunological decline with aging will be discussed in depth by other contributors to this volume and will therefore not be reviewed at this time. A crucial point, however, is that the key site of immunological decline with age appears to be in the T-cell population (i.e., thymus-derived cells) and that it is the lack of responsiveness of T-cells to novel challenges which is responsible for the increased susceptibility of aged animals and humans to death from infections and perhaps from neoplastic diseases.

"Death Clock" Theories

Finally there is a group of theories which have as their central concept the idea that a sort of "death clock" exists. This hypothetical death clock is a device of unknown location which triggers a group of deteriorative responses once an animal has reached a particular age. Examples that have been cited include the rapid change in the structure and metabolism of migrating salmon as they return to their natal mating grounds—a change which appears to be mediated by the pituitary. Other sites of death clocks have also been suggested including the neural complex called the limbic system. Alternatively, ineffectual limbic interactions with the hypothalamic-pituitary axis have been suggested or implicated. It is of interest that some diseases such as Parkinsonism, which occurs at approximately 40 to 50 years of age, are, as pointed out by Finch, in some important respects, close mimics of the aging process per se. In normal humans and laboratory animals there is a gradual decrease in the amount of dopaminergic substances produced, and it is for this reason that the administration of L-Dopa is effective in counteracting some Parkinsonian symptoms and in reversing some reproductive age changes.

SUMMARY

It seems likely that the essential sources of aging will be uncovered in the coming decades. Aging processes have a number of functions in common: (1) intrinsicality, (2) universality, (3) progressiveness, and (4) deleteriousness. The major sites of deteriorative change are in the nonreplenishing components, particularly in nondividing cells. These changes are of two major kinds: depletional and accumulational, respectively. Loss of redundant DNA, particularly of rDNA, and accumulation of age pigments are probably key examples. Aging at the molecular-cellular level also exerts itself in decreased communication efficiency between different cell types. The genetic mechanisms that determine species longevity are subject to evolutionary selection and may, in part at least, depend on loss of ability to translate specific code words as cells mature

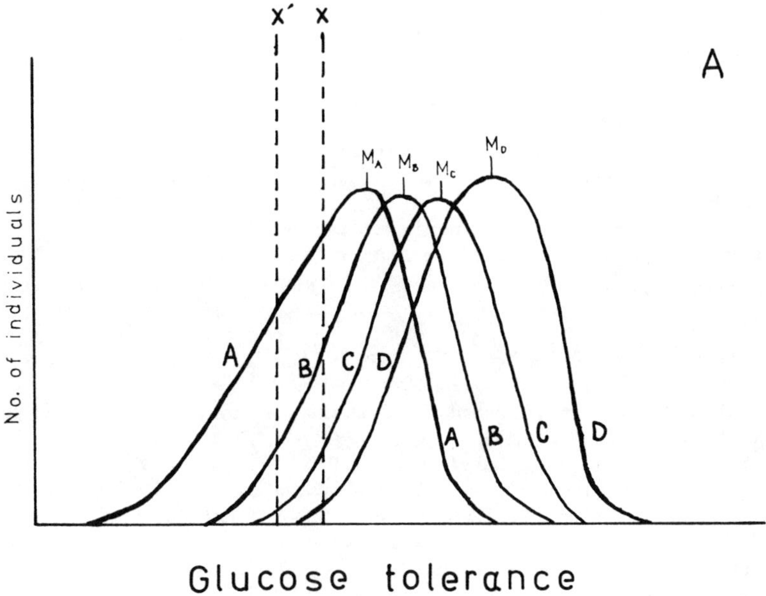

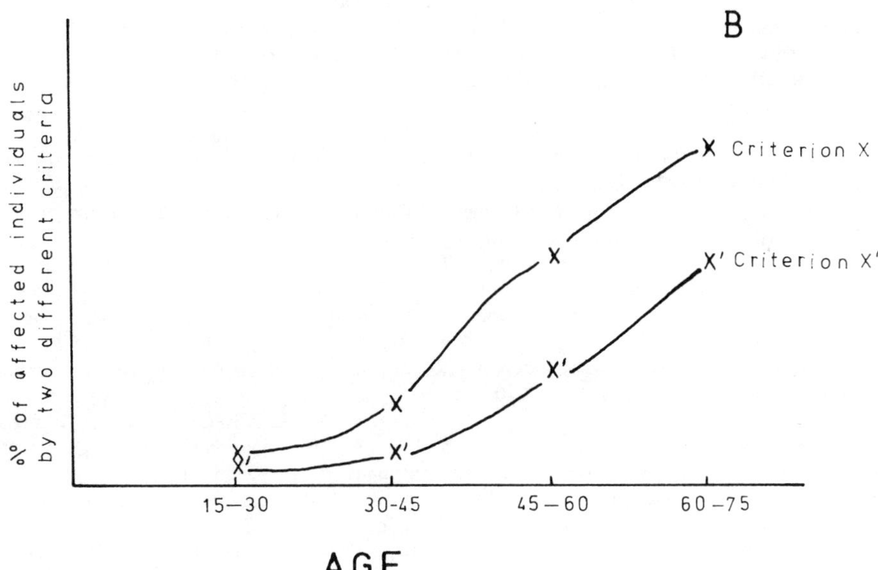

FIGURE 2. A — Diagrammatic representation of glucose tolerance test score distributions in various age groups. B — Percentage of individual diagnosed as "adult-onset" diabetics when individuals falling below criterion X′ or X are tabulated. Ages of different population groups: A — 60—75; B — 45—60; C — 30—45; D — 15—30. X′, X are "arbitrary" criteria for diabetic state. Notes: (1) Juvenile diabetics are excluded, (2) the distributions at each age group are essentially Maxwellian, (3) the mean values decrease with age, and (4) the percent of "diabetics" increases more rapidly than glucose tolerance (mean values) falls.[60]

with age. Particular sites for life-limiting "death clocks" have been proposed, but evidence regarding these hypotheses is inconclusive.

REFERENCES

1. **Medawar, P. B.,** *An Unsolved Problem of Biology,* Lewis, London, 1951.
2. **Strehler, B. L.,** Origin and comparison of the effects of time and high-energy radiations on living systems, *Q. Rev. Biol.,* 34, 117, 1959.
3. **Strehler, B.,** *Time, Cells and Aging,* 1st ed., Academic Press, New York, 1962.
4. **Weismann, A.,** *Essays Upon Heredity and Kindred Biological Problems,* Oxford University Press, New York, 1891.
5. **Comfort, A.,** *The Biology of Senescence,* Rinehart, New York, 1956.
6. **Bidder, G. P.,** The mortality of plaice, *Nature (London),* 115, 495, 1925.
7. **Williams, G. C.,** Pleiotropy, natural selection and the evolution of senescence, *Evolution,* 11, 398, 1957.
8. **Strehler, B.,** Molecular and systemic aspects of brain aging: psychobiology of informational redundancy, in *Neurobiology of Aging,* Terry, R. and Gershon, S., Eds., Raven Press, New York, 1976, 281.
9. **Campbell, B. and Campbell, E. H.,** Retention and extinction of learned fear in infant and adult rats, *J. Comp. Physiol. Psychol.,* 55, 1, 1962.
10. **Strehler, B.,** *Time, Cells and Aging,* 2nd ed., Academic Press, New York, 1977.
11. **Sacher, G. A.,** Maturation and longevity in relation to cranial capacity in hominid evolution, in *Antecedents of Man and After,* Vol. 1, Tuttle, A., Ed., Mouton, The Hague, 1975, 417.
12. **Cutler, R. G.,** Evolution of human longevity and the genetic complexity governing aging rate, *Proc. Natl. Acad. Sci. U.S.A.,* 72, 4664, 1975.
13. **Strehler, B.,** Polygamy and the evolution of human longevity, *Mech. Ageing Dev.,* 9, 369, 1979.
14. **Rubner, N.,** Probleme des Wachstums und der Lebensdauer, *Mitt. Gesch. Inn. Med. Wein.,* 7 (Suppl. 9), 58, 1908.
15. **Alpatov, W. W. and Pearl, R.,** Experimental studies on the duration of life. XII. Influence of temperature during the larval period and adult life on the duration of life of the imago of Drosophila melanogaster, *Am. Nat.,* 63, 37, 1929; *Biol. Abstr.,* 4, No. 21461, 1930.
16. **Henshaw, P. S., Riley, E. R., and Stapleton, G. E.,** The biological effects of pile radiation, *Radiology,* 49, 349, 1947.
17. **Curtis, H. J.,** *Biological Mechanisms of Aging,* Charles C Thomas, Springfield, Ill., 1966.
18. **Curtis, H. J. and Crowley, C.,** Chromosome aberrations in liver cells in relation to the somatic mutation theory of aging, *Radiat. Res.,* 19, 337, 1963.
19. **Johnson, L. K., Johnson, R. W., and Strehler, B.,** Cardiac hypertrophy, aging and changes in cardiac ribosomal RNA gene dosage in man, *J. Mol. Cell. Cardiol.,* 7, 125, 1975.
20. **Strehler, B., Johnson, L. K., and Chang, M. P.,** Substantial loss of ribosomal DNA obtained from aging human myocardium, *Mech. Ageing Dev.,* 11, 6, in press.
21. **Strehler, B., Hirsch, G., Gusseck, D., Johnson, R., and Bick, M.,** The codon-restriction theory of aging and development, *J. Theor. Biol.,* 33, 429, 1971.
22. **Efstratiadis, A., Kafatos, F., and Maniatis, T.,** The primary structure of rabbit beta-globin mRNA as determined from cloned DNA, *Cell,* 10, 571, 1977.
23. **McReynolds, L., O'Malley, B. W., Nisbet, A. D., Fothergill, J. E., Givel, D., Fields, S., Robertson, M., and Brownlee, G. G.,** Sequence of chick ovalbumin mRNA, *Nature, (London),* 273, 723, 1978.
24. **Baralle, F.,** The nucleotide sequence of human beta globin mRNA, *Cell,* 12, 1085, 1977.
25. **Shine, J., Seeburg, P., Baxter, J. D., and Goodman, H. M.,** Human Chorionic Somatomammotropin: construction and analysis of recombinant DNA, in press.
26. **Shine, J., Seeburg, P. H., Martial, J., Baxter, J. D., and Goodman, H. M.,** Nucleotide sequence of rat growth hormone mRNA and amino acid sequence of rat pre-growth hormone, *Nature (London),* 270, 489, 1977.
27. **Hayflick, L.,** The limited in vitro lifetime of human diploid cell strains, *Exp. Cell Res.,* 37, 614, 1965.
28. **Hayflick, L.,** Current theories of biological aging, *Fed. Proc. Fed. Am. Soc. Exp. Biol.,* 34, 9, 1975.
29. **Hay, R. J., Menzies, R. A., Morgan, H. P., and Strehler, B. L.,** The division potential of cells in continuous growth as compared to cells subcultivated after maintenance in stationary phase, *Exp. Gerontol.,* 35, 44, 1967.
30. **Martin, G. M., Sprague, C. A., and Epstein, C. J.,** Replicative life-span of cultivated human cells: effects of donors' age, tissue and genotype, *Lab. Invest.,* 23, 86, 1970.
31. **Doldavsky, I., Johnson, L. K., Greenburg, G., and Gospodarowicz, D.,** Vascular endothelial cells grown in the absence of fibroblast growth factor undergo structural and functional alterations that are incompatible with their in vivo differentiated properties, in press.
32. **Makinodan, T., Price, G. B., and Modak, S. P.,** *Science,* 171, 917, 1971.
33. **Bada, J. L.,** *Abs. Pap. ACS,* 30, 171, 1977.

34. **Robinson, A.**, personal communication.
35. **Gershon, H. and Gershon, D.**, Detection of inactive enzyme molecules in aging organisms, *Nature (London)*, 227, 1214, 1970.
36. **Gershon, H. and Gershon, D.**, Altered enzyme molecules in senescent organisms: mouse muscle aldolase, *Mech. Ageing Dev.*, 2, 33, 1973.
37. **Reiss, U. and Rothstein, M.**, Age related changes in isocitric lyase from the free living nematode Turbatrix aceti, *J. Biol. Chem.*, 250, 826, 1975.
38. **Rothstein, M.**, Aging and the alteration of enzymes, *Mech. Ageing Dev.*, 4, 325, 1975.
39. **Strehler, B. L.**, Studies on the comparative physiology of aging. II. On the mechanism of temperature life shortening in *Drosophila melanogaster, J. Gerontol.*, 16, 2, 1961.
40. **Strehler, B. L., Mark, D., Mildvan, A. S., and Gee, M.**, Rate and magnitude of age pigment accumulation in the human myocardium, *J. Gerontol.*, 14, 430, 1959.
41. **Reichel, W., Hollander, J., Clark, H., and Strehler, B.**, Lipofuscin pigment accumulation as a function of age and distribution in the rodent brain, *J. Gerontol.*, 23, 71, 1968.
42. **Novikoff, A. B., Beaufay, H., and DeDuve, C.**, Electron microscopy of lysosome-rich fractions from rat liver, *J. Biophys. Biochem. Cytol.*, 179 (Suppl. 2), 84, 1956.
43. **Jayne, E. P.**, Cytology of the adrenal gland of the rat at different ages, *Anat. Rec.*, 115, 459, 1953.
44. **Treff, W. M.**, Das Involutionsmuster des Nucleus dentatus cerebelli, in *Altern,* Platt, D., Ed., Schattauer, Stuttgart, 1974, 37.
45. **Mann, D. M. A. and Yates, P. O.**, Lipoprotein pigments — their relationship to aging in the human nervous system. I. The lipofuscin content of nerve cells. II. The melanin content of pigmented nerve cells, *Brain*, 97, 481, 1964.
46. **Medvedev, Sh. A.**, *Aktual Vopr. Sovr. Biol.*, 51, 299, 1961.
47. **Orgel, L. E.**, The maintenance of the accuracy of protein synthesis and its relevance to ageing, *Proc. Natl. Acad. Sci. U.S.A.*, 49, 517, 1963.
48. **Holliday, R.**, Errors in protein synthesis and clonal senescence in fungi, *Nature (London)*, 221, 1224, 1969.
49. **Popp, R. A., Bailiff, E. G., Hirsch, G. P., and Conrad, R. A.**, Errors in human hemoglobin as a function of age, *Interdiscip. Top. Gerontol.*, 9, 209, 1976.
50. **Reichel, W., Hollander, J., Clark, H., and Strehler, B.**, Lipofuscin pigment accumulation as a function of age and distribution in the rodent brain, *J. Gerontol.*, 23, 71, 1968.
51. **Adelman, R. C.**, Age dependent effects in enzyme induction—a biochemical expression of aging, *Exp. Gerontol.*, 6, 75,1971.
52. **Adelman, R. C., Freeman, C., and Karoby, K.**, Impaired availability and potency of insulin during aging, comment made at the 27th Meet. Gerontol. Soc. Am., November 1974.
53. **Kay, M. M. B.**, personal communication, January 1978.
54. **Gajdusek, D. C.**, Slow virus infection and activation of latent infections in aging, *Adv. Gerontol. Res.*, 4, 201, 1972.
55. **Miquel, J.**, Aging of male Drosophila melanogaster: histological, histochemical and ultrastructural observations, *Adv. Gerontol. Res.*, 3, 39, 1971.
56. **Verzar, F.**, Veranderungen der thermoelastischen Kontraktion von Sehnenfasern beim Altern, *Experientia*, 11, 230, 1955.
57. **Chvapil, M. and Hruza, Z.**, The influence of aging and undernutrition on chemical contractility and relaxation of collagen fibres in rats, *Gerontologia*, 3, 241, 1959.
58. **Gallop, P. M., Blumenthal, O. O., Henson, E., and Schneider, A. L.**, Isolation and identification of alpha-amino aldehydes and collagen, *Biochemistry*, 7, 2409, 1968.
59. **Sinex, F. M.**, Cross linkage and aging, *Adv. Gerontol. Res.*, 1, 165, 1964.
60. **Andres, R.**, Diabetes and aging, *Hosp. Prac.*, 2, 63, 1967.

GENETICS*

Diana M. Popp and Raymond A. Popp

Advice by Oliver Wendell Holmes on attaining long life, "The first thing to be done is, some years before birth, ...to advertise for a couple of parents both belonging to long-lived families."

INTRODUCTION

Insofar as the phenotype of an individual is the direct expression of its genome, the life span of a species must be genetically determined. Man is tailless, grows to be 85 kg, and lives to be nearly 100-years-old; mice have long tails, grow to 30 g and live nearly 3 years. If we can say with little argument that the size and tail, or lack thereof, are genetically determined, it follows that the life span also is genetically determined. Many authors accept the presumption, but definitive studies to verify this conclusion are lacking. Potential life span is a constant characteristic and can differ greatly from species to species.[1-3] Within a species such as the mouse, in which genetic homogeneity can be defined, long-lived and short-lived strains can be identified.[4] Life span is highly heritable within a colony,[5,6] and variability of life span reported by different institutions can be attributed to environmental factors.[5-8] The identification of gene control of longevity has been pursued through three approaches. Data gathered in two approaches, familial association of life span in man and animals[1,9-10] and longitudinal studies of senescent twins, support the conclusion that heredity is a significant factor in determining life span.[11,12] The third, studies with genetically defined mice, has shown a direct association of specific loci within the major histocompatibility complex (MHC) with life span.[13,14] Although the data gathered in population and twin studies have many flaws affecting the reliability of conclusion,[15] and although considerable influence of background genomic control over life span is evidenced in Smith and Walford's study,[14] these approaches have yielded evidence suggestive of heritable factors controlling life span.

In some instances genetic predisposition to longer life may represent lack of genetic susceptibility to disease; however, other more subtle gene interactions that regulate the ability to cope with external and internal environments can affect the general vigor of the individual. With remarkable prescience, Comfort[1] pointed out that the ability to survive may represent heterosis at what he called "disease loci" permitting individuals with the greatest heterogeneity the greatest capability for long life. Though senescence in the absence of specific disease does occur, chronic degenerative changes are always associated with "natural death",[7,16] and, with few exceptions, the loci controlling these conditions are the most difficult to define. They determine a variety of interacting physiological processes that have individual liability to time and changing environment, among which slight imbalances will slightly alter the survival ability of the individual. Thus, minor changes can accumulate in different ways at different rates. These loci have been described by Yunis and Greenberg[17] as a "longevity homeostasis gene complex", and others propose as few as "three or four"[18] or a "small number of genes."[19]

Many theories of aging have been proposed: wear and tear, nutrition, cross-linking of macromolecules, biological clocks, finite replicative potential, ionizing radiation, mutations, errors in transcription and translation, and waning of immunological

* Operated by Union Carbide Corporation under contract W-7405-eng-26 with the U.S. Department of Energy.

vigor;[20-22] the last is one of few to lend itself well to an analysis of aging from the point of view of genetic control. In recent years a complex of several closely linked loci (MHC) has been identified that regulates the various immune responses associated with diseases of the aged or diseases that predicate life span.[23] Because in mice these loci contain genes that control immune response and susceptibility to tumorigenesis, population studies in man have also focused on the association of disease with the analogous gene complex, HLA. A strong association was found with specific diseases, mostly nonmalignant and noninfectious but frequently autoimmune,[24] that accompany declining health in old age.[25,26] Thus, the search for MHC-associated diseases has identified an association of a number of "senescence genes" with a gene complex regulating immunological integrity of the individual. The studies of genetic control of diseases have yielded no clear evidence demonstrating simple Mendelian control of life span, but the studies suggest that genes control how effectively the individual copes with the environment, and the immunological distinction between self and nonself may also determine how long the individual lives.

Disease, immune regulation, and genetic stability are major correlates of aging. Their interrelationship with age suggests a basis for genetic determination of longevity. We will try to integrate the fundamental knowledge developed in these areas to establish the interdependent relationship between them and to discuss the relevance of the genetic regulation of these parameters to life span. New data will be presented describing a formal genetic test of linkage of life span with the MHC of the mouse.

CORRELATES OF AGING

Most if not all organisms have a finite life span. The exceptions that have been noted,[7] the redwood and the Mexican cypress, may appear to have an infinite life span only because it exceeds that of man and man's records. Some species have life spans determined by a common and cataclysmic event such as steroid toxicosis in salmon or starvation in insects.[7] Mammals suffer no such known, common life-determining event; yet dying is a certainty, and the mean age of death is characteristic for a species; and, frequently, for strains within species.

A very interesting homology in the development of aging processes over the life span of different species has been noted by several authors.[7,27-29] The life span can be divided into four quarters, which Finch[29] designates in chronological order *postnatal development, maturity, middle age,* and *senescence.* Although these divisions cover different time spans for mouse, dog, or man, alterations in physiological capacities, degenerative changes, and even increases in disease incidences occur in homologous quarters of the life span. This suggests that the appearance of age-related processes is not a random event but an orderly progression of aging and mortality that is governed by some genetic control (Figure 1).

Life span data are expressed in two ways. A survival curve depicts the percentage surviving as a function of age. The 90, 50, and 10% survival age can be determined from this form of presentation.[6,21,31] Comparisons of these parameters are valid only when the environmental influence is equivalent. Survival curves of populations of mice[6] or man[1,21] show that although improved living conditions permit a greater percentage of the populations to live to the senescence period (Figure 2), the life span remains the same, an observation referred to as "squaring the curve".

Life span data have also been expressed as the rate of mortality as a function of age. In man, the probability of dying increases after age 10 and logarithmically increases after age 35[30] (Figure 3).[32] The increasing likelihood of death with increasing age was first noted by Gompertz in 1825[33] and is referred to as Gompertz's Law. Age-

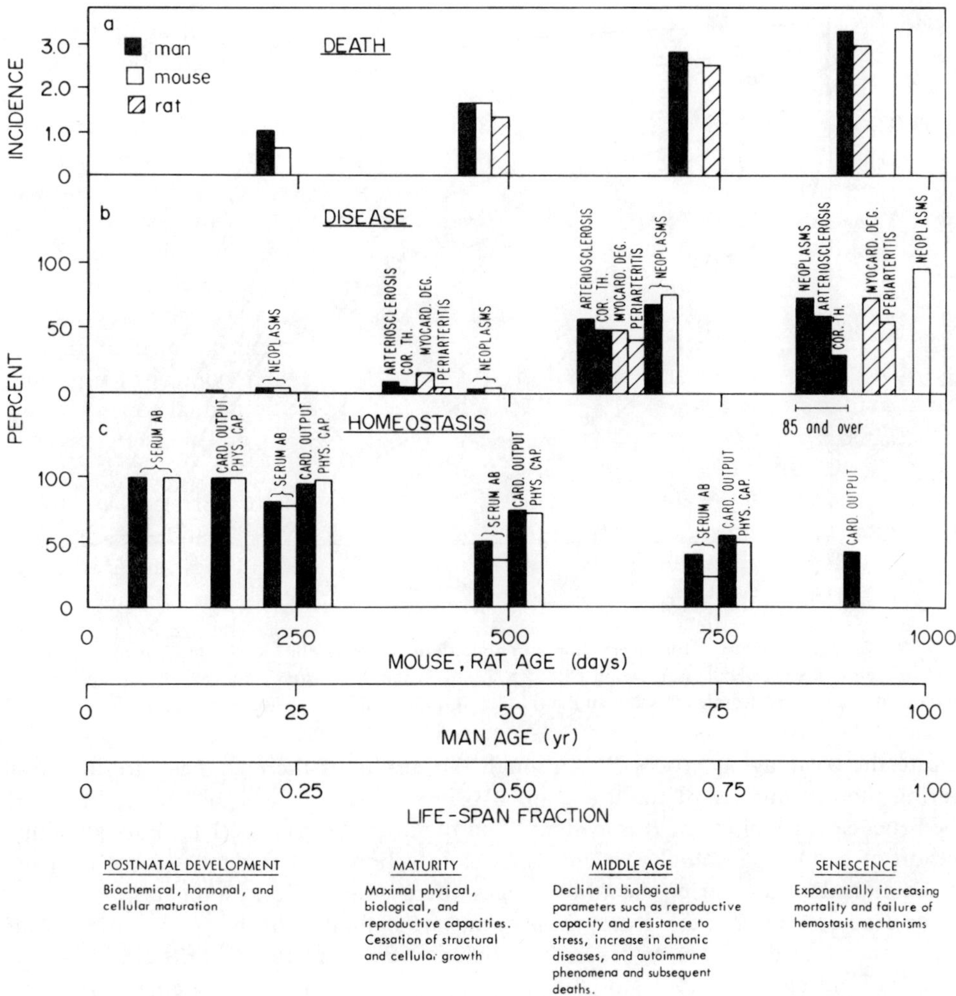

FIGURE 1. Death and neoplasms in (a) and (b) are expressed as the log of incidence per 100,000 individuals per rodent day or man month. Pathological lesions in (b) are expressed as prevalence in populations (percent) at the end of each quarter of life span. Efficiency of homeostatic mechanisms at the end of each quarter of life span are expressed as the fraction (percent) of peak value attained at indicated age in first quarter of life span.[11,21,27-30]

specific death rates have been described graphically for rats,[34] mice,[7,27,35] and lower forms of animal life,[36] and a similar logarithmic relationship is found for these species. For man, the mortality rates from different countries[11,32] and from different years[1,37] have been compared (Figure 3). Very little change is seen in death rate in the later years, and the risk of death is approximately the same in all aging populations. Such curves show that the probability of dying doubles about every 8 years. The shapes of the age-specific death rate curves are also determined by the causes of mortality; the greatest differences occur during the middle years, reflecting improved sanitation, nutrition, and health practices,[11] but the maximum life span of 90 to 95 years remains the same.[21] It is evident from both types of mortality curves that the elimination of nonage-related diseases does not alter maximum longevity.

The final phase of the life span in which the mortality rate is unaffected by mortality in earlier life is called senescense,[29] and the changes that contribute to senescence con-

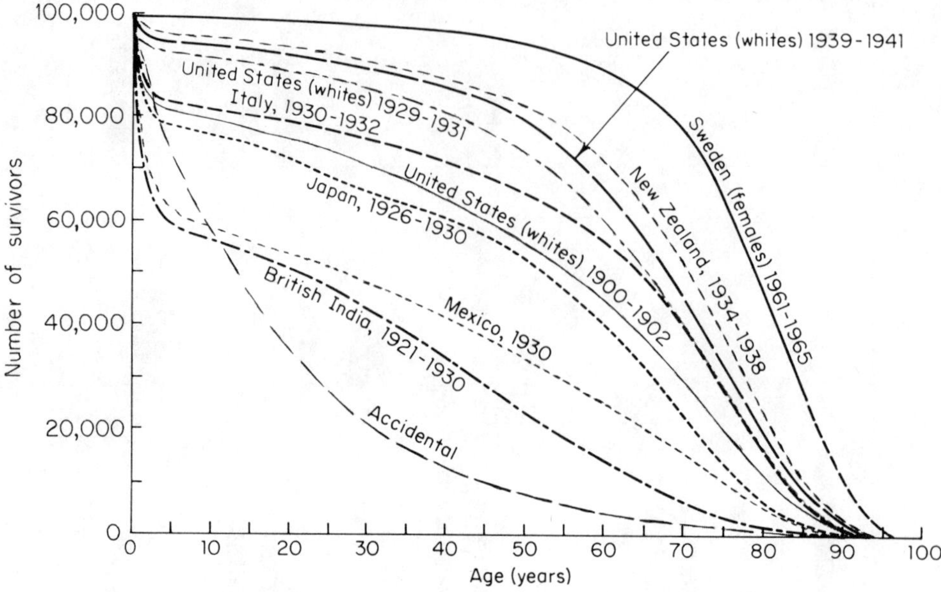

FIGURE 2. Survival curves for several human populations. (From Kohn, R. R., in *Principles of Mammalian Aging,* Prentice-Hall, Englewood Cliffs, N.J., 1978; modified from Comfort, A., in *Ageing: The Biology of Senescence,* Routledge & Kegan Paul, London, 1964. With permission.)

stitute the basic aging process.[11] Although the results of these changes are manifest during the last quarter of the life span, it is unknown at which part of the life span the processes are initiated. It is evident from the mortality curves that although elimination of certain pathological events such as infections and epidemics cause changes in the mortality rate during the middle years, there is little effect on the mortality rates in the senescence years; therefore, these events are not a part of the aging process. The major causes of death during senescence include a preponderance of degenerative diseases[38] (Figure 4). The ability of the aging individual to successfully cope with these degenerative changes is largely determined by environmental and genetic factors. The genetic endowment determines the individual's susceptibility to environmental factors, which in turn determine how severely (if at all) the degeneration of functional homeostasis (constant internal environment) will affect the normal physiology. Thus, the interactions of genetic, physiological, and environmental factors determine which homeostatic change will be preeminent or lethal and are the major determinants of mortality. Genetic regulation of this interaction is the subject of the remainder of this paper.

Disease

Aging and death are usually accompanied by multiple disease processes.[7] This observation has been made for man,[38] rats,[31] and mice.[8] Not only is disease associated with death, but the incidence of disease increases exponentially with age[30] (Figure 4). Indeed, as shown in rats the exponential increase in chronic degenerative disease parallels the exponential increase in mortality with age.[39] In man, the association of disease incidence and age-associated death is clearly seen in data tabulated by Kohn[38] (Figure 4), in which the rate of death from 16 of the most common causes of death in the human population is logarithmic after 30 years of age and mortality rates due to specific diseases show a remarkable parallelism to death from all causes. The similarity of mortality rates and disease incidence suggests a relationship, perhaps causative, be-

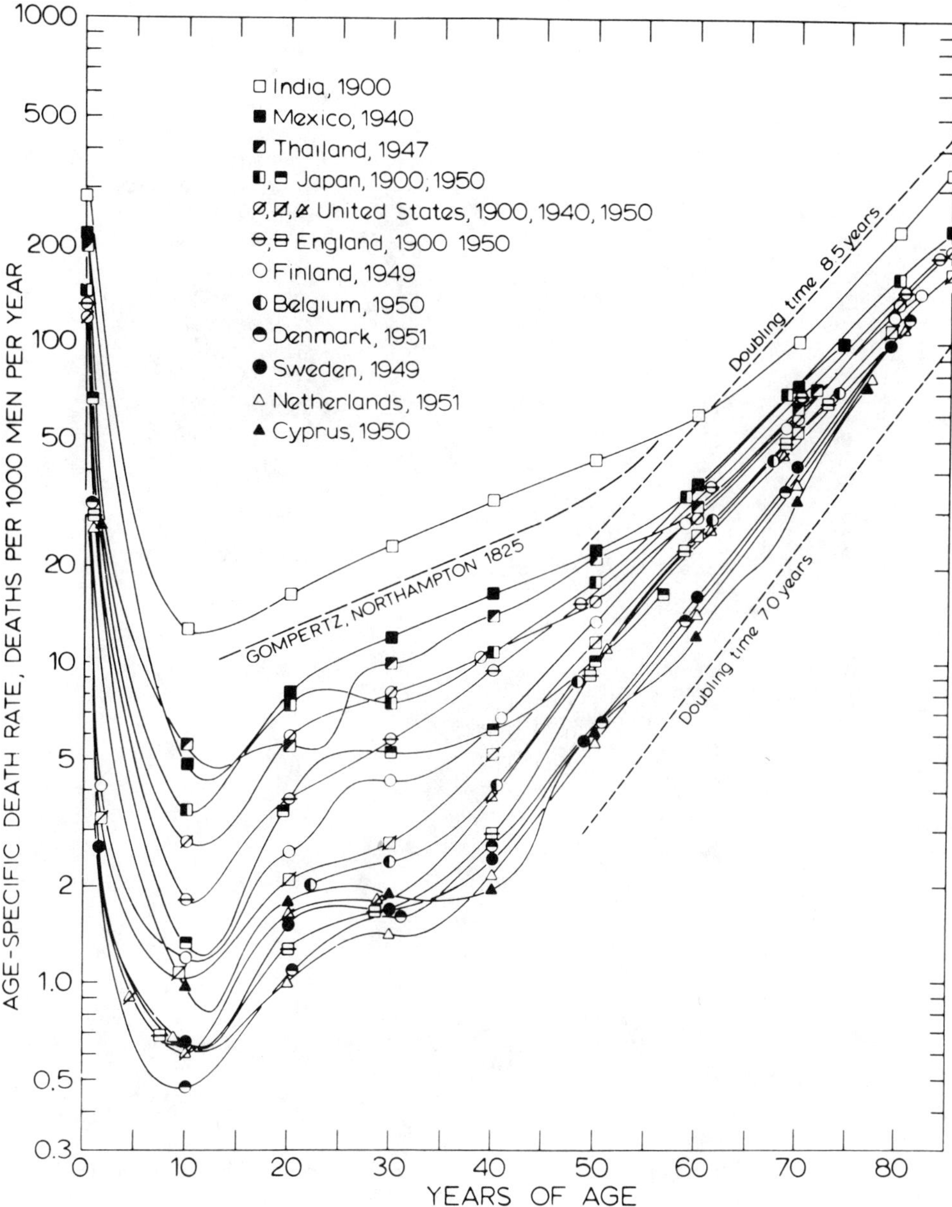

FIGURE 3. Incidences of death over the life span in different countries and years. (From Jones, H. B., in *The Biology of Aging*, Finch, C. E. and Hayflick, L., Eds., Lawrence Berkeley Laboratory, University of California, Berkeley, 1977, 514. With permission.)

tween disease and longevity. Although it is true that all deaths do not occur from any single disease and some deaths occur in apparent absence of disease, few individuals die without evidence of pathological lesions or disease processes at autopsy.[7] In all studies, the close relationship of disease with mortality is inescapable. The mortality rate is directly related to the increased probability of onset of the disease and not to a faster rate of progression once incurred.[34] Since certain disease states may contribute to mortality data but not to the aging process, the categories to be considered as diseases of aging must be selected for their contribution to the increasing rate and prob-

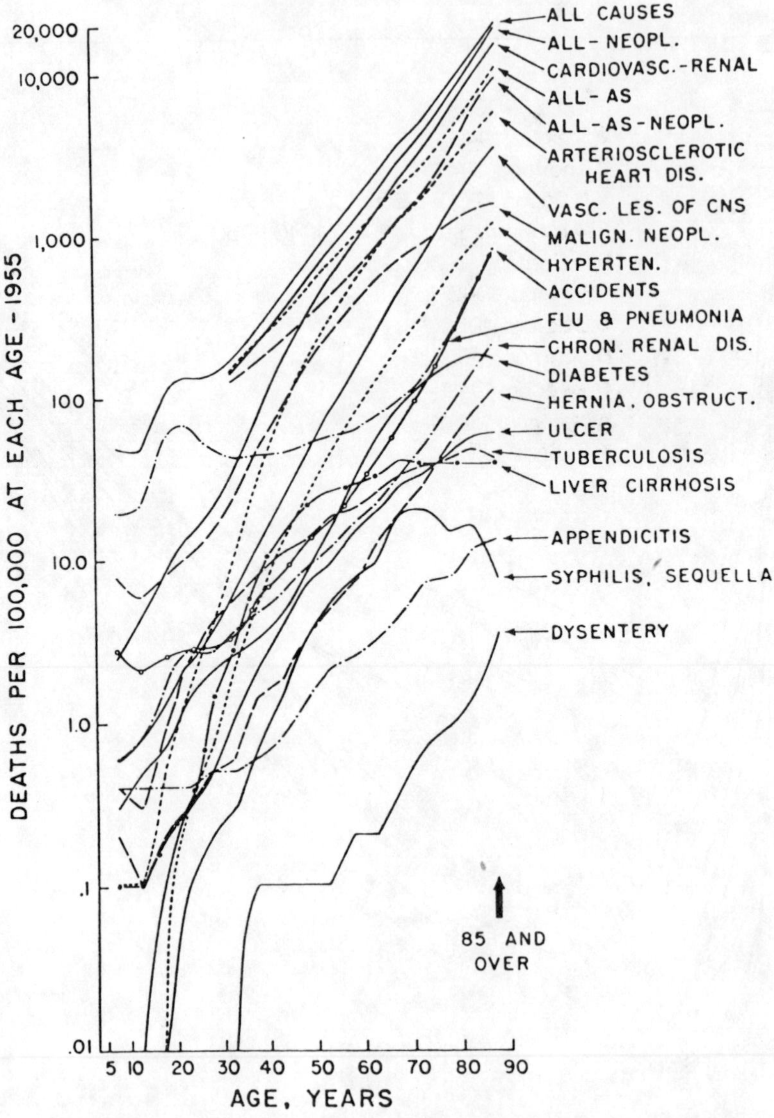

FIGURE 4. Incidences of death from major causes over the life span. (Reprinted with permission from *J. Chronic Dis., 16, Kohn, R. R., Human Aging and Disease,* 1963, Pergamon Press, Ltd.)

ability of death with increasing age. These diseases have been categorized in several ways. Kohn[38] describes two categories: (a) well-defined diseases, which show an increased incidence with age (atherosclerosis, hypertension, and malignant neoplasms) and (b) stresses, which kill the old more readily than the young (accidents and respiratory infections) (Table 1). Deaths from atherosclerosis and related diseases (cerebrovascular accidents, coronary artery occlusion, and peripheral arterial disease) double every 9 to 10 years, and those from hypertension and related diseases (cardiovascular and renal disease, heart failure, and cerebral hemorrhage) double every 7 to 8 years. The logarithmic curve derived from the age-specific death rates for these diseases is characteristic of basic age-related processes and suggests a close association between these diseases and such processes. The tendency for decreasing incidence during the final quarter of the life span makes malignancy a special case for gerontologists, but

Table 1
CAUSES OF DEATH OF THE AGED[a]

Well-Defined Diseases

A. Universal aging processes exhibiting chronic progression
   1. Atherosclerosis and related diseases (cerebrovascular accidents, coronary artery occlusion, and peripheral arterial disease)
      a. Incidence and severity increase with age
      b. Disease-related deaths double every 9 to 10 years
   2. Hypertension and related diseases (cardiovascular and renal disease, heart failure, and cerebral hemorrhage)
      a. Incidence and severity increase with age
      b. Disease-related deaths double every 7 to 8 years

B. Diseases that affect susceptible segments of the population, suggesting discrete genetic control; since only a segment of the population is affected, this is not a universal aging process
   1. Malignancies
      a. Incidence increases with age until senescence, when it declines
      b. There are different forms with variable peak incidence and age of onset for different neoplasms
      c. The diseases are frequently fatal for those afflicted, removing a segment of the population from the entire aging population
   2. Diabetes, tuberculosis, syphilis
      a. Several forms occur early in life that are fatal or controllable
      b. Peak incidence is variable

Nonspecific Causes of Death Reflecting Susceptibility to Stress

Represent failure of an individual to cope with or adapt to physiological stress and environmental insult with age. Does not occur in all individuals; incidence does not increase with age, but lethality increases in older individuals; incidence of death from these causes in senescence populations is higher than that from other diseases

A. Physiological stress
   1. Infections
      a. Bronchopneumonia
      b. Influenza
   2. General
      a. Hernia
      b. Ulcers
      c. Intestinal blockage

B. Environmental stress
   1. Accidents
   2. Changing diet, climate or emotional status

[a] Table compiled from Kohn.[38]

a general increased incidence with age is observed in studies in man[11,40] and experimental animals,[31,41] and in those individuals afflicted with the disease cancer resembles a basic aging process.

For these reasons malignancies are included in a special category that includes diseases that lack universality in that they do not occur in all aging individuals but do at some point in the life span show an increasing incidence with age. The prominent cause of death in this category is malignancy. Although there is an age-associated increase in incidence from age 10 to 50, after age 65 the probability of dying from malignancy is less than the probability of dying from other causes. The susceptibility of the individual is a genetically determined trait, and the reduced mortality due to cancer deaths is probably the result of removal of a subpopulation of genetically susceptible individuals in the earlier age spans. This is because there are variable peak ages of incidence for different neoplasms, some of which peak in the middle years.[11,21,38,40] This observation is even more significant for other diseases in this category such as diabetes, tuberculosis, and syphilis, which suggests that the severity of these diseases removes those afflicted from the general aging population. In addition, a decreased incidence of death in the last quarter may result from inclusion of several forms of a disease. For example, diabetes can occur in several forms with different age of onset and different rates of progression and may influence the other mortality rate curves, since it has been suggested that those who survive the diabetic disease become victims of atherogenesis.[42] The pathogenesis of the diseases in this category may be so severe that once an individual contracts them he is less able to cope with the more chronic disease processes that develop during subsequent age-related deficiencies.

Complications of stress is a category of diseases that includes a large number of deaths due to nonspecific causes. These diseases are seen by Kohn[38] as the result of a breakdown in homeostasis. The physiological processes that maintain homeostasis show a decreased effectiveness with age.[21,38] These diseases have several special features that make them the most interesting group of causes of death. During senescence the probability of dying from these is greater than from all causes. Individuals die with little evidence of pathological lesions and, though the incidence of these diseases is no greater in the later years, the lethality is increased with age among those afflicted, suggesting that the aging changes make the individual more sensitive to environmental insult or less able to cope or successfully adapt to the environment. This group of diseases provides the best evidence that aging is really a chronic, degenerative change in ability to function, either to defend from general or specific disease or to respond mechanically to external stimuli.

It is evident that diseases associated with mortality are very different, but they kill at approximately the same period of life and determine a characteristic life span for each species. An aging individual can have more than one disease,[31,38] and that he succumbs to one may be more fortuitious than predictive. The totality of the degenerative changes is the single, basic aging process which is manifested variously as the specific age-related diseases. This concept allows for the absence of one specific disease entity (atherosclerosis) in one species (mouse) that is a primary cause of aged death in another (man) even though both species undergo a similar aging process.

A common finding in studies reporting detailed pathology on aging populations is that degenerative changes are the leading pathological lesion. The most feared disease of aging, cancer, ranked as low as fifth in one study,[43] representing 7.8% of the deaths of an aged group older than 65 years and in another review was cited as the cause of 17% of all deaths in the U.S. in 1967.[11] The incidence of nonneoplastic, degenerative diseases was reported to be increased and the severity greater in a short-lived compared with a longer-lived strain of mouse.[8] Because of the insidious nature of the degenerative diseases, their etiology has been difficult to understand. However, several renal, cardiovascular, and chronic neurological diseases have been described as having microbial or viral etiology.[44]

It is evident that resistance or susceptibility to environmental agents, the age of susceptibility, and the efficiency with which the individual contends with the environment will depend largely upon the genome, and the resultant degenerative disease, malignancy, or disturbed homeostasis determines the life span. The basis of the genetic control of these parameters has only recently been elucidated through the extensive studies on genetic control of diseases which will be described in the next section.

Disease Susceptibility Genes

A large body of evidence in the literature suggests that expression and development of age-associated diseases are controlled by the genome. Cohen[15] has written a com-

Table 2
PHENOTYPES OF SENESCENCE[a]

Intrinsic mutagenesis
Nonconstitutional chromosomal aberrations
Susceptibility to neoplasms relevant to aging
Stem cell defect (numbers or kinetics)
Premature greying or hair loss
Dementia or degenerative neuropathology
Susceptibility to "slow virus"
Amyloid depositions
Depositions of lipofuscin pigments
Diabetes mellitus
Disorder of lipid metabolism
Hypogonadism
Autoimmunity
Hypertension
Degenerative vascular disease
Osteoporosis
Cataracts
Abnormalities of mitochondria
Regional fibrosis
Variations in amounts or distribution of adipose tissue

[a] From Martin.[48]

prehensive review of the literature showing that offspring of families with a history of degenerative diseases have a higher risk of mortality from these diseases. Studies of twins[45,46] show greater concordance for disease and longevity in monozygous than in dizygous twins. A very extensive study of the progeny of nonagenarians shows a positive relationship between age at death of the progeny and the nonlongevous parent.[10] Inbred mouse strains show great homogeneity of life span and disease incidence; both factors are changed after hybridization.[22,41,47] But what evidence is there for disease susceptibility genes, particularly age-associated-disease susceptibility genes?

In an exhaustive study of 2336 known human mutations, Martin[48] selected 162 genetic syndromes of potential relevance to the pathobiology of aging. From these figures he estimates the number of possibly relevant loci of the total mammalian genome to be 7000. If only 1% of these control major aspects of aging, 70 genes could be the principal moderators of longevity, and perhaps 10% of these would be of "extraordinary importance." When the 162 genetic syndromes phenotypically related to aging were categorized according to 20 phenotypes of senescence (Table 2), 10 syndromes were identified as "segmental progeroid syndromes" or accelerated aging syndromes. They are designated segmental because they do not bear a 100% resemblance to normal aging, but they do show many of the major characteristics of aging. No single locus in this survey of the entire genome of man was found to control life span or the physiological decline with age. The syndromes identified in this survey reflect the effect of single gene mutation on life span and affect mortality in early life, making the relationship between phenotype and genotype apparent. Since the victims of these mutations and related disease states succumb early in the normal life span, these loci may have little relevance to the universal degenerative changes seen in normal aging.

Methodologies for determining inheritance of single-gene diseases in man are available. However, diseases determined by single-factor inheritance with complete penetrance are infrequent in the aged. Age-related degenerative diseases appear to be of a heterogeneous nature, the expression and severity of which are subject to environmental factors, thus heritability is more difficult to demonstrate.[49] However, even for the major causes of death in persons over 80, atherosclerosis and hypertension, familial inheritance has been described.[50] In studying families afflicted with primary immunodeficiency diseases, Good and Yunis[51] noted apparent autosomal, dominant inheritance of arthritis and mesenchymal diseases, prominent age-related disorders. A high incidence of atherosclerosis is found as a complication of two known genetic disorders, diabetes mellitus and hypercholesterolemia.[50] Bierman[42] reported on the close association of early onset of coronary heart disease and a monogenetically controlled hyperlipidemia and atherosclerosis. This latter disease is, perhaps, a model aging disease, since it is the most common age-related disorder in the Western world and represents an intrinsic degenerative change that is influenced by environment (diet, smoking, tension) and subject to genetic control in determination of age of onset and severity of disease.[42] Superimposed on this system are risk factors that have some genetic basis in their origin, such as high blood pressure, hyperglycemia, diabetes, and obesity. The influence of so many factors on the expression of this one disease exemplifies the heterogeneous nature of the diseases of aging. However, like most age-related disorders, atherosclerosis is in itself not the basic aging process, as some human populations die at the appropriate life span with no evidence of this disease.[52]

Immune dysfunction has been suggested as having a major role in the pathogenesis of age-related diseases.[18,51,53,54] Linder et al.[55] describe similarities in autoimmune related pathological lesions found in the short-lived NZB mouse strain and at later phases of life in long-lived mouse strains. Using the short-lived immunodeficient NZB mouse as a model, Yunis and Greenberg[17] postulate separate mechanisms for the etiology and pathogenesis of aging. Cellular dysfunction (i.e., loss of suppressor function) leads to active pathological processes (i.e., autoimmunity) which culminate in life-threatening conditions. These authors propose a ''longevity homeostasis gene complex'' that regulates the immune response, self recognition, and hormonal balance. The relationship of endocrine regulation and immune cognitive-effector function of the homeostasis complex with diseases and longevity is unclear.[17] Walford was perhaps the first to describe the role of immunological systems in natural aging,[53] bringing together the concepts of histocompatibility antigens, disease states, aging, and developmental biology of the immune system into a pathogenetic theory of aging. Central to this theory are the alterations of the immune system with age. He proposes a ''limited gene theory of aging'', with as few as three or four genes, one of which is the ''mutator gene'', closely associated with and acting upon loci within the MHC.[56]

The influence of gene control on the inheritance of age-associated diseases is inescapable in the literature. However, identification of disease susceptibility or senescence genes has been elusive. Age-associated diseases influenced by multiple genetic and environmental factors exhibit incomplete penetrance. Until recently, the absence of linked genetic markers made inheritance of diseases difficult to follow. The ABO blood group antigens in man provided good genetic markers,[57] but attempts to demonstrate an association of diseases with these loci were rewarded with only a few but relatively weak associations (duodenal ulcers were associated with blood group O and stomach cancers with blood group A).[58] However, studies in mice showed that resistance to leukemogenesis was associated with a different cell surface antigen system, the histocompatibility (*H-2*) system.[59,60] These studies led to the description of leukemia in the mouse as a multiple-gene disease.[61] Subsequent reports of the association of Hodgkin's disease,[62] glomerulonephritis,[63] and human leukemia[64] with the H-2 analogue in man, HLA, as well as the identification of immune response genes closely linked with the MHC of the mouse prompted a search for association of the MHC with other diseases.[65] Although the early association of HLA with malignancies was not verified under expanded studies[66] (with the exception of a weak but constant association with acute lymphocytic leukemia and HLA-A2), the original association of disease states with HLA proved fortuitous since the highly polymorphic HLA locus provided a good marker to demonstrate heritability among progeny in subsequent studies with other diseases.

Genetics of Disease

The elucidation of the genetic nature of age-related diseases came about through the convergence of three areas of research: (a) the growing evidence that the diseases that accompany aging with certain notable exceptions are insidious, degenerative, autoimmune-type diseases, often of viral etiology; (b) evidence that decline in immunological function accompanies aging in mouse and man (see following section); and (c) identification and detailed genetic characterization of a supergene, the MHC, that controls such complex and variable immune functions as induction of B- and T-cell differentiation, cognitive and regulatory cellular interactions, viral resistance and susceptibility, regulation of the immune response to specific antigens, complement biosynthesis, and endocrine balance. The similarity between the functions that appear to fail with age and the functions controlled by the supergene made this region of the genome a likely site to look for disease susceptibility genes.

The MHC of man is identified by markers at four loci, *HLA-A, -B, -C,* and *-D* (Table 3), and by the D-related B lymphocyte determinants, DR. A note on nomenclature is advisable at this point, since many early reports used local designations for antigens that now may have a different symbol. When the segregant series A, B, C, and D were defined, the hyphen was dropped from HL-A. The number of the specificity is preceded by the relevant segregant series designation A, B, C, D, or DR and separated from HLA by a hyphen. The original specificity numbers were retained in the A and B series, thus, the numbers do not overlap; but the C, D, and DR series each begin at 1. A "w" in the designation indicates that the antigens still has a provisional definition and the relevant antibodies are still being tested in workshops,* except in the C series, in which all the C-locus specificities retain the "w" to avoid confusion with complement components C2 and C4 also coded for by genes in the HLA region. In the following summary the new designations will be used, although the references in some cases may contain old designations. The new and old designations are shown in Table 3. Presently there are 20 specificities identified at *HLA-A,* 33 at *HLA-B,* 6 at *HLA-C,* and 11 at *HLA-D,* and 7 serologically determined DR specificities.

Some MHC-linked autoimmune diseases have been noted in experimental animals,[69,70] but the most informative studies from the viewpoint of aging have been in humans. Since the first report on an association of Hodgkin's disease with HLA[62] many studies have been undertaken and summarized in the literature;[24] a recent report lists 40 diseases, of which 28 show a positive association with HLA.[49] However, these data are accumulated from population or family studies done with antisera of variable quality, and much care must be taken to assure that the associations found in a single study are real. Svejgaard et al.[49] discuss several sources of error: ascertainment of controls, diagnosis of patients, serology, and statistics. Although Hodgkin's disease does not appear on the more recent, stringently controlled lists, viral-associated autoimmune diseases do.[71] The method of establishing association of HLA with disease is to determine the incidence of particular HLA antigens in patient groups relative to the incidence in a control population. If patients have a different incidence than the general population, an association is established; increased frequencies are the most common, suggesting susceptibility is one of the genetic effects.[49] Two forms of studies are

* Cooperative exchanges, generally held every 2 years, of antisera and test cells among laboratories to obtain agreement on the specificity of antisera and the identity of antigens.

Table 3
RECOGNIZED HLA SPECIFICITIES, PROVISIONAL DESIGNATIONS, AND SYNONYMS OF THE A, B, C, AND D LOCI

A = LA = 1st Series

New[a]	Previous[a]
HLA-1	HL-A1
HLA-2	HL-A2
HLA-3	HL-A3
HLA-9	HL-A9
HLA-10	HL-A10
HLA-11	HL-A11
HLA-25	W25
HLA-26	W26
HLA-28	W28
HLA-29	W29
HLA-Aw19	Li
HLA-Aw23	W23
HLA-Aw24	W24
HLA-Aw30	W30
HLA-Aw31	W31
HLA-Aw32	W32
HLA-Aw33	W19.6
HLA-Aw34	Malay 2
HLA-Aw36	Mo^x
HLA-Aw43	BK

B = FOUR = 2nd Series

New	Previous
HLA-B5	HL-A
HLA-B7	HL-A7
HLA-B8	HL-A8
HLA-B12	HL-A12
HLA-B13	HL-A13
HLA-B14	W14
HLA-B15	W15
HLA-B17	W17
HLA-B18	W18
HLA-B27	W27
HLA-B37	TY
HLA-B40	W10
HLA-Bw4	w4,4a
HLA-Bw6	w6, 4b
HLA-Bw16	W16
HLA-Bw21	W21
HLA-Bw22	W22
HLA-Bw35	W5
HLA-Bw38	W16.1
HLA-Bw39	W16.2
HLA-Bw41	Sabell (MK)
HLA-Bw42	MWA
HLA-Bw44	B12
HLA-Bw45	TT
HLA-Bw46	HS, SIN2
HLA-Bw47	407,MO66,BW40C
HLA-Bw48	KSO,JA,Bw40.3
HLA-Bw49	Bw21.1,SL-ET
HLA-Bw50	Bw21.2, ET
HLA-Bw51	B5.1
HLA-Bw52	B5.2
HLA-Bw53	HR
HLA-Bw54	Bw22-J, SAP1

C = AJ = 3rd Series

New	Previous
HLA-Cw1	T1, AJ
HLA-Cw2	T2, 170
HLA-Cw3	T3, UPS
HLA-Cw4	T4, 315
HLA-Cw5	T5
HLA-Cw6	T7, 11P

D = MLC = LD-1 Series

New	Previous
HLA-Dw1	LD101, w5a, J
HLA-Dw2	LD102,7a
HLA-Dw3	LD103,8a
HLA-Dw4	LD104,w15a
HLA-Dw5	LD105
HLA-Dw6	LD106
HLA-Dw7	LD107, 12a
HLA-Dw8	LD108,w10a
HLA-Dw9	TB9, OH
HLA-Dw10	LD16
HLA-Dw11	LD17

DR = B Cell Antigen[b]

New	Previous
HLA-DRw1	
HLA-DRw2	
HLA-DRw3	
HLA-DRw4	
HLA-DRw5	
HLA-DRw6	
HLA-DRw7	

[a] New = most recent designations;[67] previous = earlier or provisional designations.[67,68]

[b] See Reference 67, pp. 70-76 for local equivalents of DRw specificities.

used, population (unrelated patients) and family studies, from which different information can be obtained.

Population studies permit identification of possible disease-antigen association and provide the quantitative data necessary for risk estimates. However, linkage disequilibrium must exist between the presumed disease gene and the marker, otherwise recombination would destroy evidence of an association. Since genetic disequilibrium has been noted for the MHC, population studies have provided valuable information. However, when linkage disequilibrium exists, it is not possible to determine if the HLA or a linked gene is the responsible factor. Family studies permit testing the heritability of the antigen-disease association and determination of the extent to which other elements of the MHC or genome and the contribution of environmental factors are involved.[49] In particular, family studies are helpful in determining if a disease is monogenic (one gene at one locus), multifactorial (influence of environment superimposed

Table 4
DISEASE ASSOCIATION WITH HLA ANTIGENS[a]

Disease	Class I	Class II	Both
Ankylosing spondylitis	B27		
Reiter's disease	B27		
Acute anterior uveitis	B27		
Juvenile arthritis	B27		
Subacute thyroiditis de Quervain	Bw37		
Psoriasis	B13,Bw17,Bw37,Cw6		
Behcet's disease	B5		
Recurrent herpes labialis	A1		
Systemic lupus erythematosus	B8		
Idiopathic hemochromatosis	A3,B14		
Polycystic kidney disease	A5		
Buerger's disease	Bw35		
Autoimmune hemolytic anemia	A3		
Rheumatoid arthritis		Dw4	
Optic neuritis		Dw2	
Multiple sclerosis			A3,B7,Dw2
Myasthenia gravis			B8,Dw3
Juvenile diabetes mellitus			B8,Bw15,Cw3,Dw3,Dw4
Graves' disease			B8,Dw3
Addison's disease			B8,Dw3
Chronic hepatitis			B8,Dw3
Coeliac disease			B8,Dw3
Dermatitis herpetiformis			B8,Dw3
Sjogren's disease			B8,Dw3
C2 deficiency			A10,B18,Dw2

[a] Data in table from Batchlor and Morris[73] and Dupont and Svejgaard.[74]

on genetic control),polygenic (combined action of many unlinked genes), or oligogenic (limited number of unlinked gene).

Initially, the correlations were made with series A or B antigens. A surprising number of diseases were correlated with HLA-B8. They represent conditions of antigen hypersensitivity (dermatitis herpetiformis and coeliac disease) and autoimmune disorders (Addison's disease, myasthenia gravis, and chronic aggressive hepatitis). Another B-locus allele, B27, was associated with several arthropathies (ankylosing spondylitis, acute anterior uveitis, Reiter's syndrome). Useful information can be obtained from another approach, determination of haplotype (unique combination of alleles at linked loci) frequencies among the HLA-associated diseases.[72] This type of data permits an estimate of how much of the MHC may be involved in the determination of the disease and whether certain combinations may be obligatory for the development or progression of a disease.

The types of diseases will be clinically categorized as follows, but are presented in Table 4 as being under the control of Class I (A,B,C) or Class II (D, DR) MHC loci or both.

Malignancies

Despite extensive studies, most of the malignancies have shown, at best, weak associations.[23,49,69] A major problem is that they have been primarily retrospective studies, meaning that the patients have been diagnosed for some time prior to phenotyping, therefore the increased incidence of an antigen in afflicted individuals may reflect survival value.[75-78] Accurate phenotyping of lymphocytes of individuals suffering from acute leukemias is difficult.[23] An interesting finding is that the frequency of heterozygotes is higher in long-term leukemia victims as well as a deficiency in homozygotes, suggesting a deleterious effect of homozygosity at the HLA locus.[77] The failure of neoplasms to be clearly an age-associated or a HLA-associated disease may be due to the fact that they are more greatly influenced by environmental factors than are the other diseases.

As pointed out by McDevitt and Bodmer,[79] many considerations may confound the demonstration of association of MHC with disease: (a) environmental factors may influence the severity of a disease by being present at different levels of exposure or not at all, making the phenotype of a genetically susceptible individual questionable or indistinguishable, (b) several etiologies may contribute to a similar pathology, (c) other unlinked genes may be necessary but not sufficient for the disease susceptibility, and (d) recombination may occur with MHC loci. Because of the linkage disequilibrium that exists in the MHC, recombination has not affected the association of many diseases with MHC. However, if a selective advantage exists for haplotypes associated with diseases resulting in linkage disequilibrium but not for any haplotypes associated with neoplasms permitting random recombination, associations would be contradictory and inconsistent in populations.

Rheumatoid Diseases

This group includes one of the strongest HLA associations described — ankylosing spondylitis (AS) and HLA-B27.[23,80,81] Of AS patients, 96% carry the HLA-B27 antigen, compared with 8% in the control population. Common haplotypes such as the *A1,B8* (9.8%) and *A3,B7* (5.4%) have not been reported in AS patients.[72] AS is used as the model for HLA-associated diseases. Family studies demonstrate the generally accepted concept that the loci responsible for HLA-linked diseases are not the marker loci but unidentified linked loci. One family study showed that AS can occur in a family member negative for B27, suggesting a recombination between the AS gene and the marker B27 gene.[82-84] In addition, B27 siblings of affected children can show no clinical symptoms of the disease, suggesting polygenic control, environmental influence, or both. A high rate of concordance in monozygotic twins suggests genetic control, but a small number of discordant monozygotic twins reveals environmental involvement.[85] Generally, in family studies, afflicted individuals will carry the associated antigen, but not all individuals carrying the antigen will be afflicted. Other diseases in this category demonstrating close association with HLA-B27 are Reiter's syndrome,[23,80] acute anterior uveitis,[80] and juvenile rheumatoid arthritis.[86] Rheumatoid arthritis has been associated with Dw4[73,87] and is unique in that it has never been shown in association with HLA-A or B antigens.

Skin Diseases

A higher than normal incidence of HLA antigens Bw17, B13, Bw37, and Cw6 occurs among individuals suffering from psoriasis in three racial groups.[73] It is thought that the disease is more closely associated with the C locus and that the increase in B-locus antigens is due to linkage disequilibrium with the disease-assoiated antigen Cw6. The immunological nature of this disease is suggested by cross-reactivity between B13 and a protein portion of streptococcus A[88] and an increase in immunoglobulin levels. Behçet's disease has been associated with B5.[89] Dermatitis herpetiformis, which, like the gastrointestinal coeliac disease, is characterized by a high level of antigluten antibody, is also associated with the same antigens, B8 and Dw3. Recurrent herpes labialis has an association with the A locus antigen A1.[74]

Endocrine Diseases

These diseases as a group are interesting in that a single antigen, B8 or B8-containing haplotype, is often involved. Graves' disease[90] and idiopathic Addison's disease[91] have a close association with HLA-B8. Juvenile diabetes mellitus shows an association with two haplotypes, *B8, Dw3,* and *Bw15, Cw3, Dw4,* depending on the form of the disease.[73] The effects of the two B antigens seem to be cumulative in that patients having both antigens have a higher risk than patients having either one alone.[92] This suggests that susceptibility is dominant.[49] Walford et al.[93] suggest that *B8* (or a closely linked locus) is an autoimmune-susceptibility gene and describe the associated disease, diabetes, as "one of the most characteristic diseases of aging", citing several complications of the disease such as arteriosclerosis, autoantibodies, amyloidosis, and reduced replicative potential of fibroblasts.

Neurologic Diseases

One of the first known HLA-associated diseases, multiple sclerosis (MS), was reported to be weakly associated with A3;[94] it was later reported to be more strongly associated with B7 (55%),[95] an antigen frequently found in combination with A3.[72] However, more recent studies looking for disease susceptibilities associated with the D region found MS to be even more closely associated with Dw2[96] (70% compared with 16% in the control population).[97] This disease provides an example of linkage disequilibrium, that is, an instance of several antigens appearing together in a haplotype at a frequency greater than would be predicted on the basis of the gene frequencies. The *A3,B7,DRw2* haplotype is relatively common in Caucasian populations, and disease genes closely associated with the MHC would be expected to show an association with all three. Since the antigen with the highest frequency in a population of unrelated MS patients is DRw2, the disease susceptibility gene must lie in or near the D region. The basis for linkage disequilibrium is unknown, but selection[98] and population migration[99] are the most frequently advanced theories.

Not only is there a tenfold elevated incidence of HLA-B8 among individuals afflicted with myasthenia gravis, there is also a sex effect in that the disease occurs more frequently in women, and B8 appears at the highest frequency in afflicted women with age of onset before age 40. Furthermore, this disease appears to be more prevalent in HLA-B8 homozygotes than heterozygotes.[100] The frequency of B7 and Dw2 is elevated in patients with optic neuritis associated with multiple sclerosis and only slightly elevated in patients with optic neuritis.[101] An interesting correlation between the presence of oligoclonal IgG in the cerebrospinal fluid and the presence of A7,Dw2 was noted in both patient groups.

Gastrointestinal Diseases

Coeliac disease is characterized by an increase in antigluten antibodies and in serum IgA; it has been shown to be associated with HLA-B8,[102] as has autoimmune chronic active hepatitis.[103] Idiopathic hemochomatosis has been associated with A3 and B14.[104]

Immunopathologic Diseases

Systemic lupus erythematosus (SLE) was reported to be associated with HLA antigens,[65] but Kissmeyer-Nielsen et al.[105] were unable to confirm the association. However, the association of autoaggressive antibodies in these patients makes leukocyte typing difficult.[105] Also, individuals with C2 deficiency, which is strongly linked to A10,B18, and Dw2,[106,107] frequently have SLE-like syndromes (such as glomerulonephritis and antinuclear antibodies[106]), and chronic glomerulonephritis has been weakly associated with A2 in two studies.[63,108] More recently, a weak association of B8 with

SLE has been confirmed.[106] Buerger's disease, characterized by mesangial deposits of IgA and C3, has been reported to be associated with Bw35.[106,109] Polycystic kidney disease has been reported to be associated with A5,[23] autoimmune hemolytic anemia with A3,[110] and Sjogren's disease (a rheumatoid joint disease) with B8 and Dw3.[106] Grass and ragweed allergies could be shown to have an association with B8 and A2, respectively.[86] The proposed relationship between complement deficiencies and SLE-like syndromes such as glomerulonephritis and antinuclear antibodies provides a clear causal relationship between MHC and autoimmune entities.[106]

Clearly, the diseases associated with HLA are varied. Interestingly, they do not include malignancies or overtly infectious diseases, but frequently represent chronic diseases of dubious origin that are polygenic and multifactorial, whose etiology is not defined, but in which immunological mechanisms play a major role. Many have immunological complications, even autoimmune symptoms. They have late age of onset and little influence on reproductive features.[86] In short, they resemble age-associated diseases.

More recent compilations of diseases have been published reflecting major collaborative efforts by many laboratories in different countries using common reagents aimed at establishing definitive associations. By 1977 as many as 90 diseases had been studied for possible association with HLA,[74] and the MHC of man was recognized as the most important genetic marker system for human diseases. A major objective of the Seventh Histocompatibility Testing Workshop was to determine if there are even closer associations with the serologically defined HLA D-locus-related antigens, DR.[104] Basic to this pursuit are the implications for pathogenesis, since it has been shown in the mouse that the homologous Ia antigens are controlled by a genetic region that carries genes controlling immune response, self vs. nonself discrimination, T-B-cell interactions, and suppressor cell regulation. The workshop gathered information on 25 diseases, but concentrated on 10, all of which have been mentioned above; the previous findings were confirmed as was the association with D and DR antigens. Due to linkage disequilibrium within the HLA system, population mixture, and difficulties over the selection of control populations, it was not always possible to determine if a disease was more closely associated with single antigens or haplotypes. Diseases may have associations with different antigens in different geographical regions, since some haplotypes that are frequent in one region will be infrequent in another.[111] In the U.S., myasthenia gravis and MS are associated with *B8,Drw3*. In Japan the incidence of this haplotype is infrequent, and myasthenia gravis and MS show an HLA association with *DRw4* and *Bw22,DRw5*, respectively, which are more common to that country.[104] Interestingly enough, the disease patterns change insofar as the high-titer antibodies seen in the B8-associated chronic hepatitis are not seen in the same disease among the Japanese. The association of the same disease with different antigens in different racial groups strengthens the evidence that the disease susceptibility gene is not the marker HLA gene but a linked locus. Evidence from follow-up data on leukemic patients obtained during the workshop showed a high incidence of B8 in survivors, suggesting the prognostic value of B8 in patients with acute monocytic leukemia and confirming the survival value of B8 postulated by Falk and Osoba in 1971.[75] The workshop provided definitive evidence of association of rheumatoid arthritis with DRw4. Hemochromatosis is unique in that it is more closely associated with the A locus antigen A3 than B or D antigens, and there is no known immunological basis for the disease.[104]

Association of disease with HLA-D and DR loci is important because of the homology with the I (immune response) and Ia (I-associated antigens) regions of the mouse and the relevance to pathogenesis. Diseases associated with HLA-D,DR regions show increased antibody titer such as antigluten antibody in coeliac disease and dermatitis herpetiformis, and antiadrenal antibodies in Addison's disease, suggesting an immune response determinant specific for the target. Most diseases associated with B8 have been called "immunopathic" disorders (active chronic hepatitis, SLE, thyrotoxicosis, myasthenia gravis, coeliac disease, Sjogren's syndrome, dermatitis herpetiformis, juvenile diabetes mellitus, and idiopathic Addison's disease). They have good if not hyperimmunologic activity, suggesting that the common denominator in these varied diseases is hyperimmune function, perhaps gene controlled, the target of which is controlled by other factors, genetic and environmental. That HLA-B7 may be a marker for hypoimmune reactivity is suggested by poor T-cell effector abilities,[112] B7-associated reduced cellular immunity in MS[113,114] reduced tuberculin skin test reactivity,[115] and an increased tendency to reject kidney grafts in B-positive compared with B-negative recipients.[116] These considerations caused Bias and Chase[86] to suggest a pair of allelic genes existing in balanced polymorphism in the populations conferring increased (B8) or decreased (B7) immune responsiveness.

A recent review[25] lists the diseases associated with the HLA region purported to control immune responses. MS is shown in association with *Dw2,* and all the diseases previously associated with *B8* are shown in association with *Dw3,DRw3:* the incidence of *Dw3,DRw3* is higher than that of *B8* in the patients, suggesting that the disease susceptibility gene is closer to the D region than the B region. For the reasons stated above, *B8* best resembles an autoimmune gene. Since the pathology of the diseases associated with *B8* is so varied, either another genetic factor or an environmental factor must determine which organ is involved. Rheumatoid arthritis is associated with the *Dw4*-related B-cell antigen DRw4,[87] and this disease is unique in that so far no association has been found with any other HLA locus. Juvenile rheumatoid arthritis may be determined by a different D,DR factor.

Immune Regulation

The appearance of degenerative diseases is one major correlate of aging. These diseases are either preceded by or accompany deficiencies in physiological parameters. One of the most striking physiological correlates of aging is the decline in immune function. This decline has been documented in almost all phases of immune function at the organ, systemic, and cellular levels in mouse, rat, and man. The first, and perhaps fundamental, change noted in an organ system is the involution of the thymus that occurs shortly after sexual maturity.[117] Since one of the major lymphoid populations concerned with recognition and regulation is the thymus-dependent T-cell, the implications for maintenance of immune function are evident. Shortly after an individual reaches sexual maturity, the thymic lymphoid cells are replaced by adipose tissue, but the hormone-secreting cells remain, permitting a continuous production of thymosin activity.[117] There is a high level of thymosin in young people, which falls dramatically at age 25 (Figure 5). The decrease in thymosin is inversely correlated with an increase in age-related disorders.[117]

It has been shown that the level of circulating natural antibodies declines with age in man.[54,118] The maximum response to antigenic stimulus measured by humoral antibody appears to be equivalent in aged and young people, but the level before and after the peak response is lower in the aged and declines faster. Also, delayed hypersensitivity reactions are reduced in aged population.[118] In experimental animals, the humoral antibody response declines with age to 10% of the peak response about the time of thymic involution.[119] The ability to reject skin grafts[120] and resistance to infectious disease are not as great as in the young.[38] Paralleling these declining responses is an increase in symptoms of autoimmune reactions and autoantibodies.[51,54,117,121] Increased mortality was noted among aged individuals who had little or no indication of delayed hypersensitivity reactions.[118]

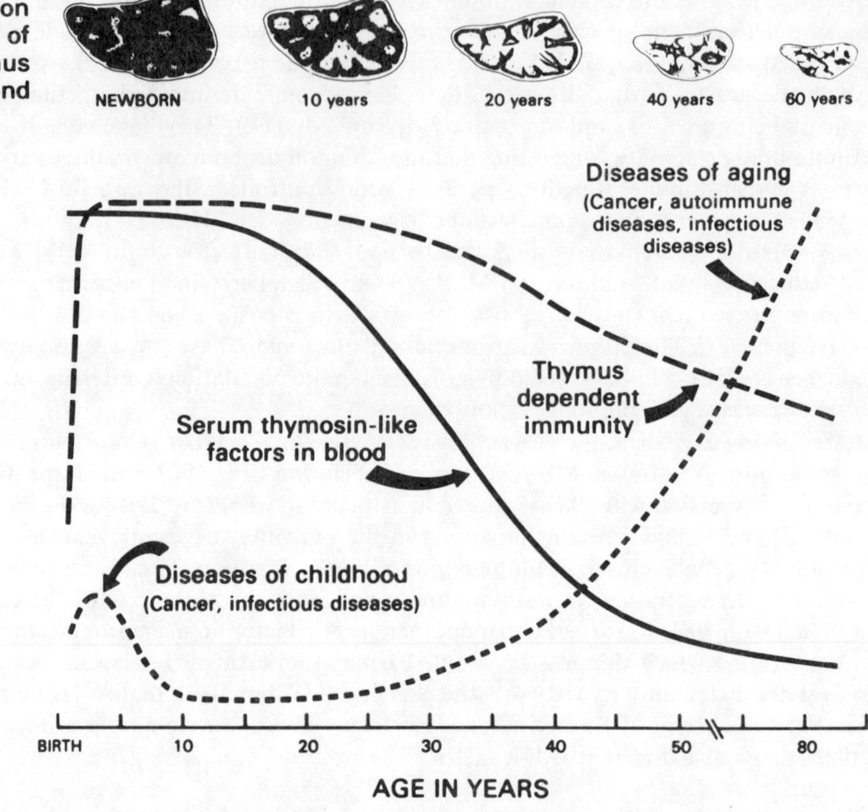

FIGURE 5. Relationship of thymus development and function with life span and disease. (From Goldstein, A. L., Thurman, G. B., Low, T. L. K., Trivers, G. E., and Rossio, J. L., in *Aging Series, Vol. 8, Physiology and Cell Biology of Aging,* Cherkin, A., Finch, C. E., Kharasch, N., Makinodan, T., Scott, F. L., and Strehler, B. S., Eds., Raven Press, New York, 1979, 51. With permission.)

For the basis of declining immune functions to be understood, the efficiencies of the various aspects of the immune reactions have to be assessed in relation to the total capacity to find where the system breaks down. Since the initial observations of declining humoral responses, much information has been obtained at the cellular level on the genetic control of the mechanisms of humoral and cellular immunity as well as the effects of age on the efficiency of these mechanisms. However, the added information has only made us more cognizant of the complexity of immunoregulation.

Experimental studies in rodents have explored the cellular basis for the reduced response to antigen with age.[121] Deficiencies have been reported in the responsible cells primarily, but environmental changes contribute to loss of efficiency of response as well.[122]

Although the sizes of lymph nodes and spleen change little with age,[121,123] histological differences have been reported[124,125] describing fewer germinal centers and an increase in plasma cells and macrophages with age. The numbers of T- and B-cells (in long-lived mice) and θ-positive cells remain the same,[122,126] but the ability of these cells to respond to mitogenic stimulus is depressed in man[118,127] and mice.[128] Although natural antibody titers (to extrinsic antigens) are low in the aged, an increase in antibody titer to intrinsic antigens such as granulocyte[129] and liver nuclei[54] has been documented in aging populations, with a greater risk of mortality from vascular disease associated with increased levels of autoantibody to liver nuclei.[54] In another study in which changes in serum levels of three classes of immunoglobin in older subjects were evaluated from cross-sectional and longitudinal data, serum levels were found to increase in a majority of aged individuals. However, a number of individuals showed a trend toward decreasing levels,[130] and an association between the group with decreasing levels and mortality was reported. Since one study deals with specific antibody and the other with total antibody levels, these observations are not irreconcilable.

The decrease in T-cell response to mitogens occurs very early in the life span, sooner than and more severely than the decline in B-cell response.[122] This differential decline in proliferative response results in a disturbed T/B cell ratio. The result of such a disturbed homeostasis may lead to immunopathology, although definitive studies on the effects of relative changes of regulatory T-cell subpopulations have not been done. The abrupt decline in proliferative response of some T-cells may be maturational effect[13] and not a parameter of the age-related decline in function. However, mixing studies show that cells from spleens of old mice actively suppress proliferative responses of spleen cells from young mice.[131,132] Another indication of deficient response, perhaps active suppression, is that a tenfold increase in antigen is required to maximally immunize old mice in vivo, although in vitro the amount is the same for both young and old.[133] Perhaps antigen presentation is deficient in old mice.[122]

Many of these studies suggest that the decline in immune function with age is due to changes in the T-cell population of lymphocytes.[123] However, some long-lived strains of mice have no detectable decrease in cell-mediated immunity even though they have detectable levels of autoantibodies.[126] Conflicting reports have appeared in the literature as well with respect to the relative ability of spleen cells from young and old mice to respond in mixed-lymphocyte culture (MLC) in an in vitro assay.[123] When the response of lymph node lymphocytes to allogenic antigens is measured in vivo, the cells respond with equal if not greater blastogenesis.[134] The in vivo test system may allow more accurate measurement of cellular capacity since it is not subject to artifacts such as cell density (relative decrease in effector cell number due to increase in inert cells) and mitomycin leakage.[123] However, the responding cells in the lymph nodes of old mice are a different population (cortisone resistant) than those from young mice (cortisone sensitive), suggesting a qualitative change in cellular composition[135] even though in the in vivo assay no change in proliferative response with age was noted.

It has been suggested from studies on the relative ability of T-cells from old and young mice to promote antibody response to T-cell-dependent antigen[133] that T helper-cell function declines with age.[119,122] However, the ability to sustain an allogeneic effect is not impaired in T-cells from mice old enough to have deficient humoral immune function.[136] Since these are similar T-cell functions, the deficiency noted in reconstitution experiments may be a function of effector cell density in the T-cell populations from aged mice. The B-cell population in middle-aged mice (12 months) was shown to be refractory to the allogeneic effect,[136] demonstrating a deficiency in function at the B-cell level. Other changes in T-cell-independent B-cell functions have also been reported, such as decreases in germinal centers (B-cell areas) in lymphatic follicles,[124,125] a decline in transformation of immunoblasts into plasma cells with age,[137] and a 3- to 3.5-fold decrease in proliferative potential in B-cell mitogenic response.[133]

Although the number of stem cells in aged mice appears to be unchanged, there must be some change in dynamic equilibrium, since the frequency of stem cells decreases but the total number of cells increases, sometimes twofold.[138] Bone marrow from old mice is capable of producing plaque-forming cells when injected with sheep red blood cells into irradiated recipients, whereas bone marrow from young mice is not.[119] Thus, the quality of the stem cells must have changed with age even if the numbers have not.

It is evident that there are inconsistencies in the literature. These conflicts are probably more artifactual than real. It is likely that they result from the use of different species, strains, and ages for experimental subjects and different experimental designs leading, at times, to different results.[123] An important consideration frequently ignored is that the maturation rates, ages of peak response, and decay rates of different immune responses differ between strains of mice.[93]

Many of the same age-related deficiencies in immune function occur following neonatal[139] and adult[140] thymectomy, resulting in shortened life span. They also occur early in the life span of short-lived autoimmune susceptible mouse strains,[139] leading some authors to postulate that these strains undergo accelerated aging.[18] However, such short-lived autoimmune mice also undergo a progressive decline with age in θ-positive cells and cell-mediated immunity that cannot be demonstrated in nonautoimmune susceptible long-lived strains.[126] It is unclear yet whether these short-lived mice are genetic aberrations with little relevance to aging[126] or whether they experience early in life the extreme of a condition which in the long-lived mice may be so slight as to be undetectable by available methodologies but sufficient to lead to chronic and debilitating autoimmunity.

Experimental studies and clinical observations show that immunodeficiencies, induced or natural, are accompanied by autoimmune reactions and autoimmune disease[51] such as rheumatoid disease, SLE, and dermatomyositis. These observations suggest that a ''precise balance of complex interacting immunological systems'' is essential for ''maintenance of health and avoidance of autoimmunity''. Regulation of these systems is controlled by genes located primarily in the MHC.

The Major Histocompatibility Gene Complex

All vertebrates examined have an MHC; experimental evidence demonstrates, to a greater or lesser degree, elements of an MHC in primates, dogs, cattle, pigs, rabbits, Syrian hamsters, guinea pigs, rats, chickens, mice, and humans.[141] Although an homologue to the MHC has not yet been described in invertebrates,[142] tissue rejection and antibody production with subsequent development of memory have been demonstrated in primitive vertebrates,[143] and histoincompatible reactions have been described in invertebrates.[141,142,144] The most completely studied MHCs are HLA of man and H-2 of mouse. Experimental work on the mouse was facilitated by the availability of congenic lines of mice that differ only at the MHC. The use of intra-H-2 recombinants permitted analysis of the effects of differences at small regions of the MHC, resulting in the identification of linked loci affecting many related and seemingly unrelated functions. Klein[145] lists as many as 59 pleomorphic effects. An abbreviated list is shown in Table 5. Much of the animal work formed the basis for the studies in man which had to depend on the more difficult approach of population genetics to characterize the human HLA system. For instance, the identification of complement factors linked to H-2 in the mouse led to the successful search for homologous loci in man.[146] However, since man is a heterogeneous species composed of an unlimited number of haplotypes and haplotype combinations living in uncontrolled and variable environments, studies on the human MHC have contributed to an understanding of the influence of the interaction of components of this gene complex with the environment on normal aging and disease.

These gene complexes lie on chromosome 6 of man[147] and 17 of mouse.[148] The genetic organization of these chromosomes is shown in Figure 6A. Genes controlling major homologous functions (Table 5) are indicated for major serological determinants and allograft target antigens *(HLA-A, -B, -C; H-2D, -K),* ability to induce an MLC response *(HLA-D; Ir-1A, Ir-1B, Ia-5),* serologically defined B lymphocyte anti-

Table 5
MHC-REGULATED FUNCTIONS[a]

Serologically detectable cell surface alloantigens
Induction of allograft reaction
Target of allograft reaction
Complement levels
Susceptibility to viral leukemogenesis
Testosterone levels
Helper and/or suppressor T-cells
Immune response to T-dependent antigens
Level of humoral antibody response
Level of antibody class
Restriction of T-B-cell collaboration
Restriction of cytotoxic effector cell
Complement receptor expression
Serologically detectable B cell antigens
Cyclic AMP levels
Maturation of immune function
T/B lymphocyte ratios
Cell-mediated immunity
Humoral immunity
Sex and lymphoid organ weights
Natural killer cells
Life span

[a] Modified from Klein.[145]

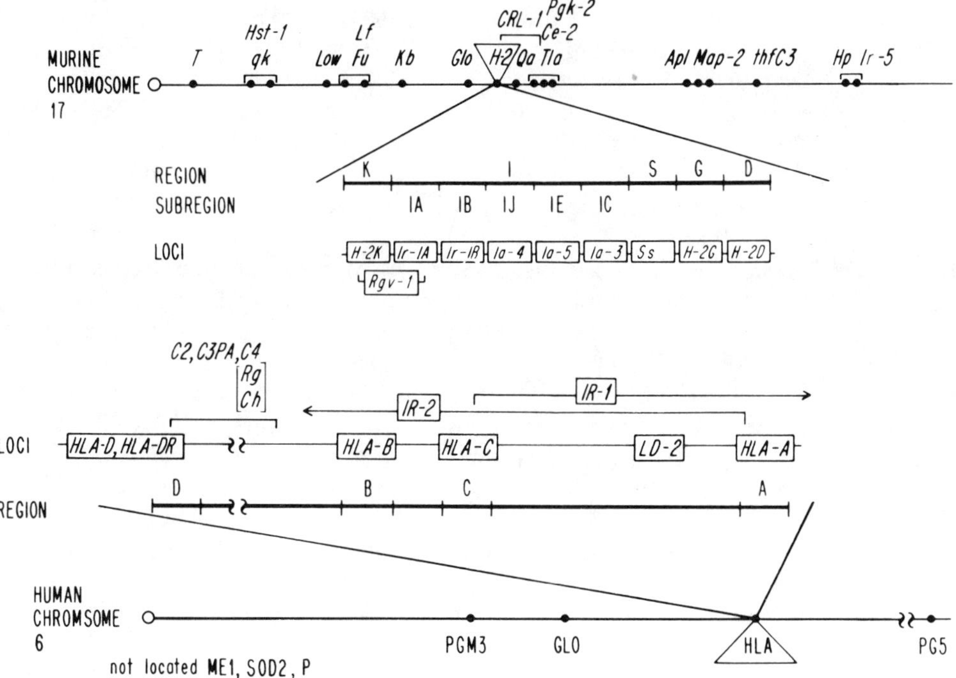

FIGURE 6A. Organization of chromosomes 17 of mouse and 6 of man on which lie the MHC. Locations of known loci and regions are indicated. Positions of HLA B and A regions are placed in relation to the homologous *H-2* regions K and D.[85,145,149-152]

gens *(HLA-DR; H-2Ia),* and levels of complement factors *(C2, C3PA, C4; C3,*[153] *Ss(C4), CRL-1*[154]*).* Though not yet appearing on the gene map, one family study suggests that C8 deficiency in man may be associated with HLA centromeric to HLA-A.[151] Other factors located on these chromosomes and perhaps related to the physiologic function of this supergene are: for the mouse; hormonal regulation of testosterone production *(Hom-1),* thymus leukemia antigen *(Tla),* and virus susceptibility *(Rgv-1),* for man; red-cell antigens *P,* Chido *(Ch),* and Rogers *(Rg);* the last two appear to be components of C4.[156] Other biochemical markers are shown [PGM_3 (phosphoglucomutase), *GLO* (glyoxylase), 21-OH-DEF (21-hydroxylase deficiency)[157] and *PG5* (urinary pepsinogen)], as are unlocated biochemical markers [*ME1*] (cytoplasmic malic enzyme) and *SOD 2* (superoxide dismutase)] for man[149] and *Ce-2* (kidney catalase-2), *Pgk-2* (phosphoglycerate kinase-2), *Apl* (acid phosphatase of the liver), *Map-2* (mannosidase processing-2), and *GLO*[153] for mouse. The complex *T/t* region, an independent gene complex controlling cell-to-cell interactions in differentiation which may have an influence on recombination within the H-2,[158] is located distally to the centromere on the mouse 17th chromosome. Evidence for the existence of a similar locus linked to HLA in man has been reported by Amos et al.[159] The mouse MHC is unique in that the region controlling the B-cell Ia antigens and immune response to specific antigens (I region) lies between the *H-2K* and *H-2D* loci, whereas in man it lies outside the homologous *HLA-A* and *HLA-B* loci. However, Amos and Ward[160] caution that the linear order may still be open to interpretation, pointing out that H and Ir loci may exist outside the limits of D and K. For more detailed review of the genetic structure of these chromosomes see reviews by Bodmer,[149] Thorsby[150] (human), Klein[145,161] Vitetta and Capra,[148] and David[162] (mouse). The combination of alleles at all loci of the MHC on the same chromosome is called the haplotype and as few as four polymorphic loci can generate a very large number of different haplotypes. In man, considering only the known alleles at the four HLA loci A, B, C, D, Lamm and Kristensen[163] estimate 13×10^3 possible haplotypes.

It can be seen from Figure 6B that in mice the MHC controls diverse functions (listed in Table 5) ranging from the original observations of susceptibility to viral leukemogenesis[59,167] and allograft recognition and rejection to more sophisticated immunological functions,[164] such as regulation of specific antibody formation,[168] T helper and suppressor cell function,[169] T-B-cell interactions,[170] *H-2* restriction of cell-mediated function,[171-173] and regulation of levels of several components of the complement cascade to gene control over nonimmunological parameters such as vesicular gland,[174] testes and thymus weight,[175] serum testosterone level,[176,177] target organ sensitivity to testosterone,[178] cAMP level in liver cells,[179] and level of a cytosol cortisone-binding protein.[180] Most of these functions have been identified in man as well.[85,149] Considering the diversity of function represented in the MHC, can this region be called a "supergene" as defined by Ceppellini?[181] The nature of the functions outlined in Table 5 suggests that this complex exerts powerful regulatory control over the maintenance of homeostasis and therefore qualifies according to Bodmer's description of a supergene[149] as a group of "closely linked genes controlling functions that are at least to some extent interrelated, and with respect to which, in some cases, selective interaction occurs in such a way as to favor close linkage." However, where the supergene starts and stops in unclear.

Genetically, the MHC has been divided into *regions, subregions,* and *loci,*[182] but the complex can be divided functionally into three classes.[141] The regions within each class have not only similar functions but also similar biochemical properties, which implies similarity in evolutionary origin.

Class I — Regions code for glycoproteins expressed on the membrane of most cells

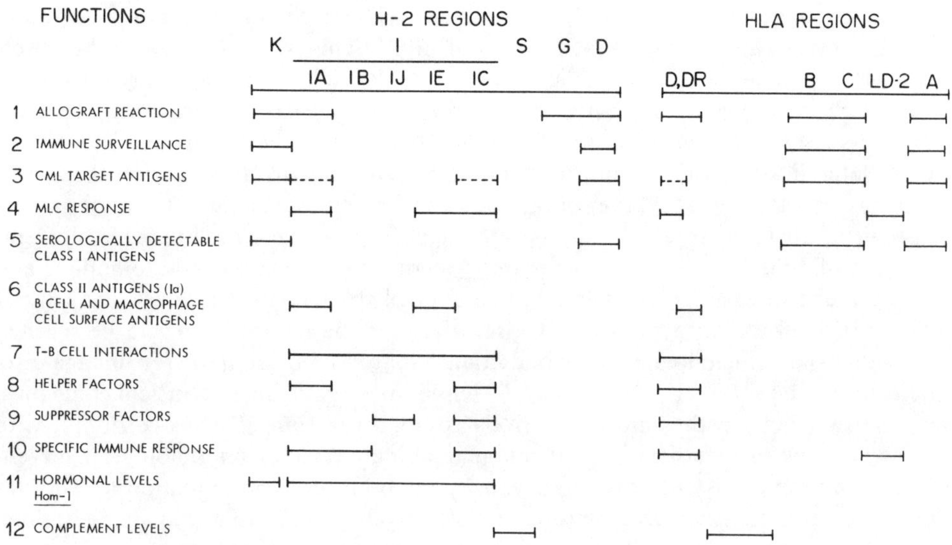

FIGURE 6B. Probable regions that control defined immune functions in the MHC of mouse and man.[145,152,161,164-166]

that readily induce antibodies, T-cell proliferation, and the generation of effector cells. They are the principal target of alloreactive cytotoxic T cells and are identifiable by serological methods. They represent the first observed MHC alloantigens described for mouse[183] and man, originally designated LA and FOUR.[184,185] The loci controlling these antigens tend to occur in pairs separated by other loci.

Class II — Regions (I for mouse and D for man) cluster in one area and are characterized by their ability to stimulate proliferation of allogeneic T-cells in vitro (MLC).[165,186,187] In the mouse this region controls the immune response to specific antigens (*Ir* genes).[168] Genes located in this region (*Ia* in the mouse and DR in man) code for glycoproteins serologically identified on macrophages and B-cells, with lesser amounts found on sperm and epidermal cells.[188-190] It is undetermined whether D and DR represent the same or different gene products.[166, 191]

Class III — Regions control components of the complement pathway. These may be regulatory rather than structural loci since they determine serum levels in the mouse, *C3* and *Ss* (C4); deficiencies in man, *C2, C3PA, C4,* and *C8;* or rate of appearance of receptors for C3, *CPL-1,* described in the mouse.[154] Distribution of several Class III loci over the MHC has not yet been determined, but it has been proposed that for man they exist between HLA-B and HLA-D.[26] This classification leaves out the loci regulating steroid function which have a role in maintenance of homeostasis by the regulation of endocrine balance.[17]

The association of diseases with a gene complex that controls immune function, T-B-cell differentiation and interaction, levels of Ig production, hormonal regulation, and complement levels suggests but does not prove cause and effect. It is not the purpose of this paper to speculate on mechanisms; however, several reviews have been written suggesting mechanisms by which the MHC may favor susceptibility to disease.[49,68,69,86,160] Nevertheless, several observations should be made on specific function to introduce the next topic, "Genetic Stability". It is paradoxical that this genetic region, which has been selected to protect the individual from environmental assault and to regulate homeostatic mechanisms, would suddenly work against the health of the individual and cause degenerative and ultimately, lethal changes in the physiology.

It has been suggested that genes that facilitate survival in the juvenile and young adult periods may be life-limiting in later stages of life.[173] This is consistent with the observation that patients with diseases associated with B8 are immunologically hyperreactive, which facilitates their survival during the early stages of the growth curve when infectious diseases account for most mortality and permits these individuals to survive to the later interval of the mortality but then succumb to autoimmune disease.[173] Svejgaard et al.[49] suggest that selection years ago for genes resistant to the major killers (influenza, tuberculosis, cholera, malaria, plague, leprosy, and even the great epidemics of the Middle Ages) renders succeeding generations susceptible to autoimmune and hyperimmune diseases. Since Class II loci control the recognition phase and Class I loci function as the target for cellular reactivity,[172] the haplotype would be selected for, rather than single loci.[66] van Rood et al.[66] suggest that the basis for linkage disequilibrium is the survival value of a *A1,B7* haplotype in resistance to ancient epidemics, i.e., the two loci together more effectively combat infections. This is consistent with the suggestions of heterozygous advantage in aging people or immunological surveillance[171] and the persistence of heterozygosity in an inbreeding population.[192] The stability of determinants which function more effectively as a group would assure optimal antibody response, albeit at the price of greater autoimmune disease later.

However, the effects of other correlates of aging, integrity of the transcription, translation, and stability of the DNA, must be considered. Within the MHC are genes that code for receptor sites on T and B cells whose structures are exquisitely defined to participate in the function of recognition of self and nonself. It was once thought that the immune system recognized and eliminated foreignness and ignored (tolerated) self. However, in view of the concepts of corecognition of self and altered self,[193] it may be that recognition of foreignness occurs only in the context of self and tolerance of foreignness occurs when self-recognition breaks down. Slight alterations and variations can change efficiency of interactions leading to reduced or enhanced responses. The loss of recognition of self is a well-known phenomenon leading to autoimmunity. Indeed, one of the major observations of aging is that immunological imbalance is followed by autoimmune reactions.[51,194] Thus, MHC determinants determine specific structures on lymphocytes and macrophages as well as on other tissues which stimulate proliferation and activation of effector cytotoxic lymphocytes that produce aggressive delayed hypersensitivity, allograft, immunoglobulin-producing plasma cells, and graft-vs.-host reactions. Included within this complex are also genes controlling viral susceptibility as well as regulating T-T-cell interactions that determine cell-mediated responses to viral altered membrane components. Therefore, minor alterations in the structural integrity of the DNA or in the fidelity of transcription and translation can conceivably disturb these delicate homeostatic mechanisms. Obviously, the maintenance of genetic stability with time is important in maintaining balanced immunoregulatory and endocrine function.

Genetic Stability

Biological processes must be precise for complex steps of cellular differentiation to proceed sequentially resulting in differentiated cells equipped with the appropriate gene products required for their function. Each unique protein or molecule that governs a biological reaction or becomes a structural component of cells is encoded by a unique nucleotide sequence within a gene. Although DNA polymerases are highly accurate, errors in replication and transcription do occur, and translation of the genetic message is even less accurate. In this section we present known facts and implications of the effects of mutations in DNA and errors in protein synthesis as they pertain to cell surface antigens, immunogenetics, and aging.

Germinal and Somatic Mutations

In a discussion of mutations it is important to note that although germinal mutations affect the quality of cellular antigens, all the cells of a mutant organism express the same altered antigens, so germinal mutations do not affect the recognition of self vs. nonself among cells of the mutant organism. In contrast, mutations of individual somatic cells would cause the expression of new cell surface antigens only on the mutant cells so that the mutant cells would be easily recognized as nonself and eliminated. Furthermore, infrequent errors in the incorporation of amino acids during protein synthesis would change only a few of numerous cell surface antigens, which may minimize the chance that the minute quantity of the new antigen will promote nonself recognition; although the latter cells may not be eliminated immediately, the cumulative effect of minute quantities of such altered antigens could cause the induction of antibodies or the stimulation of immunocytes that become involved in antitumor protection or the late development of autoimmunity. Thus, genetic stability is important in the maintenance of homeostasis, and mutations in somatic cells and errors in protein synthesis could disturb the balance of interacting systems and promote the aging process. If DNA polymerases in tissues of aged animals commonly permit a higher frequency of errors in DNA replication and transcription, and if protein synthesis becomes more error-prone in old animals, such errors in genes located within the MHC could be a molecular basis for a breakdown in immunoregulation, resulting in the higher frequency of cancer and other degenerative diseases in older animals.

As stated above, germinal mutations per se are not important in self and nonself discrimination; however, data on the frequency of germinal mutations are useful in estimating an expected frequency of mutations in somatic cells if one assumes that the same genes mutate at similar frequencies in germinal and somatic cells. The natural frequency of germinal mutations at 36 different biochemical loci in man is not greater than 2.24×10^{-5} mutations per locus per generation for electrophoretically detectable protein variants,[195,196] which corresponds well with the spontaneous frequency of 5×10^{-6} deleterious mutations per locus per cell generation in human somatic cells.[197,198] McKusick[199] has estimated that there are approximately 10^5 structural genes in the DNA of human cells. Martin[48] has noted that as many as 162 of the 2336 genetic loci listed by McKusick may affect the life span of humans. Although one may generalize on the total risk by multiplying mutation rate by loci at risk, the risk to the individual of mutations at different loci is not the same for several reasons. Ohno and Nagai[200] have suggested that the accumulation of mutations in single-copy genes is not likely to accelerate the aging process, but that mutations in multiple-copy genes (i.e., genes for 5s, 18s, and 28s rRNA; the tRNAs; and the five species of histones) have the potential to affect the performance of the entire genome. A few single-copy genes (i.e., genes for DNA and RNA polymerases and DNA repair enzymes) would show a similar pervasive effect.[200] The histocompatibility loci should be added to the group of genes that affect the aging process.[13,14] Klein[145] has tabulated published data on the spontaneous frequency of mutations at several loci in laboratory mice, and cumulative data from several laboratories show that relative to other loci the H-2 locus has a very high frequency of 4.0×10^{-5} spontaneous mutations per gamete. While the average frequencies of mutation at dominant and recessive visible loci in mice are 4.4×10^{-7} and 3.8×10^{-6} mutations per locus gamete, respectively, the frequency of germinal mutations for all histocompatibility loci combined is 2.3×10^{-3} per gamete.[145] This exceedingly high frequency of germinal mutations at the histocompatibility loci is significant if a comparable high frequency of spontaneous mutations occurs at the histocompatibility loci of somatic cells, because alleles at the histocompatibility loci have an important role in the recognition of self and nonself, the induction of cytotoxic cells, and the elimination of cells that express variant antigens on their cell surface.

Data on the susceptibility of alterations at the *H-2* loci by environmental insult have been reported in studies that show that chemicals and viruses are able to induce the expression of nonisogenic H-2 as well as non-H-2 transplantation antigens involved in antitumor protection.[201,202] Newly expressed tumor-associated transplantation antigens may appear as a result of mutations or the derepression of specific genes that are a part of a polygenic system. Very different mechanisms must be invoked to bring about these diverse alternatives. The mutation theory suggests that a new allele arises either through base substitutions, frameshifts, and insertions or deletions in the DNA, whereas the derepression theory suggests that cells of an organism have the entire spectrum of structural genes of a given species but that normally most of these genes are repressed. Data bearing on which alternative is correct have been obtained by Brown et al.[203] who compared the column chromatographic properties of tryptic peptides obtained from the histocompatibility antigens of parental B10.D2 mice and one of their mutant offspring,B10.D2-$H\text{-}2^{dml}$ (M504). Although *H-2D* and *H-2K* molecules differed at 40% of their tryptic peptides, only a few peptides of the $H\text{-}2^{da}$ molecules of the mutant were altered, which suggests that the new antigens in M504 resulted from recent bona fide alterations in DNA rather than from derepression of silent *H-2* alleles.

Repair of genetic lesions resulting from physical and chemical insults to DNA is one mechanism for maintaining genetic stability. The observations that the incidence of spontaneous chromosome aberrations is increased in persons with Fanconi's anemia and ataxia telangiectasia, and that DNA-repair is deficient in persons with xeroderma pigmentosum led to the proposal that aging may result from an accumulation of DNA lesions in cells.[204] However, patients with progeria or Werner's syndrome do not have defective DNA repair, thus defective DNA repair as the universal cause of aging seems doubtful.

Present data on mutations involve structural loci only; the area of mutations at regulatory loci is basically untapped, but they may be equally important with respect to the onset of debilitating diseases. Regulatory genes are those which coordinate the levels of expression of different genes during development, maturation, and senescence as cells respond to their internal and external environments. The role of regulatory genes in aging must await improved methods for the study of regulatory genes in higher eukaryotes.

Polymerase Errors

Molecular mechanisms which permit errors to occur during the replication and transcription of DNA and the translation of mRNA have been identified largely through the use of enzymatic systems of *Escherichia coli* and bacteriophage, and we shall draw on this literature to discuss such mechanisms. Microorganisms are often used because of the relative ease of identifying relationships between the altered genome and enzymic processes in simple organisms. More limited studies on the fidelity of biological systems in higher eukaryotes, however, indicate that similar mechanisms and degrees of fidelity are expressed in higher organisms.

The spontaneous frequencies of mutations in *E. coli* and T-4 bacteriophage are in the order of 10^{-6} to 10^{-8}, which indicates that the fidelity of polymerase in the replication of DNA is very high. The fidelity of polymerase in in vitro systems is in the order of 2.5×10^{-6}, which is only slightly less than that found in vivo. Studies on polymerases in L56 and L88 indicate that the accuracy of DNA replication is controlled in part by the structure of DNA polymerase. L56 and L88 have defective structural genes for DNA polymerase which permit a three- to fourfold increase in the misincorporation of thymidine (T) into polydeoxyguanosine nucleotide (poly dG) during the in vitro replication of polydeoxycytidine nucleotide. Normally misincorporation of T into poly dG occurs at a frequency of about 2.4×10^{-6}, but the polymerase from the mutant phage allowed misincorporation of T at a frequency of 8.3×10^{-6}.[205] Although misincorporation of T was relatively similar for a number of factors tested, substitution of 2.0 m*M* Mn^{2+} for 0.2 m*M* Mn^{2+} increased the polymerase error frequency from 2.7×10^{-6} to 61×10^{-6} for the wild type and from 14×10^{-6} to 240×10^{-6} for L56 phage.[205] Observations that DNA polymerases have a reduced fidelity in the presence of Mn^{2+} are significant because Mn^{2+} has been shown to increase the frequency of mutations in *E. coli* and T-4 bacteriophage.[206,207]

Observations of a decreased fidelity of DNA polymerase in *E. coli* and T-4 bacteriophage suggested a mechanism whereby the accumulation of defective polymerases might constitute a molecular basis for aging. Indeed, the low-molecular-weight DNA polymerase isolated from the liver of 24- to 30-month-old BALB/c mice was more error-prone than that of 3- to 6-month-old BALB/c mice.[208] Moreover, DNA polymerase isolated from aging human fibroblasts in culture showed a decreased level of activity with increasing passage, and the fidelity of polymerase using synthetic templates was more error-prone for late-passage cells.[209]

The reduced fidelity of replication could be the basis for the increased frequency of somatic mutations at the glucose-6-phosphate dehydrogenase locus[210] and the higher incidence of observed chromosomal abnormalities near the end of the life span of human fibroblasts in culture.[211]

Translation Errors: Misacylation

The stability of DNA may be affected indirectly via errors in the translation of mRNA. In 1963, Orgel[212] proposed that infrequent translation errors could produce variant proteins, such as polymerases and ribosomal proteins, that could subsequently permit the occurrence of an even higher frequency of errors of replication, transcription, and translation. Cells must have mechanisms to remove most error-containing proteins or else additional errors could increase exponentially until their cumulative effects would exceed the homeostasis required for cell survival.

Misincorporation of amino acids into proteins is a fairly easy end point to measure. Amino acid misincorporation is defined as the incorporation of an amino acid that does not correspond to the codon in the mRNA. Such errors can occur through two basic mechanisms: the appropriate tRNA can be acylated by the wrong amino acid (misacylation), or tRNA that is correctly acylated can associate with an incorrect mRNA codon during peptide elongation (decoding error).

Misacylated tRNA binds to ribosomes, accepts peptides, and transfers its amino acid to the growing polypeptide as efficiently as does the correctly acylated tRNA, so the quantity of misacylated tRNA available for protein synthesis must be kept low. This is accomplished through kinetic proofreading and editing mechanisms during the aminoacylation of tRNA. Misacylated Val-$tRNA^{Ile}$ is rapidly deacylated[213] or much of its precursor, the isoleucyl-tRNA synthetase-Val adenosine monophosphate complex, is destroyed before valine is transferred to $tRNA^{Ile}$.[214] Either of these mechanisms, or a combination, coupled with a 100-fold discrimination of amino acids to associate with their proper aminoacyl synthetase,[215] permits a 1.8×10^4 greater likelihood that the properly charged amino acid will be available for the association of aminoacyl-tRNA with the codons of the mRNA.

Loftfield and Vanderjagt[216] have reported that valine is misincorporated in place of isoleucine specifically at positions 10 and 17 in the alpha chain of rabbit hemoglobin at frequencies of 2×10^{-4} and 6×10^{-4}, respectively. Adult hemoglobins of humans, marmosets, sheep, and cows do not contain coded isoleucine in their globin chains,[217] but chemical analyses of these highly purified hemoglobins showed that isoleucine replaced other amino acids at an average frequency of 3×10^{-5} to 5×10^{-5}.[218-220] Analyses of isoleucine misincorporation in the tryptic peptides of the alpha chain of pig hemoglobin,[221] and in the first 20 residues of amino acids at the amino terminus of the beta chain of rabbit hemoglobin,[219] establish that isoleucine tends to be incorporated preferentially at specific amino acid residues. The substitution frequency for specific amino acids may be tenfold higher than the average substitution frequency, as already suggested by comparison of data reported by Loftfield and Vanderjagt,[216] Popp et al.,[218,219] and Hirsch et al.[220] It is important to note that misincorporation of isoleucine is not significantly higher (less than twofold) in old than in young animals regardless of the species studied.[220]

Hirsch et al.[222] have studied the incorporation of α-aminoisobutyric acid (AIBA) into proteins to investigate the extent of misacylation. AIBA has no isoaccepting tRNA, thus misincorporation of AIBA must proceed first through misacylation. The frequency of incorporation of [^{3}H]AIBA was found to be in the order of 7×10^{-5}. The presence of [^{3}H]AIBA in the protein and not in a conversion production of AIBA, e.g., another amino acid, was confirmed by the recovery and quantitation of [^{3}H]AIBA from hydrolysates of newly synthesized protein. Estimation of errors of aminoacylation of tRNA in 3- and 33-month-old C3H mice through AIBA misincorporaton indicated that misacylation did not increase by more than twofold with age. No attempt was made to localize AIBA at specific amino acid residues, so we do not know if a higher level of misacylation of certain tRNAs occurred under the conditions used. Their studies also showed that spontaneous hepatomas incorporated up to seven times as much AIBA as did adjacent normal liver tissue.[222] Elevated misincorporation of AIBA likewise occurs in transplanted hepatomas,[223] but additional studies are required to determine the significance of the higher misincorporation of AIBA in hepatomas to the incidence of other degenerative diseases.

Translation Errors: Decoding

In contrast to the studies above where misincorporation of amino acids in the studies cited above was most likely primarily through misacylation, Edelmann and Gallant[224] have shown that misincorporation of cysteine into flagellin probably results from errors in decoding. When cultures contained streptomycin, which induces an increased frequency of mistakes in the recognition of pyrimidines at the first position of CGU and CGC codons of Arg so that they are read as UGU and UGC codons for Cys,[225] they found a fivefold increase over the average misincorporation of 6 pmol [^{35}S] cysteine per 10,000 pmol of flagellin. Moreover, *relA*$^-$ mutants of *E. coli,* which normally exhibit a fivefold increase of misincorporation of cysteine during arginine starvation,[226] misincorporated three times again as much [^{35}S] cysteine into flagellin during arginine starvation in the presence of streptomycin. Since only two of the six codons of Arg can be misread as UGU or UGC codons of Cys, a decoding error of 10^{-4} can be expected for these two Arg codons in normal exponentially growing cells of *E. coli.*

The fidelity of codon-anticodon associations has also been studied in vitro by adding the deficient aminoacylated tRNAs to mutant strains that have defective tRNA synthetases. In such a system valine codons are read as two-letter code words,[277] and leucine codons must be misread frequently since a complete coat protein can be synthesized in the presence of only one (Leu-tRNA$_3^{Leu}$) of the five isoaccepting leucine tRNAs commonly found in cells.[228]

The likelihood of improper binding of aminoacylated tRNA with codons in mRNA during the decoding phase has also been investigated through studies on the relative stabilities of association between the complementary anticodons of two tRNAs.[229] Correct pairings of anticodons between tRNAs have longer complex lifetimes (usually greater than 100 msec) than those for incorrect pairings (usually less than 10 msec), which suggests that correct pairings of mRNA codons and tRNA anticodons are more stable and should result in favorable binding of the appropriate amino acid during chain elongation. If the complex lifetimes between anticodons of two tRNAs are similar to those between mRNA codons and tRNA anticodons, the ribosome must be involved in some editing function to reduce the frequency of misincorporation of amino acids when an inappropriate but rather stable mRNA codon-tRNA anticodon complex is formed.

Ribsome Editing

Menninger[230] has demonstrated that the growing but incomplete polypeptide chain can be removed from ribosomes during protein synthesis. He has suggested that this may occur preferentially as an editing function of ribosomes when there is an inappropriate association of mRNA codons and tRNA anticodons, and he has also discussed how ribosome editing could delay the onset of error catastrophe during cellular aging.[231]

Thus, there is ample opportunity for the genome to be expressed less than perfectly. It appears, however, that much genetic instability can be tolerated quite well and that alterations only at certain sites provide the cumulative disruptions that disturb homeostasis. The remainder of this report will describe experimental attempts to define the portion of the genome most sensitive to age-associated alterations.

LIFE SPAN AS A PHENOTYPE

The family studies mentioned earlier showed that there is a genetic determination of longevity, but the nature of the control was not determined. In the Abbott et al.[10] study, in which the life span of progeny of nonagenarians increased with the life span of nonproband parent, the increase in mean life span appeared to be due to a decrease in deaths in the middle years rather than to an extension of range of life (i.e., ''squaring the curve''). Since diseases determine the shape of the mortality curve, particularly degenerative diseases, and disease susceptibility genes are located in or near the MHC, what evidence is there that the genetic region in and around the MHC regulates or predicates longevity? If the life-limiting disease susceptibility genes are the MHC genes, one could look for haplotypes that favor longevity. If they are closely linked genes, one could expect that there would be some degree of disassociation of MHC from life span unless linkage disequilibrium exists between MHC and life-limiting genes, as has been shown for diseases and the MHC; in that case one might expect to find associations with age of death and haplotypes of HLA loci. Several reports show that the incidence of HLA antigens does not change when young and old groups are compared; however, Greenberg and Yunis[232] reported a deficiency of *HLA-B8* in older females when the sexes were analyzed separately.

An interesting observation has been made, however, that does suggest an MHC influence over life span. The number of HLA-homozygous individuals was shown to be deceased in older groups[233,234] showing that although no one particular haplotype favors longevity, heterozygosity does. Data from subsequent studies indicate that B locus heterozygosity is most important,[235,236] which suggests that, as with the disease susceptibility genes, the functional heterozygosity may be at the closely linked D locus which controls immune responses. The advantage of heterozygosity for survival has been shown in independent studies from four different geographical areas. The survival value of heterozygosity may be the effect of complementing immune response genes providing the individual with a more efficient humoral immune system which would be responsive to more antigens[169] and/or enhance the recognitive and effector function by increasing the range of T-cell response.[171]

Since the diseases related to MHC show association with several alleles at all the HLA-A, -B, -C, -D loci (Table 4), it would be difficult to find any unique haplotype that has survival value. Since man dies of or with multiple diseases that are associated with different haplotypes, the results of population studies of unrelated people cannot be definitive. Man is a genetically heterogeneous species in which association of a pleiomorphic end point that is under multifactorial and polygenic control with any single locus or gene complex would be a statistical nightmare. Individual HLA antigens have been shown to be associated with particular diseases, but since the MHC is associated with a majority, if not all, the diseases of aging, no one particular haplotype will be discernible as related to aging. To identify the association, one would have to demonstrate in a family study the heritability of a particular haplotype with the phenotype of long or short life. In man, except for very isolated populations, such a study is not possible since changing life style and standard of living over the years from one generation to the next obviate controlled comparisons of age of death.

Studies with animals may be of value in that controlled genetic experiments can be carried out under constant environmental conditions and the effects of discrete segments of the genome on life span can be determined. The MHC has been identified as a likely candidate for Yunis and Greenberg's[17] "longevity homeostasis gene complex".[18,194] The MHC controls the maturation rate of immune responses and maintenance of the functional integrity of the immune system in the mouse.[237] Aging is associated with marked alteration in MHC-associated immune function,[123,132] particularly in mechanisms for distinguishing self from nonself leading to autoimmunity.[238,239] If these represent the primary pathogenetic processes in the aging process,[54] one would expect the supergene that regulates such functions, the MHC, to be responsible for the time of onset, target, progression, and rate of the aging process.[14]

For genetic control of life span in mice to be studied, variants of life span must exist. Different strains of mice show different mean, 50%, or tenth decile mean survivorship.[240] In studies of this kind, however, one must be sure that the shorter life span is the result of accelerated and not precocious aging. If the strain is burdened with genetic defects (e.g., nude, motheaten, dwarf, and NZB mice), individuals will begin life with age-limiting deficiencies, and the life span will be short even though the aging rate is normal.[17,194] The short-lived autoimmune susceptible NZB mice have been described both as a model of accelerated aging[18] and as a model of autoimmunity.[139] They develop a premature T-cell maturation along with hyperimmune humoral responses, followed by typical autoimmune pathology and early death.[239] The pathological syndrome resembles SLE, Sjogren's syndrome, and Waldenstrom's macroglobulinemia.[239] However, Stutman[126] argues that the NZB-like autoimmunity is a genetic defect predisposing to deficient cell-mediated immunity which predicates early death, and the relevance to normal aging which occurs in the presence of an intact cell-mediated immune system is unclear. The T-cell deficit described in NZB mice may be a mechanism for acute NZB-like autoimmunity associated with short life, but it may not be the mechanism involved in chronic, age-related, and multidisease-associated autoimmunity seen in aged long-lived individuals. Also, in these mouse models the association of age-related pathology and the MHC has not been determined, but Talal[239] proposes an interesting hypothesis that suggests endogenous C-type virus in NZB mice contributes to the disruption of regulatory equilibrium by altering the MHC- or Ir-recognitive function on lymphocyte surface membranes.

The availability of congenic strains[241] of mice (that have identical genetic backgrounds but differ at restricted regions) permits a more direct analysis of the effect of restricted genetic loci on life span. There are a large number of strains congenic for *H-2*.[242] Smith and Walford[14] compared the effects on longevity of different *H-2* genotypes on a similar background and similar *H-2* genotypes on different backgrounds. These authors looked at seven *H-2* alleles on B10, C3H, and A backgrounds. Strains carrying three different *H-2* alleles *(m,b,r)* on the B10 background had mean survival times (99 to 141 weeks) that represented as great a range as a single allele *(b)* on three backgrounds (84 to 134 weeks). This observation is true for the mean age of death in the tenth decile as well. The range of mean age of death is as great as that observed among inbred but noncongenic strains.[41] If MHC exerts a singular influence over life span, one would have expected greater uniformity in mean age of death in the three lines with the same *H-2* allele. However, when the background genome was identical, different life spans were seen with a change in the MHC component. For the B10 and A congenic lines the longest-lived strains (B10.RIII and A/WySn, respectively) also had the highest phytohemagglutinin response (T-cell specific) throughout the life span;[237] but this relationship did not hold for the C3H congenic lines. It is evident from these surveys that there is significant interaction between MHC and the genome in life span determination, and that one has to isolate the effects of the MHC from the other unlinked genetic factors in order to identify the controlling loci. Two methods have been used to determine the effect of MHC or its component parts on the age-related functions.

One approach is to look at the genetic basis of age-associated alterations in immune function. The contribution of polygenic effects is avoided by use of congenic mice that differ at the *H-2* locus and recombinant congenic mice that differ from one another at restricted segments of the *H-2* complex.[13] Using these strains it was possible to show a difference in the immune response of lymph node lymphocytes directed against antigens controlled by the *H-2D* and *H-2K* ends of the MHC.[243] It is important to note that in these experiments the *H-2K* end also included differences at the *I* region. Differences at either the *H-2* or *H-2K* end of the MHC induced in vivo lymphocyte transformation earlier than differences at the *H-2D* end (Figure 7). Lymphocytes from 4-month-old donors responding to *H-2D*-end antigens are cortisone sensitive (Figure 7c); however, the cells responding to *H-2K*-end antigens are cortisone resistant (Figure 7b).[135] The differential in time of blastogenesis and sensitivity to cortisone acetate suggested that there are two populations of T lymphocytes responding to MHC cell surface antigens: cortisone-resistant cells responsible for antigen recognition leading to cell-mediated immunity and cortisone-sensitive cells involved in antigen recognition leading to humoral immunity.[13,135] However, these data are subject to reinterpretation, as will be discussed in the following section.

The above methodology was used to analyze the efficiency of immune recognition with age. Studies have documented the decline of primary humoral immunity as early as 12 months of age in mice, falling as low as 20% of the peak response by 24 months.[244] In order to look at the cellular basis of declining humoral immunity in mice with age, particularly antigen recognition, Popp[134] compared in vivo lymphocyte transformation by use of lymphocytes from young and old mice. Allogeneic lymphocytes from old mice (27 months) transformed as well as did allogeneic lymphocytes from young mice (Figure 7a). When the responses to *D*-end and *K*-end antigens were studied, however, it was found that although there was no difference in the ability to respond to *H-2*- or *K*-end antigens (Figure 7a,b), there was a reduction in the ability of lymphocytes from 12- and 20-month-old donors to respond to antigens at the *D* end[134] (Figure 7c). Thus, although a difference in immune function with age could not be detected across the total MHC, a difference with age could be demonstrated when the antigenic

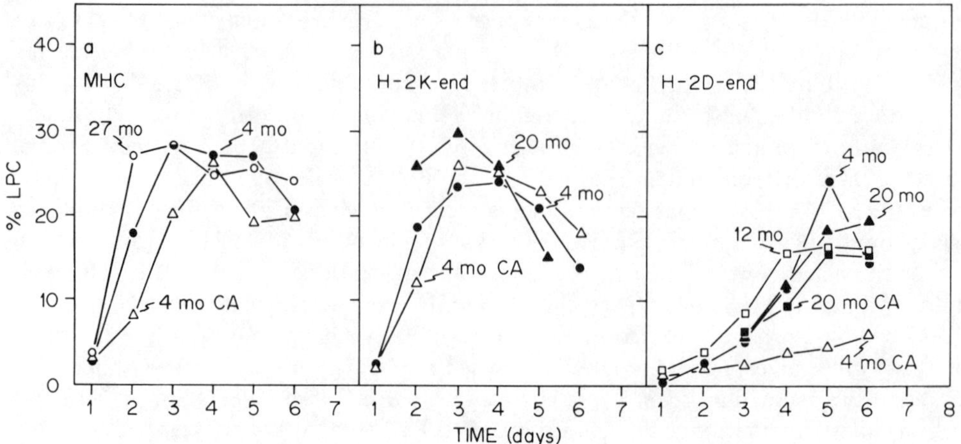

FIGURE 7. In vivo lymphocyte transformation in spleens of irradiated recipient of lymph node lymphocytes from normal or cortisone acetate-treated donors of various ages that differ at the MHC or segments thereof. CA = cortisone acetate treated; LPC = large pyrininophilic lymphocyte (immunoblast).

difference was restricted to a discrete region within the MHC. However, whereas *D*-region responsive lymphocytes from young donors are cortisone acetate sensitive, the lymphocytes that do respond to *D*-region antigens in old mice are cortisone acetate resistant[135] (Figure 7c). These observations are consistent with the model proposed by Popp[13] which says that as the mouse ages, the recognitive function of T-cells does not decline, but certain subpopulations change in relative distribution of component cells. The lymphocytes from young mice that respond are not the same as lymphocytes from old mice responding to the same antigen, but are, instead, a new population of antigen-educated cells that replace the first with time. It has been proposed that environmental antigens are responsible for the accumulation of a store of memory cells which regulate subsequent immune reactivity.[13] The interpretation of these observations in the light of current concepts of the MHC is unclear.

The interpretation that the early and late blastogenesis peaks represented cell-mediated and humoral immunity, respectively, is no longer tenable in the light of modern knowledge of the role of MHC in cellular interactions. Particularly since it has been shown that in MLC the *I*-region gene products induce clonal proliferation of T helper and suppressor precursors, and *D*- and *K*-region gene products induce cytotoxic T effector cells and are the target antigens in cell-mediated lympholysis.[165] The lymphocyte subpopulation responding to *I*-region antigens bears Ly T-cell differentiation marker Lyl, and the *D,K*-region-responsive cytotoxic effector cells bear Ly2,3.[245, 246] The Lyl cells provide helper activity during primary antibody responses[245] and amplify the killer activity of the Ly2,3 cells.[246] Since the MHC can be used to functionally differentiate lymphoid populations based on the region of the MHC to which they respond, some judgments concerning the status of T-cell populations with age can be made.

The conclusion that the cortisone-sensitive blastogenesis induced in recipient spleens on day 5 by *D*-region differences (Figure 7c) represented antigen recognition leading to humoral immunity (T helper cells) was based on the reported cortisone acetate sensitivity of T helper cells.[247] Although the conditions of that study (they used spleen cells and exogenous antigen) may make their results not comparable to lymphocyte viability in the in vivo lymphocyte transformation experiments, the discordance of the characterization of the T helper populations in their experiments with the genetic restriction placed on the MLC-responsive populations is perplexing. There may be more than one cortisone acetate-sensitive population of T-cells, and the splenic "T helper" cell identified by their system may be a different T-cell population from the alloreactive population identified in the MLC.

If the lymphocytes are classified according to Cantor and Boyse,[245] the lymphocytes responding in the late peak might be characterized as Ly2,3 cells. However, Cantor and Boyse[245] have indicated that some Ly2,3 cells are cortisone resistant, and on this basis they cannot be the cells participating in the delayed blastogenesis. These authors showed, however, that the Ly1,2,3 cell is cortisone sensitive and represents as much as 50% of the total peripheral lymphoid population. The cortisone-sensitive, *D*-responsive, delayed blastogenesis in the in vivo lymphocyte transformation assay may be the result of stimulation of the Ly1,2,3 cell population in young mice; with age these cells may change in quality (differentiate?) or be supplanted by cortisone acetate-resistant but responsive cells. This interpretation is supported by the observation that the Ly1,2,3 cell appears within the first week after birth and declines with age, while the percentage of cortisone acetate-resistant *D,K*-alloreactive Ly2,3 cells increases with age (and increasing exposure to antigen).[245] Consistent with these observations is the suggestion by McKenzie et al.[248] that in vivo priming of Ly1,2,3 cells by a high incidence of mutant *H-2* molecules[145] generates increasing numbers of alloreactive Ly2,3 cells.

It is obvious that the lack of uniformity in sources of cells and culture and assay methodology makes comparisons of data difficult and interpretations of specific functions of cell populations from different studies hazardous. Although it is not clear which population of lymphocytes changes with age, perhaps the antigen with which they react is the more significant observation. It is apparent from in vivo lymphocyte transformation data that there is an age-associated change in the lymphocytes responding to *D*-region antigens and that no change in the response to *H-2K*-end antigens of lymphocytes from young and old donors can be detected. Since the *H-2K*-end differences includes the *I*-region as well as the *K*-region, it is likely that the difference between the early and late response is due to *I*-region differences and the *H-2K*-end responding cell population reflects lymphocytes sensitive to *I*-region differences. Thus, no detectable change in lymphocyte responsiveness to Class II antigens is seen with age, while lymphocytes that respond to Class I antigens, in these experiments *H-2D* antigens, decline with age or are supplanted by cortisone-resistant cells.

These observations are reinforced by the results of a study of the influence of *D*- and *K*-end loci on the ability of young and old lymphocytes to support an allogeneic effect.[136] In these studies it was shown that *H-2K*-end (*H-2K* plus *IR-IA*, and *IR-IB*) antigens elicit the allogeneic effect and *H-2D*-end antigens do not, and that lymphocytes from 4- and 20-month-old mice are equally effective. However, the allogeneic effect could not be induced in mice as young as 12-months-old. Again, the recognitive function of the *I*-region antigens remains intact, but the secondary interaction or effector phase of successful immune response becomes deficient with time. There are not enough data to postulate a basis for the age-related reduced ability to recruit additional antibody-forming cells.[136]

There is general agreement that the major function of T lymphocytes is to recognize and react with MHC gene products.[249] Thorsby[250] suggests that alloreactivity of lymphoid cells to MHC differences is a reflection of the ability of T-cells to combine with antigen-modified self-MHC or self-MHC complexed with antigen. Class I antigens are the MHC-determined cell membrane components that function as self-markers, which in combination with foreign antigens become targets for cytotoxic cells in nonself surveillance.[150,193] These studies suggest, therefore, that the mature to aged immune system accumulates a population of cortisone-resistant memory cells alloreactive with

Class I antigens (memory cells induced by environmental antigens). Cross-reactivity of such cells with self and/or altered self would allow for a low-grade autoimmune process concomitant with a deficit in ability to recognize newly infected (i.e., viruses) antigen-MHC targets.[150] The result would be chronic low-grade viral infections such as are prevalent in the aged. These two phenomena do not have to be mutually exclusive, as indeed, the pathobiology of aging individuals appears to be an autoimmune reactivity in the face of depressed ability to resist disease.[51,173]

Although the relevance of alloreactivity of lymphocytes to general immune processes is still being debated,[251] a close functional relationship between virus elimination and immune surveillance of tumor cells is favored. These processes are proposed to occur by corecognition of Class I and foreign antigen structures on the cell surface. Thus, foreign MHC antigens would be seen as "altered self" and be responded to in like manner.[150] This reasoning suggests that Class I antigens are the target antigens in the autoimmune phenomena associated with aging, which is supported by several observations. Mutants at the *D* and *K* loci are more easily detected by cell-mediated than serological techniques.[252] Antiself, *H-2*-restricted cytotoxic cells can be generated during exposure to non-*H-2* antigenic differences or heterologous serum.[253] In an attempt to determine the basis for nonresponsiveness to multiple HLA-D antigens in some individuals, Kristensen and Jorgensen identified cytotoxic lymphocytes specific for Class I antigens HLA-A2.[254] The authors speculate that these naturally occurring cytotoxic lymphocytes may be related to the presence of streptococcal M antigens that cross-react with A2. Viral and chemical modification of the cell membrane can elicit a cytotoxic T-cell response that requires recognition of Class I antigens.[193,255] Thus, environmental alterations of self-MHC with age can be detected and reacted against by lymphoid cells alloreactive to Class I antigen.

Another approach to assess the effect of MHC on longevity is a genetic study in which the association of MHC antigens and life span are determined in segregating progeny. We have used a congenic strain that has been equally useful in studying the immunology and genetics of aging. Strain C57BL/10.F-*H-2* (B10.F) is congenic with B10 and carries the *H-2ⁿ* allele from strain F/St. The B10.F is a model of accelerated aging in that the mice suffer an early appearance of usual aging characteristics (greying and loss of hair, severe weight loss, and thin fragile skin).[13] The B10.F have a greatly shortened life span compared with the inbred partner (50% life span of 15 months compared with 24 months for strain B10) (Figure 8a). Offspring do not appear to be born with any severe life-limiting genetic defects, since the reproductive characteristics (litter size, birth weight, and weaning efficiency), infant and juvenile growth rate, and adult weight are equivalent to those of B10.[13] However, deficiencies associated with aging occur in the B10.F at an earlier age. The number of antibody-forming cells to sheep red blood cells declines from a peak at 4 months to 20% of peak value at 12 months.[13] T-cell function measured by Simonsen[256] assay and popliteal lymph node assay are diminished at an earlier age than in the B10.[257] Serum immunoglobulin IgA levels are very different between the strains; the B10 has a three- to fourfold higher level which increases with time.[258] However, since most inbred strains have a level comparable to that of B10.F, it is not clear that this observation has any relevance to the aging differences seen between the strains. The B10.F mouse expresses the degenerative symptoms of old age without any gross pathologic event predicating early death.

This congenic pair is ideal for a study of the genetic control of the aging process, because the life span differences are great enough to be differentiated in progeny and the genetic difference is restricted to the region in and near the MHC, the region already implicated in determining the aging process. Gene control can be assessed by

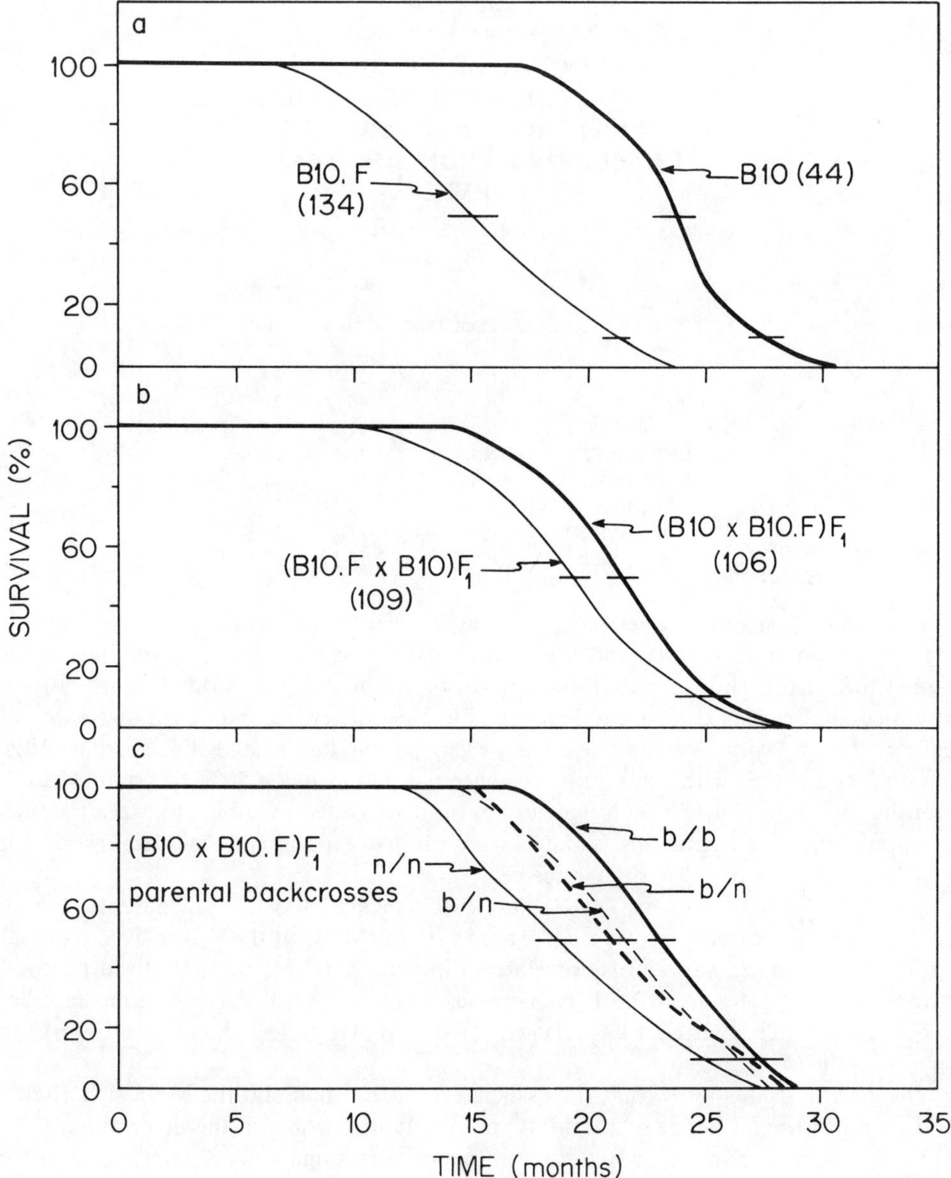

FIGURE 8. Survival curves of the congenic pair B10 and B10.F (a), reciprocal F_1 hybrids (b), and back-cross progeny segregating for the *H-2* genotype (c).

raising F_1, F_2, and backcross progeny from both inbred lines and determining the life span of the progeny carrying the $H\text{-}2^{b/b}$, $H\text{-}2^{b/n}$, and $H\text{-}2^{n/n}$ genotypes. Survival curves of the inbred strain B10 and the congenic B10.F, the reciprocal hybrids (B10 × B10.F)$_1$ and (B10.F × B10)F_1, and *H-2* segregants of progeny of (B10 × B10.F)F_1 backcrossed to the long-lived B10 and the short-lived B10.F parents are shown in Figure 8.

In Figure 8a, the survival curves of the inbred lines demonstrate the dramatic difference in survival between these two strains. The 50% and 10% survival ages are 15 and 21 months, respectively, for B10.F. The 50% survival age for B10 is 24 months and the 10% survival is 26½ months. In an earlier study on a smaller population, the

Table 6
COMPARISON OF 50 AND 10% SURVIVAL OF B10, B10.F RECIPROCAL F_1 HYBRIDS, AND (B10 × B10.F)F_1 BACKCROSS PROGENY DETERMINED FROM SURVIVAL CURVES

		Survival (months)	
Strain	*H-2* genotype	50%	10%
B10	*b/b*	24	27.5
B10.F	*n/n*	15	21
(B10 × B10.F)F_1	*b/n*	21.5	25.5
(B10.F × B10)F_1	*b/n*	19.5	24.5
(B10 × B10.F)F_1	*b/n*	21	27
× B10 ♂	*b/b*	23	27.5
(B10 × B10.F)F_1	*b/n*	21.5	26.5
× B10.F ♂	*n/n*	18.5	25

observation was made that heterozygotes may have different survival patterns depending on the maternal parent, and a maternal effect was suggested.[13] Experiments designed to test this show that survival curves of reciprocal F_1 hybrids (Figure 8b) are intermediate between the parental strains, but they differ depending on the maternal parent. The F_1 with the short-lived maternal parent has a 50% life span of 19½ months, and the F_1 with the long-lived maternal parent has a 50% life span of 21½ months. A maternal effect on longevity has been suggested by others to explain trends in population data,[10] but this is the first controlled experiment that demonstrates a maternal influence over life span in mice.

Survival curves of progeny of (B10 × B10)F_1 backcrossed to both parents (Figure 8c) show that increased survival is correlated with the MHC of the longer-lived parental strain and shortened survival is correlated with the MHC of the short-lived parental strain. Heterozygotes from both backcrosses have a survival curve intermediate between the two. The 50 and 10% survivals (Table 6) also reflect the association of life span with the MHC.

The genetic studies show that the association of life span and the MHC is heritable and establish the influence of the MHC or closely linked loci in the determination of life span. They also suggest a maternal influence over longevity. A maternal influence has been demonstrated in the regulation of basal serum levels of IgA, a phenotype also linked to the MHC.[259]

Although the mechanism of gene control over the regulation of homeostasis governed by the MHC has not yet been defined, it has been established that the MHC does regulate powerful and lethal processes that can cause cell death and destruction, potentially as lethal to a multicellular organim as any drug or toxic chemical. Perhaps more so since they are endogenous, and, as yet, we have little or no control over them. These capabilities are necessary for survival against environmental assault, but with time they become imbalanced and, when directed against self to a more or lesser degree, result in acute or chronic degenerative processes with the ultimate and certain fate of death. MHC-determined molecules participate directly in the immune response, and it is not difficult to see how slight imbalances caused by mutation, transcriptional or translational error, or misdirected accumulated memory can cause the process of immune recognition and aggression to fail to distinguish altered self from self with the required precision.

Aging and, indeed, the diseases of the aged are determined by many factors; other loci as well as environmental factors influence the progress and processes of aging, particularly at the level of interaction with the environment. However, these factors interact with the supergene, whose sensitive monitoring system picks up deviations from normal and responds accordingly. The end result is that the MHC still mediates the pathology and disease processes that have been induced, triggered, or initiated by events controlled by other unlinked genes.

REFERENCES

1. **Comfort, A.,** The influence of genetic constitution on senescence and longevity, in *Aging,* Routledge & Kegan Paul, London, 1964, chap. 4.
2. **Rockstein, M., Chesky, J. A., and Sussman, M. L.,** Comparative biology of aging, in *Handbook of the Biology of Aging,* Finch, C. E. and Hayflick, L., Eds., Van Nostrand Reinhold, New York, 1977, 3.
3. **Sacher, G. A.,** Life table modification and life prolongation, in *Handbook of the Biology of Aging,* Finch, C. E. and Hayflick, L., Eds., Van Nostrand Reinhold, New York, 1977, 582.
4. **Russell, E. S.,** Lifespan and aging patterns, in *Biology of the Laboratory Mouse,* Green, E. L., Ed., McGraw-Hill, New York, 1966, 511.
5. **Meyers, D. D.,** Review of disease patterns and life span in aging mice: genetic and environmental interactions, in *Genetic Effects on Aging,* Bergsma, D. and Harrison, D. E., Eds., Alan R. Liss, New York, 1978, 41.
6. **Abbey, H.,** Survival characteristics of mouse strains, in *Development of the Rodent as a Model System of Aging,* Book II, Gibson, D., Ed., Publ. No. (National Institute Health) 79-161, Department of Health, Education and Welfare, Bethesda, Md., 1979, 1.
7. **Finch, C. E.,** Comparative biology of senescence: evolutionary and developmental considerations, in *Animal Models for Biomedical Research IV,* National Academy of Sciences, Washington, D.C., 1971, 47.
8. **Cosgrove, G. E., Satterfield, L. C., Bowles, N. D., and Klima, W. C.,** Diseases of aging untreated virgin female RFM and BALB/c mice, *J. Gerontol.,* 33, 178, 1978.
9. **Pearl, R. and Pearl, R. de W.,** *The Ancestry of the Long-Lived,* Johns Hopkins Press, Baltimore, 1934.
10. **Abbott, M. H., Murphy, E. A., Bolling, D. R., and Abbey, H.,** The familial component in longevity. A study of offspring of nonagenarians. II. Preliminary analysis of the complete study, *Johns Hopkins Med. J.,* 134, 1, 1974.
11. **Upton, A. C.,** Pathobiology, in *Handbook of the Biology of Aging,* Finch, C. E. and Hayflick, L., Eds., Van Nostrand Reinhold, New York, 1977, 513.
12. **Bank, L. and Jarvik, L. F.,** A longitudinal study of aging human twins, in *The Genetics of Aging,* Schneider, E. L., Ed., Plenum Press, New York, 1978, 303.
13. **Popp, D. M.,** Use of congenic mice to study the genetic basis of degenerative disease, in *Genetic Effects on Aging,* Bergsma, D. and Harrison, D. E., Eds., Alan R. Liss, New York, 1978, 261.
14. **Smith, G. S. and Walford, R. L.,** Influence of the H-2 and H-1 histocompatibility systems upon life span and spontaneous cancer incidences in congenic mice, in *Genetic Effects on Aging,* Bergsma, D. and Harrison, D. E., Eds., Alan R. Liss, New York, 1978, 281.
15. **Cohen, B. H.,** Family patterns of mortality and life span, *Q. Rev. Biol.,* 39, 130, 1964.
16. **Korenchevsky, V.,** *Physiological and Pathological Ageing,* Hafner Publishing, New York, 1961, 1.
17. **Yunis, E. J. and Greenberg, L. G.,** Immunopathology of aging, *Fed. Proc.,* 33, 2017, 1974.
18. **Walford, R. L.,** Immunologic theory of aging; current status, *Fed. Proc.,* 33, 2020, 1974.
19. **Cutler, R. G.,** Evaluation of human longevity and the genetic complexity governing aging rate, *Proc. Natl. Acad. Sci. U.S.A.,* 72, 4664, 1975.
20. **Rockstein, M., Sussman, M. L., and Chesky, J.,** *Symposium on Theoretical Aspects of Aging,* Academic Press, New York, 1974, 1.
21. **Kohn, R. R.,** Aging of animals: observations and questions, in *Principles of Mammalian Aging,* Prentice-Hall, Englewood Cliffs, N.J., 1978, chap. 6.
22. **Lints, L. A.,** *Genetics and Ageing,* S. Karger, New York, 1978, 1.

23. **Dausset, J. and Hors, J.,** Some contributions of the HL-A complex to the genetics of human diseases, *Transplant. Rev.*, 22, 45, 1975.
24. **Ryder, L. P., Nielsen, L. S., and Svejgaard, A.,** Associations between HL-A histocompatibility antigens and non-malignant diseases, *Humangenetik*, 25, 251, 1974.
25. **Bernoco, D. and Terasaki, P. I.,** HL-A and disease, in *Genetic Control of Autoimmune Disease,* Rose, N. R., Bigazzi, P. E., and Warner, N. L., Eds., Elsevier/North Holland, New York, 1978, 3.
26. **Dupont, F., O'Neill, G. J., Yang, S. Y., Pollack, M. S., and Levine, L. S.,** Genetic linkage of disease-genes to HLA, in *Genetic Control of Autoimmune Disease,* Rose, N. R., Bigazzi, P. E., and Warner, N. L., Eds., Elsevier/North Holland, New York, 1978, 15.
27. **Grahn, D.,** Biological effects of protracted low dose radiation exposure of man and animals, in *Late Effects of Radiation,* Fry, R. M., Grahn, D., Greim, M. L., and Rust, J. H., Eds., Taylor and Francis, London, 1970, 129.
28. **Makinodan, T., Perkins, E. H., and Chen, M. G.,** Immunologic activity of the aged, *Adv. Gerontol. Res.*, 3, 171, 1971.
29. **Finch, C. E.,** The regulation of physiological changes during mammalian aging, *Q. Rev. Biol.*, 51, 49, 1976.
30. **Simms, H. S.,** Logarithmic increase in mortality as a manifestation of aging, *J. Gerontol.*, 1, 13, 1946.
31. **Burek, J. D.,** *Pathology of Aging Rats,* CRC Press, Boca Raton, Fla., 1978.
32. **Jones, H. B.,** *A Special Consideration of the Aging Process, Disease, and Life Expectancy,* University of California Radiation Laboratory, Berkeley, 1955.
33. **Gompertz, B.,** On the nature of the function expressive of the law of human mortality and on a new mode of determining the value of life contingencies, *Philos. Trans. R. Soc. London,* 115A, 513, 1825.
34. **Simms, H. S.** Longevity studies in rats. I. Relation between life span and age of onset of specific lesions, in *Pathology of Laboratory Rats and Mice,* Cotchin, E. and Roe, F. J. C., Eds., Blackwell, Oxford, 1967, 733.
35. **Upton, A. C., Kastenbaum, M. A., and Conklin, J. W.,** Age-specific death rates of mice exposed to ionizing radiation and radiomimetic agents, in *Cellular Basis and Aetiology of Late Somatic Effects of Ionizing Radiation,* Harris, R. J., Ed., Academic Press, New York, 1963, 285.
36. **Strehler, B. L.,** Origin and comparison of the effects of time and high energy radiations on living systems, *Q. Rev. Biol.*, 34, 117, 1959.
37. **Jones, H. B.,** The relation of human health to age, place, and time, in *Handbook of Aging and the Individual,* Birren, J. E., Ed., University of Chicago Press, Chicago, 1959, 336.
38. **Kohn, R. R.,** Human aging and disease, *J. Chronic Dis.*, 16, 5, 1963.
39. **Simms, H. S. and Berg, B. M.,** Longevity and the onset of lesions in male rats, *J. Gerontol.*, 12, 244, 1957.
40. **Doll, R.,** Cancer and aging: the epidemiological evidence, in *Tenth International Cancer Congress,* Year Book Medical Publishers, Chicago, 1970, 133.
41. **Smith, G. S., Walford, R. W., and Mickey, M. R.** Lifespan and incidence of cancer and other diseases in selected long-lived inbred mice and their F_1 hybrids, *J. Natl. Cancer Inst.*, 50, 1195, 1973.
42. **Bierman, E. L.,** Atherosclerosis and aging, *Fed. Proc.*, 37, 2832, 1978.
43. **Nielsen, J., Homma, A., and Biorn-Heinbiksen, T.,** Followup 15 years after a geronto-psychiatric prevalence study, *J. Gerontol.*, 32, 554, 1977.
44. **Abinanti, R. R.,** Chronic and degenerative diseases of man: the value of natural and experimentally induced diseases of animals, in *Animal Models for Biomedical Research IV,* National Academy of Sciences, Washington, D.C., 1971, 31.
45. **Jarvik, L. F. and Falek, A.,** Comparative data on cancer in aging twins, *Cancer,* 15, 1009, 1962.
46. **Kallmann, F. J. and Sander, G.,** Twin studies on aging and longevity, *J. Hered.*, 39, 349, 1948.
47. **Chai, C. K.,** Life span in inbred and hybrid mice, *J. Hered.*, 50, 203, 1959.
48. **Martin, G. M.,** Genetic syndromes in man with potential relevance to the pathobiology of aging, in *Genetic Effects on Aging* (Birth Defects: Original Article Series, Vol. 14, No. 1), Bergsma, D. and Harrison, D. E., Eds., Alan R. Liss, New York, 1978, 5.
49. **Svejgaard, A., Platz, P., Ryder, L. P., Nielsen, L. S., and Thomson, M.,** HL-A and disease associations — a survey, *Transplant. Rev.*, 22, 3, 1975.
50. **Knudson, A. G., Jr.,** Degenerative disease and aging, in *Genetics and Disease,* The Blakiston Division, McGraw-Hill, New York, 1965, chap. 8.
51. **Good, R. A. and Yunis, E.,** Association of autoimmunity, immunodeficiency and aging in man, rabbits, and mice, *Fed. Proc.* , 33, 2040, 1974.
52. **Goldrick, R. B., Sinnett, P. F., and Whyte, H. M.,** An assessment of coronary heart disease and coronary risk factors in a New Guinea Highland population, in *Atherosclerosis, Proceedings of the Second International Symposium,* Jones, R. J., Ed., Springer-Verlag, New York, 1970, 366.

53. **Walford, R. L.,** *The Immunologic Theory of Aging,* Munksgaard, Copenhagen, 1969.
54. **Mackay, I. R.,** Ageing and immunological function in man, *Gerontologia,* 18, 285, 1972.
55. **Linder, E., Pasternack, A., and Edgington, T. S.,** Pathology and immunology of age-associated disease of mice and evidence for an autologous immune complex pathogenesis of the associated renal disease, *Clin. Immunol. Immunopathol.,* 1, 104, 1972.
56. **Walford, R. L.,** Antibody diversity, histocompatibility systems, disease states and aging, *Lancet,* 2, 1226, 1970.
57. **Ford, E. B.,** Polymorphism, *Biol. Rev.,* 20, 73, 1945.
58. **Vogel, F. and Helmbold, W.,** Blutgruppen — Populationsgenetik und Statistik, in *Humangenetik,* Becker, P. E., Ed., Ein kurzes Handbuch in funf Banden, Band I/4, 129, 1972.
59. **Lilly, F., Boyse, E. A., and Old, L. J.,** Genetic basis of susceptibility to viral leukemogenesis, *Lancet,* 2, 1207, 1964.
60. **Lilly, F.,** The effect of histocompatibility-2 type on response to the Friend leukemia virus in mice, *J. Exp. Med.,* 127, 465, 1968.
61. **Lilly, F.,** Mouse leukemia: a model of a multiple-gene disease, *J. Natl. Cancer Inst.,* 49, 927, 1972.
62. **Amiel, J. F.,** Study of the leucocyte phenotypes in Hodgkin's disease, in *Histocompatibility Testing,* Curtoni, E. S., Mattiuz, P. L., and Tosi, R. M., Eds., Munksgaard, Copenhagen, 1967, 79.
63. **Mickey, M. R., Kressler, M., and Terasaki, P. I.,** Leukocyte antigens and disease. II. Alterations in frequencies of haplotypes associated with chronic glomerulonephritis, in *Histocompatibility Testing,* Terasaki, P. I., Ed., Munksgaard, Copenhagen, 1970, 237.
64. **Walford, R. L., Smith, G. S., and Waters, H.,** Histocompatibility systems and disease states with particular reference to cancer, *Transplant. Rev.,* 7, 78, 1971.
65. **Grumet, F. C., Conkell, A., Bodmer, J. G., Bodmer, W. F., and McDevitt, H. O.,** Histocompatibility (HL-AO antigens associated with systemic lupus erythematosus: a possible genetic predisposition to disease, *N. Engl. J. Med.,* 285, 193, 1971.
66. **van Rood, J. J., van Hooff, J. P., and Keuning, J. J.,** Disease predisposition, immune responsiveness and the fine structure of the HL-A supergene, *Transplant. Rev.,* 22, 74, 1975.
67. *Histocompatibility Testing 1977, Report of the 7th International Histocompatibility Workshop and Conference,* Bodmer, W. F., Batchelor, J. R., Bodmer, J. G., Festenstein, H., and Morris, P. J., Eds., Villadsen & Christensen, Copenhagen, 1978.
68. **Svejgaard, J., Hauge, M., Jersild, C., Platz, P., Ryder, L. P., Staub Nielsen, L., and Thomsen, M.,** The HLA system, an introductory survey, in *Monographs in Human Genetics,* Beckman, L. and Hauge, M., Eds., S. Karger, Basel, 1975, 1.
69. **Snell, G. D., Dausset, J., and Nathenson, S.,** *Histocompatibility,* Academic Press, New York, 1976, chap. 12.
70. **Gunther, E. and Stark, O.,** The major histocompatibility system of the rat (Ag-B or H-1) system, in *The Major Histocompatibility System in Man and Animals,* Gotze, D., Ed., Springer-Verlag, New York, 1977, 207.
71. **Thomsen, M., Platz, P., Andersen, O. O., Christy, M., Lyngsoe, J., Nerup, J., Rasmussen, K., Ryder, L. Pl., Staub Nielsen, L., and Svejgaard, A.,** MLC typing in juvenile diabetes mellitus and idiopathic Addison's disease, *Transplant. Rev.,* 22, 125, 1975.
72. **Terasaki, P. I. and Mickey, M. R.,** HL-A haplotypes of 32 diseases, *Transplant. Rev.,* 22, 105, 1975.
73. **Batchlor, J. R. and Morris, P. J.,** HLA and disease, in *Conference and Workshop on Histocompatibility Testing,* Bodmer, W. F., Batchlor, J. R., Bodmer, J. G., Festenstein, H., and Morris, P. J., Eds., Munksgaard, Copenhagen, 1977, 205.
74. **Dupont, B. and Svejgaard, A.,** HLA and disease, *Transplant. Proc.,* 9, 1271, 1977.
75. **Falk, J. and Osoba, D.,** HL-A antigens and survival in Hodgkin's disease, *Lancet,* 2, 1118, 1971.
76. **Rogentine, G. N., Trapani, R. J., Yankee, R. A., and Menderson, E. S.,** HL-A antigens and acute lymphocytic leukemia: the nature of the HL-A2 association, *Tissue Antigens,* 3, 470, 1973.
77. **Kissmeyer-Nielsen, F., Kjerbye, K. E., and Lamm, L. U.,** HL-A in Hodgkin's disease. III. A prospective study, *Transplant. Rev.,* 22, 168, 1975.
78. **Lawler, S. D., Klouda, P. T., Smith, P. G., Till, M. M., and Hardisty, R. M.,** Survival and the HL-A system in acute lymphoblastic leukaemia, *Br. Med. J.,* 1, 547, 1974.
79. **McDevitt, H. O. and Bodmer, W. F.,** HL-A, immune-response genes, and disease, *Lancet,* 1, 1269, 1974.
80. **Brewerton, D. A., Caffrey, M., Hart, F. D., Nicholls, A., James, D. C. O., and Sturrock, R. D.,** Ankylosing spondylitis and HL-A27, *Lancet,* 1, 904, 1973.
81. **Schlosstein, L., Terasaki, P. I., Bluestone, R., and Pearson, C. M.,** High association of an HL-A antigen W27, with ankylosing spondylitis, *N. Engl. J. Med.,* 288, 704, 1973.
82. **Strosberg, J. M., Harris, E. D., Calabro, J. J., and Allen, F. H.,** Ankylosing spondylitis: clinical and genetic studies of a kindred, *Arthritis Rheum.,* 16, 774, 1973.
83. **Dick, H. M., Sturrock, R. D., Dick, W. C., and Buchanan, W. W.,** Inheritance of ankylosing spondylitis and HL-A antigen W27, *Lancet,* 2, 24, 1974.

84. **Dick, H. M., Sturrock, R. D., Goel, G. K., Henderson, N., Canesi, B., Rooney, R. J., Dick, W. C., and Buchanan, W. W.**, The association between HL-A antigens, ankylosing spondylitis and sacro-ileitis, *Tissue Antigens*, 5, 26, 1975.
85. **Albert, E. and Gotze, D.**, The major histocompatibility system in man, in *The Major Histocompatibility System in Man and Animals*, Gotze, D., Ed., Springer-Verlag, New York, 1977, 7.
86. **Bias, W. B. and Chase, G. A.**, Genetic implications of HLA and disease associations, *Transplant. Proc.*, 9, 531, 1977.
87. **Stastny, P.**, Association of the B-cell alloantigen BRw4 with rheumatoid arthritis, *N. Engl. J. Med.*, 298, 869, 1978.
88. **Hirata, A. A., McIntire, F. C., Terasaki, P. I., and Mittal, K. K.**, Cross-reactions between human transplantation antigens and bacterial lipopolysaccharides, *Transplantation*, 15, 441, 1973.
89. **Ohno, S., Aoki, K., Sugiura, S., Nakayama, E., Italsura, K., and Aizawa, M.**, HL-A5 and Behcet's disease, *Lancet*, 2, 1383, 1973.
90. **Grumet, F. C., Konishi, J., Payne, R., and Kriss, J. P.**, Association of Graves' disease with HL-A8, *Clin. Res.*, 21, 439, 1973.
91. **Platz, P., Ryder, L., Nielsen, L., Svejgaard, A., Thomsen, M., Nerup, J., and Christy, M.**, HL-A and idiopathic Addison's disease, *Lancet*, 2, 289, 1974.
92. **Nerup, J., Platz, P., Ortved Andersen, C. M., Lyngsoe, J., Poulsen, J. E., Hyder, L. P., Staub Nielsen, L., Thomsen, M., and Svejgaard, A.**, HL-A antigens and diabetes mellitus, *Lancet*, 2, 864, 1974.
93. **Walford, R. L., Smith, G. S., Meredith, P. J., and Cheney, K. E.**, Immunogenetics of aging, in *The Genetics of Aging*, Schneider, E. L., Ed., Plenum Press, New York, 1978, 383.
94. **Bertrams, J., Kuwert, E., and Liedke, U.**, HL-A antigens and multiple sclerosis, *Tissue Antigens*, 2, 405, 1972.
95. **Bertrams, J., Hoher, G., and Kuwert, E.**, HL-A antigens in multiple sclerosis, *Lancet*, 1, 1287, 1974.
96. **Jersild, C., Dupont, B., Fog, T., Platz, P. J., and Svejgaard, A.**, Histocompatibility determinants in multiple sclerosis, *Transplant. Rev.*, 22, 148, 1975.
97. **Jersild, C., Svejgaard, A., Fog, T., and Amnitzboll, T.**, HL-A antigens and diseases. I. Multiple sclerosis, *Tissue Antigens*, 3, 243, 1973.
98. **Bodmer, W. F., Cann, H., and Piazza, A.**, Differential genetic variability among polymorphisms as an indicator of natural selection, in *Histocompatibility Testing*, Dausset, J. and Colombani, J., Eds., Munksgaard, Copenhagen, 1972, 753.
99. **Degos, L. and Dausset, J.**, Human migrations and HL-A linkage disequilibrium, *Immunogenetics*, 1, 195, 1974.
100. **Feltkamp, T. E. W., Van den Berg-Loonen, P. M., Nijennuis, L. E., Engelfriet, C. P., Van Rossum, A. L., Van Loghem, J. J., and Oosterhuis, H. J. G. H.**, Myasthenia gravis, autoantibodies and HL-A antigens, *Br. Med. J.*, 1, 131, 1974.
101. **Moller, E., Link, H., Matell, G., Olhagen, B., and Stendahl, L.**, LD alleles in ankylosing spondylitis, myasthenia gravis, multiple sclerosis, and optic neuritis, in *Histocompatibility Testing*, Kissmeyer-Nielsen, F., Ed., Munksgaard, Copenhagen, 1975, 778.
102. **Falchuck, S. M., Rogentine, G. N., and Strober, W.**, Predominance of histocompatibility antigen HL-A8 in patients with gluten-sensitive enteropathy, *J. Clin. Invest.*, 51, 1602, 1972.
103. **Mackay, I. R. and Morris, P.**, Association of autoimmune active chronic hepatitis with HL-A1, 8, *Lancet*, 2, 793, 1972.
104. **Morris, P. J. and Batchlor, J. R.**, Summary and conclusions, in *HLA and Disease, Conference and Workshop on Histocompatibility Testing*, Bodmer, W. F., Batchlor, J. R., Bodmer, J. G., Festenstein, H., and Morris, P. J., Eds., Munksgaard, Copenhagen, 1977, 369.
105. **Kissmeyer-Nielsen, F., Kjerbye, K. E., Andersen, E., and Halberg, P.**, HL-A antigens in systemic lupus erythematosus, *Transplant. Rev.*, 22, 164, 1975.
106. **Dupont, B., Good, R. A., Hauptmann, G., Schreuder, I., and Seligmann, M.**, Immunopathology, immunodeficiencies, and complement deficiencies, in *HLA and Disease*, Dausset, J. and Svejgaard, A., Eds., Williams & Wilkins, Baltimore, 1977, 233.
107. **Fu, S. M., Stern, R., Kunkel, H. G., Dupont, B., Hansen, J. A., Day, N. K., Good, R. A., Jersild, C., and Fotino, M.**, LD-7a association with C2 deficiency in five of six families, in *Histocompatibility Testing*, Kissmeyer-Nielsen, F., Ed., Munksgaard, Copenhagen, 1975, 933.
108. **Jensen, H., Ryder, L. P., Staub Nielsen, L., Clausen, E., Jorgensen, F., and Jorgensen, H. E.**, HLA antigens and glomerulonephritis, *Tissue Antigens*, 6, 368, 1975.
109. **Dausset, J.**, HLA complex in human biology in the light of associations with disease, *Transplant. Proc.*, 9, 523, 1977.
110. **Clauvel, J. P., Marcelli-Barge, A., Coggia, I. G., Poirier, J. C., Benajam, A., and Dausset, J.**, HL-A antigens and idiopathic autoimmune hemolytic anemias, *Transplant. Proc.*, 6, 447, 1974.

111. **Pickbourn, P., Piazza, A., and Bodmer, W. F.,** Population analysis, in *Conference and Workshop on Histocompatibility Testing,* Bodmer, W. F., Batchlor, J. R., Bodmer, J. G., Festenstein, H., and Morris, P. J., Eds., Munksgaard, Copenhagen, 1977, 259.
112. **Petranyi, G. G., Benczur, M., Onody, C. E., and Hollau, S. R.,** HL-A3,7 and lymphocyte cytotoxic activity, *Lancet,* 1, 736, 1974.
113. **Untermohlen, V. and Zabreski, J. B.,** Suppressed cellular immunity to measles antigen in multiple sclerosis patients, *Lancet,* 2, 1147, 1973.
114. **Platz, P., Dupont, B., Fog, T., Yrder, L. P., Thomsen, M., Svejgaard, A., and Jersild, C.,** MLC determinants, measles infection and multiple sclerosis, *Proc. R. Soc. Med.,* 67, 1133, 1974.
115. **Persson, I., Ryder, L. P., Staub Nielsen, L., and Svejgaard, A.,** The HL-A histocompatibility antigen in sarcoidosis in relation to the tuberculin skin test, *Tissue Antigens,* 6, 50, 1975.
116. **Kissmeyer-Nielsen, F., Jorgenson, F., and Lamm, L. U.,** The HL-A system in clinical medicine, *Johns Hopkins Med. J.,* 131, 385, 1972.
117. **Goldstein, A. L., Thurman, G. B., Low, T. L. K., Trivers, G. E., and Rossio, J. L.,** Thymosin: the endocrine thymus and its role in the aging process, in *Aging Series, Vol. 8, Physiology and Cell Biology of Aging,* Cherkin, A., Finch, C. E., Kharasch, N., Makinodan, T., Scott, F. L., and Strehler, B. S., Eds., Raven Press, New York, 1979, 51.
118. **Roberts-Thomson, I. C., Whittingham, S., Young-chaiyud, U., and Mackay, I. R.,** Aging, immune response, and mortality, *Lancet,* 2, 368, 1974.
119. **Nordin, A. A. and Makinodan, T.,** Humoral immunity in aging, *Fed. Proc.,* 33, 2033, 1974.
120. **Teller, M. N.,** Interrelationships among aging, immunity and cancer, in *Tolerance, Autoimmunity and Aging,* Sigel, M. M. and Good, R. A., Eds., Charles C Thomas, Springfield, Ill., 1972, 18.
121. **Makinodan, T.,** Immunity and aging, in *Handbook of the Biology of Aging,* Finch, C. E. and Hayflick, L., Eds., Van Nostrand Reinhold, New York, 1977, 379.
122. **Makinodan, T. and Adler, W. H.,** Effect of aging on the differentiation and proliferation potentials of cells of the immune system, *Fed. Proc.,* 34, 153, 1975.
123. **Kay, M. M. B. and Baker, L. S.,** Cell changes associated with declining immune function, in *Aging Series, Vol. 8, Physiology and Cell Biology of Aging,* Cherkin, A., Finch, C. E., Kharasch, N., Makinodan, T., Scott, F. L., and Strehler, B. S., Eds., Raven Press, New York, 1979, 27.
124. **Chino, F., Makinodan, T., Lever, W. H., and Peterson, W. J.,** The immune systems of mice reared in clean and dirty conventional laboratory farms. I. Life expectancy and pathology of mice with long life-spans, *J. Gerontol.,* 26, 497, 1971.
125. **Peter, C. P.,** Possible immune origin of age-related pathological changes in long-lived mice, *J. Gerontol.,* 28, 265, 1973.
126. **Stutman, O.,** Cell-mediated immunity and aging, *Fed. Proc.,* 33, 2028, 1974.
127. **Hallgren, H. M., Buckley, C. E., III, Gilbertsen, V. A., and Yunis, E. J.,** Lymphocyte phytohemagglutinin responsiveness, immunoglobulins and autoantibodies in aging humans, *J. Immunol.,* 111, 1101, 1973.
128. **Konen, T. G., Smith, G. S., and Walford, R. L.,** Decline in mixed lymphocyte reactivity of spleen cells from aged mice of a long-lived strain, *J. Immunol.,* 110, 1216, 1973.
129. **Rowley, M. J., Buchanan, H., and Mackay, I. R.,** Reciprocal change with age in antibody to extrinsic and intrinsic antigens, *Lancet,* 2, 24, 1968.
130. **Buckley, C. E., III, Buckley, E. G., and Dorsey, F. C.,** Longitudinal changes in serum immunoglobulin levels in older humans, *Fed. Proc.,* 33, 2036, 1974.
131. **Halsall, M. H., Heidrick, M. L., Dietchman, J. W., and Makinodan, T.,** Role of suppressor cells in age-related decline in the proliferative capacity of spleen cells, *Gerontologist,* 13, 46, 1973.
132. **Gerbase-DeLima, M., Meredith, P., and Walford, R. L.,** Age-related changes, including synergy and suppression, in the mixed lymphocyte reaction in long-lived mice, *Fed. Proc.,* 34, 159, 1975.
133. **Price, G. B. and Makinodan, T.,** Immunologic deficiencies in senescence. I. Characterization of intrinsic deficiencies, *J. Immunol.,* 108, 403, 1972.
134. **Popp, D. M.,** The effect of age on antigen-sensitive cells, *Mech. Aging Dev.,* 4, 221, 1975.
135. **Popp, D. M.,** Qualitative changes in immunocompetent cells with age: reduced sensitivity to cortisone acetate, *Mech. Ageing Dev.,* 6, 355, 1977.
136. **Popp, D. M. and Francis, M.,** Age-associated changes in T-B cell cooperation demonstrated by the allogeneic effect, *Mech. Ageing Dev.,* 10, 341, 1979.
137. **Beregi, E.,** Morphology of antibody-forming cells in young and aged experimental animals, *Mech. Ageing Dev.,* 1, 233, 1972.
138. **Chen, M. G.,** Age-related changes in hematopoietic stem cell populations of a long-lived hybrid mouse, *J. Cell. Physiol.,* 78, 225, 1971.
139. **Yunis, E. J., Fernandes, G., Teague, P. O., Stutman, O., and Good, R. A.,** The thymus, autoimmunity and the involution of the lymphoid system, in *Tolerance, Autoimmunity and Aging,* Sigel, M. M. and Good, R. A., Eds., Charles C Thomas, Springfield, Ill., 1972, 62.

140. **Jeejeebhoy, H. F.**, Decreased longevity of mice following thymectomy in adult life, *Transplantation,* 12, 525, 1971.
141. **Klein, J.**, Evolution and function of the major histocompatibility system: facts and speculations, in *The Major Histocompatibility System in Man and Animals,* Gotze, D., Ed., Springer-Verlag, New York, 1977, 340.
142. **Cohen, N. and Collins, N. H.**, Major and minor histocompatibility systems of ectothermic vertebrates, in *The Major Histocompatibility System in Man and Animals,* Gotze, D., Ed., Springer-Verlag, New York, 1977, 313.
143. **De Ioannes, A. E., and Hildemann, W. H.**, Preliminary structural characterization of Pacific hagfish immunoglobulin, in *Immunologic Phylogeny,* Hildeman, H. H. and Benedict, A. A., Eds., Plenum Press, New York, 1975, 151.
144. **Hildemann, W. H.**, Phylogenetic and immunogenetic aspects of aging, in *Genetic Effects on Aging,* Bergsma, D. and Harrison, D. E., Eds., Alan R. Liss, New York, 1978, 97.
145. **Klein, J.**, H-2 mutations: their genetics and effect on immune functions, *Adv. Immunol.,* 26, 55, 1978.
146. **O'Neill, G. J. and Dupont, B.**, Serum C4 levels, Chido, Rodgers, and allotypes of C4 component of complement, *Transplant. Proc.,* 11, 1102, 1979.
147. **Lamm, L. U., Friedrich, U., Petersen, G. B., Jorgensen, J., Nielsen, J., Therkelsen, A. J., and Kissmeyer-Nielsen, F.**, Assignment of the major histocompatibility complex to chromosome no. 6 in a family with a pericentric inversion, *Hum. Hered.,* 24, 243, 1974.
148. **Vitetta, E. S. and Capra, J. D.**, The protein products of the murine 17th chromosome: genetics and structure, *Adv. Immunol.,* 26, 147, 1978.
149. **Bodmer, W. F.**, HLA: a super supergene, in *The Harvey Lectures, Series 72,* 1976-1977, Academic Press, New York, 1978, 91.
150. **Thorsby, E.**, The human major histocompatibility complex HLA: some recent developments, *Transplant. Proc.,* 11, 616, 1979.
151. **Meyer, M. M.**, Complement, past and present, in *The Harvey Lectures, Series 72,* 1976-1977, Academic Press, New York, 1978, 139.
152. **Taussig, M. M.**, Mapping immune response genes in man using the antigen-specific T-cell factor in *Ir Genes and Ia Antigens,* McDevitt, H. O., Ed., Academic Press, New York, 1978, 493.
153. **Rubinstein, P., Vienne, K., and Hoecker, G. F.**, The location of the *C3* and *GLO* (Glyoxalase 1) loci of the IXth linkage group in mice, *J. Immunol.,* 122, 2584, 1979.
154. **Gelfand, M. C., Sachs, D. H., Lieberman, R., and Paul, W. E.**, Ontogeny of B lymphocytes III. *H-2* linkage of a gene controlling the rate of appearance of complement receptor lymphocytes, *J. Exp. Med.,* 139, 1974, 1142.
155. **Merritt, A. D., Peterson, B. H., Biegel, A. A., Meyers, D. A., Brooks, G. F., and Hotes, M. E.**, Chromosome 6: linkage of the eighth component of complement (C8) to the histocompatibility region (HLA), in *Human Gene Mapping 3,* Baltimore Conference, Bergsma, D., Ed., S. Karger, New York, 1976.
156. **O'Neill, G. J., Yang, S. Y., and Dupont, B.**, Two *HLA*-linked loci controlling the fourth component of human complement, *Proc. Natl. Acad. Sci. U.S.A.,* 75, 5165, 1978.
157. **Levine, L. S., Zachman, M., New, M. I., Prader, A., Pollack, M. S., O'Neill, G., Yang, S. Y., Oberfield, S. E., and Dupont, B.**, Genetic mapping of the 21-hydroxylase-deficiency gene within the HLA linkage group, *N. Engl. J. Med.,* 299, 1978, 911.
158. **Bennett, D. and Dunn, L. C.**, Transmission ratio distorting genes on chromosome IX and their interactions, *Proc. Symp. Immunogenetics of the H-2 System,* Lengerova, A. and Vojtiskiva, M., Eds., S. Karger, Basel, 1971, 90.
159. **Amos, D. B., Rudeman, R., Mendell, N. R., and Johnson, A. H.**, Linkage between HL-A and spinal development, *Transplant. Proc.,* 7, 93, 1975.
160. **Amos, D. B. and Ward, F. E.**, Theoretical consideration in the association between HLA and disease, in *HLA and Disease,* Dausset, J. and Svejgaard, A., Eds., Williams & Wilkins, Baltimore, 1977, 269.
161. **Klein, J.**, Genetics of H-2-linked loci, in *Biology of the Mouse Histocompatibility-2 Complex,* Springer-Verlag, New York, 1975, chap. 11.
162. **David, C. S.**, The major histocompatibility system of the mouse, in *The Major Histocompatibility System in Man and Animals,* Gotze, D., Ed., Springer-Verlag, New York, 1977, 255.
163. **Lamm, L. U. and Kristensen, T.**, Formal genetics of the HLA system, in *HLA System - New Aspects,* Ferrara, G. B., Ed., North-Holland, Amsterdam, 1977, 1.
164. **David, C.**, Role of Ia antigens in immune response, *Transplant. Proc.,* 11, 677, 1979.
165. **Bach, F. H., Bach, M. L., and Sondel, P. M.**, Differential function of major histocompatibility complex antigens in T-lymphocyte activation, *Nature (London),* 259, 273, 1976.
166. **Balner, H.**, Are D and DR antigens identical? A review of available data for man and the Rhesus monkey, *Transplant. Proc.,* 11, 657, 1979.

167. **Lilly, F.,** The inheritance of susceptibility to the Gross leukemia virus in mice, *Genetics,* 53, 529, 1966.
168. **Benacerraf, B. and Katz, D. H.,** The histocompatibility-linked immune response genes, *Adv. Cancer Res.,* 21, 121, 1975.
169. **Benacerraf, B. and Germain, R. N.,** The immune response genes of the major histocompatibility complex, *Immunol. Rev.,* 38, 70, 1978.
170. **Katz, D. H. and Benacerraf, B.,** The function and interrelationships of T-cell receptors, Ir genes and other histocompatibilty gene products, *Transplant. Rev.,* 22, 173, 1975.
171. **Doherty, P. C. and Zinkernagel, R. M.,** Enhanced immunological surveillance in mice heterozygous at the H-2 gene complex, *Nature (London),* 256, 50, 1975.
172. **Doherty, P. C., Blanden, R. V., and Zinkernagel, R. M.,** Specificity of virus-immune effector T-cells for H-2K or H-2D compatible interactions: implications for H-antigen diversity, *Transplant. Rev.,* 29, 89, 1976.
173. **Zinkernagel, R. M.,** Association of disease susceptibility to major histocompatibility antigens, *Transplant. Proc.,* 11, 624, 1979.
174. **Ivanyi, P. and Mickova, M.,** Further studies on genetic factors in the ninth linkage group influencing reproductive performance in male mice, in *Proc. Symp. Immunogenetics of the H-2 System, Liblice-Prague, 1970,* Lengerova, A. and Vojtiskova, M., Eds., S. Karger, Basel, 1971, 104.
175. **Ivanyi, P., Gregorova, S., and Mickova, M.,** Genetic differences in thymus lymph node, testes and vesicular gland weights among inbred mouse strains. Association with the major histocompatibility (H-2) system, *Folia Biol. (Prague),* 18, 81, 1972.
176. **Ivanyi, P., Hampl, R., Starka, L., and Mickova, M.,** Genetic association between H-2 gene and testosterone metabolism in mice, *Nature (London) New Biol.,* 238, 280, 1972.
177. **Ivanyi, P., Hampl, R., Mickova, M., and Starka, L.,** The influence of the H-2 system and blood serum testosterone level, *Folia Biol. (Prague),* 22, 42, 1976.
178. **Mickova, M. and Ivanyi, P.,** Influence of the H-2 system on the sensitivity of vesicular glands to testosterone hormone, *Folia Biol. (Prague),* 21, 435, 1975.
179. **Meruelo, D. and Edidin, M.,** Association of mouse liver adenosine 3′,5′-cyclic monophosphate (cyclic AMP) levels with histocompatibility-2 genotype, *Proc. Natl. Acad. Sci. U.S.A.,* 72, 2644, 1975.
180. **Goldman, A. S., Katsumata, M., Yaffe, S. J., and Gasser, D. L.,** Palatal cytosol cortisal-binding protein associated with cleft palate susceptibility and H-2 genotype, *Nature (London),* 265, 643, 1977.
181. **Ceppellini, R.,** Old and new facts and speculations about transplantation antigens of man, in *Progress in Immunology,* Vol. 1, Amos, D. B., Ed., Academic Press, New York, 1971, 973.
182. **Klein, J., Bach, F. H., Festenstein, F., McDevitt, H. O., Shreffler, D. C., and Stimpfling, J. H.,** Genetic nomenclature for the *H-2* complex of the mouse, *Immunogenetics,* 1, 184, 1974.
183. **Gorer, P.,** The detection of antigenic differences in mouse erythroyctes by the employment of immune sera, *Br. J. Exp. Pathol.,* 17, 42, 1936.
184. **Dausset, J.,** Iso-leuco-anticorps, *Acta Haematol.,* 20, 156, 1958.
185. **Kissmeyer-Nielsen, F., Svejgaard, A., and Hauge, M.,** Genetics of the human HL-A transplantation system, *Nature (London),* 219, 1116, 1968.
186. **Yunis, E. and Amos, D. B.,** Three closely linked genetic systems relevant to transplantation, *Proc. Natl. Acad. Sci. U.S.A.,* 68, 3031, 1971.
187. **Thorsby, E., Albrechtsen, D., Hirschberg, H., Kaalomem, A., and Solheim, B. G.,** MLC-activating HLA-D determinants: identification, tissue distribution, and significance, *Transplant. Proc.,* 9, 393, 1977.
188. **Hammerling, G. J.,** Tissue distribution of Ia antigens and their expression on lymphocyte subpopulations, *Transplant. Rev.,* 30, 64, 1976.
189. **van Rood, J. J., van Leeuwen, A., Termijtelen, A., and Keuning, J. J.,** B-cell antibodies, Ia-like determinants, and their relation to MLC determinants in man, *Transplant. Rev.,* 30, 122, 1976.
190. **Walford, R. L.,** Human B-cell alloantigenic systems: their medical and biological significance, in *HLA System — New Aspects,* Ferrara, G. B., Ed., North-Holland, Amsterdam, 1977, 105.
191. **Amos, D. B. and Kostyu, D. D.,** HLA-A central immunological agency of man, in *Advances in Human Genetics,* Harris, H. and Hirschhorn, K., Eds., Plenum Press, New York, 1980, 137.
192. **Chaventre, A., Bengtson B., and Jacquard, A.,** Selective pressure on HL-A polymorphism, *Nature (London),* 249, 62, 1974.
193. **Zinkernagel, R. M. and Doherty, P. C.,** The concept that surveillance of self is mediated via the same set of genes that determines recognition of allogenic cells, *Cold Spring Harbor Symp. Quant. Biol.,* 41(2), 505, 1977.
194. **Yunis, E. J., Fernandes, G., and Greenberg, L. J.,** Immune deficiency, autoimmunity, and aging, in *Immunodeficiency in Man and Animals,* Bergsma, D., Good, R. A., Finstad, J., and Paul, N. W., Eds., Sinauer Associates, Sunderland, Mass., 1975, 185.
195. **Harris, H., Hopkinson, D. A., and Robson, E. B.,** The incidence of rare alleles determining electrophoretic variants: data on 43 enzyme loci in man, *Ann. Hum. Genet.,* 37, 237, 1974.

196. **Neel, J. V.**, Some trends in the study of spontaneous and induced mutation in man, *Human Genetics*, Int. Congr. Ser. 411, Excerpta Medica, Elsevier, Amsterdam, 1976, 19.
197. **Albertini, R. J. and DeMars, R.**, Somatic cell mutation. Detection and quantification of x-ray-induced mutation in cultured, diploid human fibroblasts, *Mutat. Res.*, 18, 199, 1973.
198. **DeMars, R.**, Resistance of cultured human fibroblasts and other cells to purine and pyrimidine analogues in relation to mutagenesis detection, *Mutat. Res.*, 24, 335, 1974.
199. **McKusick, V. A.**, *Mendelian Inheritance in Man*, 4th ed., Johns Hopkins University Press, Baltimore, 1975.
200. **Ohno, S. and Nagai, Y.**, Genes in multiple copies as the primary cause of aging, *Birth Defects: Original Article Series*, 14, 501, 1978.
201. **Parmiani, G.**, Foreign histocompatibility determinants as tumor-associated transplantation antigens of chemically induced murine fibrosarcomas, in *HLA System - New Aspects*, Ferrara, G. B., Ed., North-Holland, Amsterdam, 1977, 45.
202. **Festenstein, H.**, The major histocompatibility system, tumors, and viruses, in *HLA System — New Aspects*, Ferrara, G. B., Ed., North-Holland, Amsterdam, 1977, 53.
203. **Brown, J. L., Nairn, R., and Natheson, S. G.**, Structural differences between the mouse H-2D products of the mutant BIO.D2.M504 (H-2da) and the parental nonmutant strain BIO.D2 (H-2^{d}), *J. Immunol.*, 120, 726, 1978.
204. **Tice, R. R.**, Aging and DNA-repair capability, in *The Genetics of Aging*, Schneider, E. L., Ed., Plenum Press, New York, 1978, 53.
205. **Hall, Z. W. and Lehman, I. R.**, An *in vitro* transversion by a mutationally altered T4-induced DNA polymerase, *J. Mol. Biol.*, 36, 321, 1968.
206. **Demerec, M. and Hanson, J.**, Mutagenic action of manganous chloride, *Cold Spring Harbor Symp. Quant. Biol.*, 16, 215, 1951.
207. **Orgel, A. and Orgel, L. E.**, Induction of mutations in bacteriophage T4 with divalent manganese, *J. Mol. Biol.*, 14, 453, 1965.
208. **Barton, F. W., Waters, L. C., and Yang, W. K.**, *In vitro* DNA synthesis by low-molecular-weight DNA polymerase-increased infidelity associated with aging, *Fed. Proc. Abstr.*, 33, 1419, 1974.
209. **Linn, S., Kairis, M., and Holliday, R.**, Decreased fidelity of DNA polymerase activity isolated from aging human fibroblasts, *Proc. Natl. Acad. Sci. U.S.A.*, 73, 2818, 1976.
210. **Fulder, S. J. and Holliday, R.**, A rapid rise in cell variants during the senescence of populations of human fibroblasts, *Cell*, 6, 67, 1975.
211. **Thompson, K. V. A. and Holliday, R.**, Chromosome changes during the *in vitro* ageing of MRC-5 human fibroblasts, *Exp. Cell Res.*, 96, 1, 1976.
212. **Orgel, L. E.**, The maintenance of the accuracy of protein synthesis and its relevance to aging, *Proc. Natl. Acad. Sci. U.S.A.*, 49, 517, 1963.
213. **Hopfield, J. J., Yamane, T., Yue, V., and Coutts, S. M.**, Direct experimental evidence for kinetic proofreading in amino acylation of $tRNA^{Ile}$, *Proc. Natl. Acad. Sci. U.S.A.*, 73, 1164, 1976.
214. **Fersht, A. R.**, Editing mechanisms in protein synthesis. Rejection of valine by the isoleucyl-tRNA synthetase, *Biochemistry*, 16, 1025, 1976.
215. **Loftfield, R. B. and Eigner, E. A.**, The specificity of enzymic reactions. Aminoacyl-sRNA ligases. *Biochim. Biophys. Acta*, 130, 426, 1966.
216. **Loftfield, R. B. and Vanderjagt, D.**, The frequency of errors in protein biosynthesis, *Biochem. J.*, 1, 1353, 1972.
217. **Dayhoff, M. D., Hunt, L. T., McLaughlin, P. J., and Barker, W. C.**, Genetics, in *The Atlas of Protein Sequence and Structure*, National Biomedical Research Foundation, Silver Spring, Md., 1972, D51.
218. **Popp, R. A., Bailiff, E. G., Hirsch, G. P., and Conrad, R. A.**, Errors in human hemoglobin as a function of age, *Interdiscip. Top. Gerontol.*, 9, 209, 1976.
219. **Popp, R. A., Hirsch, G. P., and Bradshaw, B. S.**, Amino acid substitution: its use in detection and analysis of genetic variants, *Genetics*, 92, s39, 1979.
220. **Hirsch, G. P., Popp, R. A., Francis, M. C., Bradshaw, B. S., and Bailiff, E. G.**, Aging, cancer and cell membranes, in *Advances in Pathobiology*, Vol. 7, Borek, C., Fenoglio, C. M., and King, D. W., Eds., Thieme-Stratton, New York, 142.
221. **Owens, S. A. and Popp, R. A.**, unpublished data, 1979.
222. **Hirsch, G. P., Holland, J. M., and Popp, R. A.**, Amino acid analog incorporation into protein in dimethyl sulfoxide and mutagen-treated aging mice, *Birth Defects, Orig. Art. Ser.*, 14, 431, 1978.
223. **Hirsch, G. P., Popp, R. A., and Holland, M.**, unpublished data, 1979.
224. **Edelmann, P. and Gallant, J.**, Mistranslation in *E. coli*, *Cell*, 10, 131, 1977.
225. **Davies, J., Gorini, L., and Davis, B. D.**, Misreading of RNA codewords induced by aminoglycoside antibiotics, *Mol. Pharmacol.*, 1, 93, 1965.
226. **Hall, B. and Gallant, J.**, Defective translation in RC^- cells, *Nature (London) New Biol.*, 237, 131, 1972.

227. **Mitra, S. K., Florentyna, L., Akesson, B., Lagerkuist, U., and Strid, L.**, Codon-anticodon recognition in the valine codon family, *J. Biol. Chem.*, 250, 471, 1977.
228. **Holmes, W. M., Hatfield, G. W., and Goldman, E.**, Evidence for misreading during tRNA-dependent protein synthesis *in vitro*, *J. Biol. Chem.*, 252, 3482, 1978.
229. **Grosjean, H. J., de Henau, S., and Crothers, D. M.**, On the physical basis for ambiguity in genetic coding interactions, *Proc. Natl. Acad. Sci. U.S.A.*, 75, 610, 1978.
230. **Menninger, J. R.**, Peptidyl transfer RNA dissociates during protein synthesis from ribosomes of *Escherichia coli*, *J. Biol. Chem.*, 251, 3392, 1976.
231. **Menninger, J. R.**, Ribosome editing and the error catastrophe hypothesis of cellular aging, *Mech. Ageing Dev.*, 6, 131, 1977.
232. **Greenberg, L. J. and Yunis, E. J.**, Genetic control of autoimmune disease and immune responsiveness and the relationship to aging, in *Genetic Effects on Aging*, Bergsma, D. and Harrison, D. E., Eds., Alan R. Liss, New York, 1978, 249.
233. **Bender, K., Rutter, G., Mayerova, A., and Hiller, C.**, Studies on the heterozygosity at the HL-A gene loci in children and old people, in *Int. Symp. HL-A Reagents*, Regamey, R. H. and Sparck, J. V., Eds., S. Karger, Basel, 1973, 287.
234. **Gerkins, V. R., Ting, A., Menck, H. T., Terasaki, P. I., Pike, M. C., and Henderson, B. E.**, HL-A heterozygosity as a genetic marker of long-term survival, *J. Natl. Cancer Inst.*, 52, 1909, 1974.
235. **Macurova, H., Ivanyi, P., Sajdlova, H., and Trojan, J.**, HL-A antigens in aged persons, *Tissue Antigens*, 6, 269, 1975.
236. **Converse, P. J. and Williams, D. R. R.**, Increased HLA-B heterozygosity with age, *Tissue Antigens*, 12, 275, 1978.
237. **Meredith, P. and Walford, R. L.**, Effect of age on response to T and B cell mitogens in mice congenic at the *H-2* region, *Immunogenetics*, 5, 109, 1977.
238. **Gleichmann, E., Gleichmann, H., and Wilke, W.**, Autoimmunization and lymphomagenesis in parent-F_1 combinations differing at the major histocompatibility complex: model for spontaneous disease caused by altered self-antigens?, *Transplant. Rev.*, 31, 156, 1976.
239. **Talal, N.**, Disordered immunologic regulation and autoimmunity, *Transplant. Rev.*, 31, 240, 1976.
240. **Storer, J. B.**, Longevity and gross pathology at death in 22 inbred mouse strains, *J. Gerontol.*, 21, 404, 1966.
241. **Snell, G. D.**, Histocompatibility genes of the mouse. II. Production and analysis of isogenic resistant lines, *J. Natl. Cancer Inst.*, 21, 843, 1958.
242. **Klein, J.**, List of congenic lines of mice. I. Lines with differences at alloantigen loci, *Transplantation*, 15, 137, 1973.
243. **Popp, D. M.**, *In vivo* lymphocyte transformation induced by H-2D and H-2K components of the H-2 locus, *Transplant. Proc.*, 5, 281, 1973.
244. **Makinodan, T. and Peterson, W. J.**, Growth and senescence of the primary antibody forming potential of the spleen, *J. Immunol.*, 93, 886, 1964.
245. **Cantor, H. and Boyse, E. A.**, Functional subclasses of T lymphocytes bearing different Ly antigens. I. The generation of functionally distinct T-cell subclasses is a differentiative process independent of antigen, *J. Exp. Med.*, 141, 1376, 1975.
246. **Cantor, H. and Boyse, E. A.**, Functional subclasses of T lymphocytes bearing different Ly antigens. II. Cooperation between subclasses of Ly^+ cells in the generation of killer activity, *J. Exp. Med.*, 141, 1390, 1975.
247. **Segal, S., Cohen, I. R., and Feldman, M.**, Thymus-derived lymphocytes: humoral and cellular reactions distinguished by hydro-cortisone, *Science*, 175, 1126, 1972.
248. **McKenzie, I. F. C., Pang, T., and Blanden, R. V.**, The use of H-2 mutants as models for the study of T cell activation, *Immunol. Rev.*, 35, 181, 1977.
249. **Paul, W. E. and Benacerraf, B. B.**, Functional specificity of thymus-dependent lymphocytes, *Science*, 195, 1293, 1977.
250. **Thorsby, E.**, Biological function of HLA, *Tissue Antigens*, 11, 321, 1978.
251. **Snell, G. D.**, T cells, T cell recognition structures, and the major histocompatibility complex, *Immunol. Rev.*, 38, 3, 1978.
252. **Berke, G. and Amos, D. B.**, Cytotoxic lymphocytes in the absence of detectable antibody, *Nature (London) New Biol.*, 242, 237, 1972.
253. **Peck, A. B., Wigzell, H., Janeway, C., Jr., and Andersson, L. C.**, Environmental and genetic control of T cell activation *in vitro*: a study using isolated alloantigen-activated T cell clones, *Immunol. Rev.*, 35, 146, 1977.
254. **Kristensen, T. and Jorgensen, F.**, False HLA-D assignments may be caused by cytotoxic responder lymphocytes, *Tissue Antigens*, 11, 443, 1978.
255. **Shearer, G. M., Rehn, T. G., and Schmitt-Verhulst, A.**, Role of the murine major histocompatibility complex in the specificity of in vitro T-cell-mediated lympholysis against chemically modified autologous lymphocytes, *Transplant. Rev.*, 29, 222.

256. **Simonsen, M.,** Graft-versus-host reactions: their natural history and applicability as tools of research, *Prog. Allergy*, 6, 349, 1962.
257. **Perkins, E. H. and Popp, D. M.,** unpublished data, 1979.
258. **Popp, D. M.,** Basal serum immunoglobulin levels. I. Evidence for genetic control in B10 and B10.F mice, *Immunogenetics*, 9, 125, 1979.
259. **Popp, D. M.,** Basal serum immunoglobulin levels. II. Interaction of genetic loci and maternal effect on regulation of IgA, *Immunogenetics*, 9, 281, 1979.

BODY HOMEOSTATIC MECHANISMS AND AGING OF THE IMMUNE SYSTEM

Nicola Fabris

INTRODUCTION

It is now well established that the immune function is the result of a complex cooperation among different cell types and, within the lymphoid system itself, among different subsets of lymphocytes.[1,2] The complexity of such a working pattern of the immune system has been interpreted as a major self-regulating mechanism, developed by evolution in order to achieve the most efficient defense response with the minimal involvement of other body organs and apparatus. Following this line of thought, it has also been suggested that it is the disruption of such a complex self-regulatory mechanism which causes the immunodeficiency state and the immunopathological sequence occurring with advancing age.[3-7]

Since a general feature, at least of higher organisms, is that their organs and apparatus are controlled not only through self-regulation but also by supervisor homeostatic mechanisms mediated by the neuroendocrine system, it is unlikely that the immune system would function in the autonomous manner thus far proposed.

This consideration gains even further relevance when the immune function is investigated during its development and decline, or during periods of life, such as pregnancy, when the neuroendocrine balance is more or less far from the "maturity-state".[8]

It may be reasonable to neglect the possibility of interference to immune efficiency by extraimmunological homeostatic mechanisms during maturity on the basis of an equilibrium within which different and perhaps opposite pressures mutually counteract one another. However, these extraimmunological homeostatic mechanisms should be taken into account after maturation when these pressures operate in an unbalanced condition.

Unfortunately, neither the microenvironmental factors which can physiologically influence the immune system nor their alteration with advancing age are not well enough understood to draw a comprehensive picture. Nevertheless, some consistent evidence has been reported in recent years. This chapter will try to present it, to show what we still need in terms of further investigation, rather than the conclusions which can be drawn from the present state of knowledge.

MICROENVIRONMENTAL FACTORS IN IMMUNOREGULATION

Since the main function of the homeostatic mechanisms (supported in higher organisms by the central nervous system and the endocrine system) is concerned with the restoration of body balance, when suddenly disrupted by external noxae, a general premise is that a strict distinction between external and internal factors acting upon immunoregulation is somewhat academic. Moreover, due to the fact that the "internal milieu" is the result of the interaction of very complex homeostatic mechanisms, and that the vast majority of experimental studies have been performed in vivo, it is difficult to discriminate the effects directly dependent on a given internal regulatory mechanism from those supported by other homeostatic mechanisms frequently recruited in the same reaction.

Psychosocial Factors

The idea that extrinsic noxae may influence the immune efficiency is supported by a number of clinical and experimental observations, primarily related to the physical and psychosocial environment. Alterations in immunological functions have been induced by substantial variations in diet[9] and in environmental temperature.[10] In addition, it has been suggested that psychological stresses, such as those related to avoidance learning procedures, overcrowding and exposure to complex stimulation, may modify susceptibility to viral and parasitic infections, to the development and course of experimentally induced tumors, and to serum levels of antibodies directed towards various antigens.[11]

Since the experimental models used generally reflect the animal facilities and the immune parameters available in different laboratories, information is frequently fragmentary. Nevertheless, it seems that the immunological modifications induced by psychological manipulation may differ according to the psychosocial stimulus chosen and the immune parameter measured.

Thus, increased susceptibility to viral and parasitic infections has been reported in mice submitted to avoidance learning procedures or housed in groups, while segregation decreases parasitic infections and increases susceptibility to encephalomyocarditis virus. Infantile handling and mild electric shock increase the development of Walker 256 sarcoma and lymphoid leukemias.

Daily handling of mice early in life increases both primary and secondary immune responses to flagellin immunization[12] whereas overcrowding in adult age reduces both of them. From these fragmentary findings, the suggestion emerges that behind the psychological experience there exsits a still unknown number and quality of forces able to change the actual potentiality of the immune system. Such a suggestion finds even more substantial support in the observation that, within the same group of animals, dominant individuals show higher antibody responses than all the other animals of the group. This fact is shown in the empirical criterion used in choosing rabbits for antisera preparation: the more aggressive the rabbit, the higher the antiserum titer obtained.

If, according to this premise, the idea is accepted that psychosocial conditions modulate the immune system, the mechanisms by which they operate are far from being understood. While the phenomenon of psychologically induced immunodepression may in fact be interpreted as the consequences of an increased stress-dependent output of corticosteroids, it is unlikely that the same mechanism is responsible for those cases, in which an increased immune response is observed.

Since the central nervous system (CNS) represents the primary organ which filters, through its peripheral sensory apparatus, the majority of psychosocial information and coordinates (through the involvement of hypothalamic regions), the most appropriate response is that it may also mediate the psychosocially induced immunological modifications.

Central Nervous System

Since the pioneering work at the beginning of this century on the relationship between the CNS and anaphylactic reactions, a renewed interest in the field has only recently appeared and has focused its attention on the relevance of different brain regions on both humoral and cellular immune responses. This research has profited by the technical possibility of inducing electrolytic focal lesions on selected areas of the brain, which allows a definition of the functional role of different brain formations[11,13] such as hypothalamus, reticular formation, thalamus, superior colliculus, caudate nucleus, and amigdaloid complex.[20,21]

The most relevant finding of these experiments is that only lesions of hypothalamus and reticular formation induce depressed Arthus and delayed skin reactions of bovine serum albumin, together with a reduction of circulating antibody titers.[13] Hypothalamic lesions also cause reduction of spleen cellularity with disappearance of germinal centers. Marked involution of the thymus is observed in brain lesioned rats independently from the area, although more pronounced changes have been documented in rats with lesions in hypothalamic, reticular formation, and superior colliculus areas.[14]

The interpretation of these findings is quite difficult since interconnections between brain areas, the autonomic nervous system (ANS), and the endocrine system,[15] which are known to influence the immune system, are complex and not well understood. All authors interested in the field agree on the idea that more than one mechanism may be involved. Two major possibilities should be taken into account: first, that in the hypothalamic areas there are cells involved in the elaboration of the various releasing factors controlling the secretion of hypophysial hormones, and second, that the same areas, in particular the anterior hypothalamus and reticular formation, are also involved in the central control of the ANS. According to the first explanation, an increased output of releasing factors for ACTH and/or pituitary gonadotropins may activate the pituitary-adrenal and/or the pituitary-sexual gland axis with peripheral increase in immunosuppressive hormonal steroids. Alternatively, a diminished secretion of releasing factors for somatotropic (STH) or thyrotropic (TTH) hormones may reduce the peripheral level of somatotropic hormone or of thyroxine, which are known to exert a developmental action on the immune system.[16] Following the second explanation, an imbalance may occur between the parasympathetic and the sympathetic nervous system, the action of which is mediated at the periphery by different catecholamines, with a predominance of the β-adrenergic receptor AMP activity on the gamma-receptor-cGMP system. Both mechanisms may justify the modifications observed in the immune responses, since either the endocrine or the autonomic nervous system may affect the immune efficiency (see below).

The Endocrine System

The assumption that the endocrine system may exert a consistent modulator action on the immune functioning is supported now by a considerable body of experimental evidence.[16] All the endocrine glands seem to be involved, although a definite role has not yet been established for each hormone produced by them. Such an assumption is based on findings obtained either from endocrine gland deprivation experiments (hypofunctional states) and sucessive reconstitution therapy, or from exogenous administration of a given hormone in otherwise normal animals (hyperfunctional states). Further support comes from the identification of receptors for different hormones on the membrane of lymphoid cells.[17] Specific binding has been documented for the somatotropic hormone,[18] insulin,[19] calcitonin,[17] T_3 and T_4,[20] and steroid hormones.[21]

Without examining the information about each hormone and its properties as an immunoregulating agent, a general picture of immune-endocrine system relationships should include the following deductions. The effect of a single hormone, as measured by the alterations induced in different immune parameters, may be positive, i.e., may increase the efficiency of the immune system or reduce it. A positive action is exerted by developmental hormones, such as somatotropic hormone,[22] thyroxine,[23,24] and insulin.[25] Depression of immune functions has been observed, besides corticosteroids with gonadotropins,[26,27] progesteroids,[28] and testosterone.[29]

Due to the concomitant presence of both stimulator and antagonist hormones, the efficiency of the immune system in a given moment should be interpreted, therefore, as that one which is permitted by the actual hormonal balance.

The hormonal action may be revealed with intensity, dependent on the age of the animal: during development a higher hormonal supply or a more critical hormone concentration seems to be required than that needed in older age.[30] Such a phenomenon is probably linked to the relevance that some hormones have for the proliferation rate of lymphoid cells. Periods of life characterized by a high turnover of cells are more sensitive to modification of the hormonal balance[31,32] than periods in which such proliferation is relatively low.[33] It must be noted, however, that even in adult age, hormone-dependent modification of the immune efficiency may be demonstrable, provided the period of experimental observation is long enough,[23,34] or the pool of mature lymphocytes is partially depleted by cortisonization[35] or irradiation,[36] and, also likely, by aging.[37]

The effect of hormones is not equally exerted on all kinds of lymphoid cells. On a functional basis, insulin and gonadotropins seem to act differently on humoral or cell-mediated immune responses.[25,27] Many hormones are quite active on thymocyte differentiation[38] while their requirement by mature lymphocytes is extremely limited. Such a differential action may be caused, in some instances, by a different concentration of hormone receptor on the surface of different subpopulations of lymphocytes. Thus, insulin receptors are found with greater concentration on B- than on T-cells.[17] Higher binding of somatotropic hormone occurs on thymocytes than on mature lymphocytes.[39]

Moreover, even within different steps of the same immune response, the sensitivity to hormones may vary: thus, corticosteroids may play a positive role during the sensitization phase of the immune response, whereas in the following periods they are not required or even harmful.[40] Insulin receptors, which are not usually found on the membrane of lymphocyte capable of responding to Con A, appear during the early phase after mitogen stimulation.[41]

In the context of endocrine modulators of immunity, a prominent role has been gained in recent years by the humoral factors produced by the thymus.[42] Although definite biochemical sequences have not yet been reached, the capacity of thymic factors to substitute for the entire gland in many experimental models has collected a considerable body of evidence.[43-46] Much less attention has been paid to the fact that it is unlikely that thymic factors, in contrast with all other known hormones, would act in an autonomous manner. Preliminary information in this field has revealed that at least those thymic-dependent factors which are measurable in the serum[47] depend on the integrity of hypophysial[48] and thyroid[49] function.

Moreover, it should be taken into account that thymic factors act on the lymphoid cell by means of the same second messengers, the intracellular cyclic-nucleotides, which mediate the majority of neuroendocrine stimulations.[50] Therefore, in the action of thymic factors at cellular level, possible interferences by the basal equilibrium between cAMP and cGMP as determined by neuroendocrine homeostasis[51] should be taken into consideration.

The Autonomic Nervous System (ANS)

The assumption that the ANS may influence lymphoid cells comes from two main lines of observation: first, that receptors for vasoactive amines have been found on the membrane of rodents and human leukocytes, and second, that the two intracellular second messengers, which mediate the action of vasoactive amines, have been demonstrated to play a primary role in the response of lymphoid cells to specific stimuli.

The first line of evidence has gained recognition from the early 1970s.[52] In particular, the presence on lymphoid cells of receptors for low-molecular-weight hormones, such as histamine. β-mimetic catecholamines, and prostaglandins has been demonstrated, while the existence of α-adrenergic receptors and of γ-acetylcholine-sensitive receptors is, at present, supported only by indirect experimental findings.

The receptors for these low-molecular-weight hormones are not present in all lymphocyte subpopulations, so that columns of hormone coated beads may remove from a heterogenous population only those lymphocytes which possess the specific receptors for the hormone itself. With these techniques it has been possible to analyze the target of different low-molecular-weight hormones and their ultimate effect on the economy of the immune system. Thus, it has been demonstrated that β-mimetic amines, histamine, and prostaglandin E, in addition to their known effect on the inflammatory process, act on both B- and T-derived cells; in particular they inhibit both the cytolytic functions and the production of lymphokines by T-effector cells (also antibody-dependent lymphocyte-mediated cytotoxicity seems to be inhibited as well) and T-cell suppressor activity. They can also, with the exception of histamine, inhibit production and release of specific antibody by B-cells.

On the other hand, cholinomimetic drugs, particularly of the muscarinic type, increase T-cell proliferation under mitogen stimulation and T-cell mediated cytolysis.

These findings have been interpreted in light of the role played by cyclic nucleotides, cAMP and cGMP, in the physiological control of proliferation and differentiation of lymphocytes.[53] The effect of drugs acting on adenyl-cyclase and on guanyl-cyclase-dependent receptors can be substituted, in fact, by cAMP and cGMP, respectively.

The exact role of these two cyclic nucleotides in immune function is far from known. While on mature cells, their effect is similar to that caused by stimulation of adenyl-cyclase or guanyl-cyclase (inhibition or facilitation, respectively), on thymocytes both cAMP and cGMP appear to be mitosis-inducers, although the action seems to be exerted on different subsets of thymocytes.[52]

Future work will certainly elucidate this complex cellular autoregulatory system. It should be noted, however, that the majority of these findings have been obtained in vitro. By trying to translate this information to the in vivo situation, the picture may become even more complex.[54] The physiological balance between cAMP and cGMP is, in fact, regulated by the level of activity of parasympathetic and sympathetic limbs of the ANS and by the action of different endocrine glands. Hormones, such as insulin, growth hormone, thyroxine sex hormones, and thymic hormones probably act on lymphoid cells through the mediation of cyclic nucleotides. The effect of in vivo experimental manipulation of ANS on the immune system, although supported by recent findings,[54] should take into account all these possible interrelationships.

Influence of Immune Reactions on Body Homeostatic Mechanisms

One of the main biological characteristics of homeostatic regulation is that a continuous flow of information occurs between the homeostatic mechanisms and their targets and that such a flow is bidirectional: in other words feedback mechanisms have been developed in order to avoid regulation excess or defect. If the idea is accepted that various body homeostatic mechanisms act on immune efficiency, it would be reasonable to assume that the immune functioning may also send information to the homeostatic mechanisms themselves. A recent study to coordinate the knowledge in this field has focused attention on the fact that various kinds of disturbances in antigen handling result in modification of the neuroendocrine system: thus germ-free mice,[55,56] neonatally thymectomized and thymic nude mice,[57] display a profoundly disturbed endocrine system. Moreover, physiological antigenic challenge in otherwise normal animals induces, in addition to the early and more obvious alteration of cyclic nucleotide and prostaglandin synthesis,[58] late modifications of the hormonal balance[59] and of hypothalmic neuronal firing rate.[60]

While the biological mediators of this information which flows from the activated immune system to the homeostatic regulatory mechanisms remains unknown at present, the relevance of a network of immune-neuroendocrine interactions in terms of the regulation of the immune system itself should not be underestimated.

AGE-DEPENDENT ALTERATIONS OF HOMEOSTATIC MECHANISMS

In assessing the functional decline with advancing age of the mechanisms of body homeostasis, a preliminary distinction should be made between the alterations which appear as the consequence of cumulative defects and those modifications which may have their cause in phenomena occurring a long time before the onset of aging, namely, during developmental stages. It is, in fact, obvious that the degree of functional failure in old age is measured on the maturity-steady state level and that the latter depends not only on the genetic background, but also on the environmental stimuli experienced during ontogeny. An interesting example in this context is the fact that very short treatments with hormones during prenatal age or during the first days of life may induce permanent modifications, which lead to an altered maturity-steady state; thus, prenatal treatment with growth hormone enhances learning ability;[61] treatment, during the first days of life, with sexual hormones causes modified sexual behavior,[62] while treatment with thyroxine causes abnormalities in hypothalamopituitary, thyroidal, and gonadal functions, which not only persist throughout life, but may even be transmitted to F_1 and F_2 progeny.[60]

In addition to hormonally induced biological "imprinting", there is dietary imprinting which can, for example, extend life span in mice and rats by caloric restriction, provided the treatment begins very early in life and although it lasts relatively few months.[64]

The biological mechanisms supporting these phenomena are, at present, unknown. Some of the experimental designs reported above have suggested the idea of irreversible modifications of the sensitivity to the homeostatic regulation systems occurring both at a central or peripheral level. Permanent alterations of the hormone receptors in hypothalamic neurons have been proposed in order to explain the modifications of mating behavior after early treatment with estrogens;[62] on the other hand, an irreversible loss of peripheral growth hormone receptors has been documented in hypopituitary growth hormone deficient dwarf mice[65] (dw). In between these two extremes of receptor modification following excess or defect of hormonal stimulation, it is conceivable to put an indefinite number of intermediate physiological situations, occurring during developmental stages, which would condition the future performance in adult life and its decline with advancing age.[24]

While the relevance of these phenomena for the aging of the homeostatic regulation system remains to be established, it is well documented that progressive alterations with advancing age do affect all the organs and apparatus for which a connection with the immune efficiency has been suggested.

Aging of the Central Nervous System

Deterioration of axonal and dendritic terminal processes, followed by the disintegration of the whole body of nerve cells, accumulation of age pigment and other metabolic substances, alteration in basic anabolic functions, through the loss of enzymes controlling carbohydrate, intermediate protein, and lipid metabolism, and modification of synthesis, release, and uptake of neurotransmitters, particularly in the dopaminergic and colinergic systems, are the most common detrimental processes observed in nearly all anatomical districts of the CNS.[66-68] According to the degree of gravity reached in different parts of the CNS, these alterations in addition to a concomitant more or less deep defect of the sensory system[83] cause a number of disfunctional biases toward a Parkinson or a senile dementia state,[67] or, when mild, to a slowing information process.[67,69]

While these changes within high CNS functions certainly interfere with the psychosocial behavior of the elderly and generally restrict their capacity to accommodate new or unfair situations, it is likely that both these changes and their psychosocial consequences would affect the functional pattern of hypothalamic regions, where the majority of homeostatic regulation systems have their central control.

There is consistent evidence that the central regulation of both the ANS and of the endocrine system becomes less adequate in old age to meet the needs of the organism.[70,71] The excitability of central neurons as well as of peripheral fibers of the ANS is reduced with advancing age.[72] On the other hand, hypothalamic neurosecretory cells, which control, through their releasing factors, the synthesis and secretion of pituitary hormones, show with advancing age a reduction of their activity.[73,74,85] Moreover, alterations in the sensitivity of these neuronal cells to the humoral substances which constitute the feedback mechanisms have also been described, although observations are controversial. An increased sensitivity to circulating corticosterone[75] has been proposed as the cause for the low resting corticosterone level observed in old age. On the other hand, an increased hypothalamic threshold level to negative feedback mechanisms has been postulated in order to explain a number of age-related disorders in homeostatic stability, such as the decreased glucose, the increased body weight and serum-colesterol, and the climacteric.[76] The possibility that such an increased hypothalamic threshold may be due to a decrease in peripheral hormone receptor density has also been investigated.[77]

Although such findings are somewhat conflicting, it is likely that the magnitude of variations, which can be compensated by central hypothalamic control, is certainly reduced in old age and/or requires more time in order to be corrected.[70]

In addition to central defects, it should be taken into account that age-related deterioration also affects the target of such a control.

Aging of the Endocrine System

In the endocrine system, failure of the pituitary gland or of its satellite glands, in addition to alterations in peripheral responsiveness to hormonal stimuli, has been taken into consideration.

Abnormalities with advancing age have been detected in nearly all endocrine glands. In part, deficiencies have been observed in pituitary-gonadal interactions,[78,79] in the pituitary-adrenal axis,[80] and in thyroid hormone secretion.[73-81] However, it is difficult to estimate the exact relevance of such findings and the extent to which these deficiencies may exert a secondary influence on body aging.[71-82]

More impressive or at least provocative are some recent findings related to pituitary changes and to peripheral responsiveness to humoral factors with advancing age. At pituitary level, in addition to minor and likely secondary defects in hormone synthesis and release, it seems that a factor is secreted, with the ability to antagonize the peripheral effects of thyroxine and that such a factor shows an increased effectiveness or is secreted in higher amounts with advancing age.[83] Hypophysectomy in old age, by removing the source of such a factor, restores the peripheral sensitivity to thyroid hormones. To a certain extent these findings are reminiscent of some old views, according to which hypofunctioning of the hypophysis might decelerate some aging processes.[85]

On the other hand, altered sensitivity of old peripheral tissues to the hormonal action has been described in many experimental models.[86] Decline of peripheral target tissue responsiveness has been ascribed to thyroid hormones, to insulin, to male and female sex steroids, and to glucocorticoid.[87]

In the majority of these cases the age-dependent variation of peripheral responsiveness seems to depend more on alterations in hormone uptake and/or binding by peripheral cells[86] rather than on fluctuations of hormone circulating levels, which, with few exceptions, remain remarkably constant throughout life.[88] Such a defect, which is probably due to the alteration of hormone receptor density, and not of their binding affinity,[89] is generally irreversible, although in a few instances, recovery by prolonged treatment with exogenous administration of the specific hormone may be achieved.[90]

Aging of the Autonomic Nervous System

Within the ANS-dependent homeostatic regulation, aging affects both ganglionic trasmission and peripheral sensitivity to the humoral mediators of ANS. At ganglionic level the reduced capacity to perform their role probably depends on the same degenerative processes, which affect neuronal systems.[68] At a peripheral level, a general insensitivity to the stimulation with synthetic or natural catecholamines has been reported,[86] and such a defect, as for protein hormones, is probably due to loss of receptor sites on the cell membrane,[89] although in some cases defective adenyl cyclase activity has been detected.[91] The ultimate consequences of these alterations involve, obviously, the intracellular level of cyclic nucleotides and the biological functions which are turned on or off by them.[87] This point is, however, more intriguing since the action of catecholamine on cyclic nucleotides is mediated through membrane enzymes, adenyl and guanyl cyclases, whose synthesis is influenced by other endocrine factors, such as thyroid hormones.[15] Age-dependent alterations of thyroid hormone level or of peripheral cell sensitivity to thyroid hormone[83] may also influence the cell responsiveness to catecholamines.

HOMEOSTATIC REGULATION AND AGING OF THE IMMUNE SYSTEM

If it is difficult, at present, to draw a comprehensive picture either of neuroendocrine-immune systems or of the aging of neuroendocrine homeostasis, it may seem nearly pure speculation to discuss the relevance that the latter has for the aging of the immune system itself. Although very little is known in this field it is likely, however, that a role in immunological aging should be assigned to the complex regulatory mechanisms, which, at least during development and maturity, have been shown to modulate some immune reactions. This assumption is supported by two orders of observations.

First, lymphoid cells may survive well beyond the life span of the species from which they derive, provided that cells are serially transplanted into syngeneic young recipients. Survival of functionally active mouse lymphoid cells has reached 5 years in length before cells were exhausted or developed into aneuploid lines.[92]

On the other hand, the lack of appearance with advancing age of immunodeficiencies in caloric restricted animals refutes that the immune system is delayed in its rate of aging in these animals, in contrast to what occurs in other tissues, such as bone, which become more fragile in long-surviving undernourished rats than in physiologically-aged animals.[93] On the contrary, caloric restriction seems to slow the rate of age-dependent decline of immune efficiency, although such an effect may depend in part on the longer period required in order to achieve full development.[9,94]

These two observations strongly support the idea that the life expectancy of lymphocytes can be appreciably modified and that such a modification may markedly depend on internal environmental conditions. The last assumption is in agreement with the finding that old cells perform better when inoculated into a young environment whereas young cells transplanted into old individuals are partially inhibited, although the functional variations achieved in both transfer systems are of limited extent.[95]

The higher efficacy of serial transplants in respect to short-term transfer of lymphoid cells in modifying their functional efficiency may indicate that the alterations with aging of the relationships between the immune system and the "internal milieu" is a chronic, and probably irreversible, process which can be substantially prevented by continuous maintenance of cells into a young environment rather than corrected by a transfer of cells into a young animal.

In order to assess the relevance of the age-related modifications of the "internal milieu" for immunological aging, both developmental events, which might condition the future performance of the immune system, and the age-related deterioration itself, should be taken into consideration.

Relevance of Developmental Phenomena

One of the primary developmental modifications of the neuroendocrine system, which may influence future performance of the immune system, is sex. It has been shown that femininity is accompanied by increased thymus size[96] and augmented efficiency of the immune system.[29] In some species, as in hamster, femininity appears to prevent post-thymectomy wasting-disease.[97]

Moreover, since femininity implies pregnancy, the ultimate effect of the latter on the immune economy should not be underestimated. Repeated pregnancies increase the life span of neonatally thymectomized female mice[98] and, in otherwise untreated mice, leave a higher plaque-forming-cell capacity than that recorded in age-matched virgin females.[99]

Congenital or experimentally induced alteration of the balance among developmental hormones during the early postnatal period also causes modifications of the immune sytem efficiency, which can be prevented by substitutive therapy, provided, however, treatment begins early enough.[16,100] In other words, the lack of some hormones for relatively short periods of developmental life may induce irreversible changes on their target organs. Thus the immunodeficiency documented in the hypopituitary dwarf mice can be prevented if hormonal therapy begins not later than the 60th day of life; in this case not only the immunological deficiencies are corrected, but also some early aging processes, which usually affect dwarf mice, are prevented.[100,101] It is to be noted that the timing of hormonal therapy required in order to reconstitute the immunodeficient dwarf mouse is similar to that needed by neonatal thymus grafts in order to recover neonatally thymectomized mice from their immune disturbances.[102] Whether the irreversibility of these phenomena depends on a progressive exhaustion of some specific target cells[103] or, alternately, on the loss of receptor sites for the hormonal action[65] is, as yet, unknown.

Permanent modifications of immune efficiency have been observed not only as negative, but also as positive phenomena. Thus, handling of rodents during developmental stages increases their immune performance when adult.[12] Treatment of mice during the early postnatal period with developmental hormones accelerates the rate of ontogenetic maturation.[104] Caloric restriction has a higher effect in terms of prolongation of life span when treatment begins during the ontogenetic period than thereafter.[64]

All these observations suggest that the maturation steps of immune system should be more closely evaluated in relation to the concomitantly developing complex mechanisms of neuroendocrine homeostasis. Furthermore, special consideration should be given to the peculiar sensitivity to environmental stimuli the immune system shows during this period of life, which can provoke profound effects on its performance in later periods of life.

Relevance of Age-Related Phenomena

Among the numerous factors which may influence the immune system, only a few have been investigated in relation to their potential relevance as co-factors in the aging of the immune system. Thus, the role of psychosocial factors, which are so relevant in old age, particularly in the modern society, has been completely neglected. An isolated observation[105] places attention on the fact that the loss of the partner, an event doubtless more frequent in old age, causes a depression of the PHA response of peripheral lymphocytes, for which a clear-cut explanation is still lacking. Similarly, the relevance of the age-related degenerative processes of both the central and autonomic nervous system has not yet received substantial experimental attention.

The majority of data regards the influence of the neuroendocrine system on immunological aging; the following hormonal aspects have been investigated in a more in-depth fashion.

Thymic Factors

With advancing age a progressive decline of thymic-dependent factors detectable in the serum has been documented.[106] The capacity of neonatal thymus grafted into old individuals to recover some age-related immunodeficiencies may depend, at least in part, on a reconstitution of the hormonal secretion. In few instances has such an interpretation achieved experimental support by the observation that treatment of old mice with thymic factor preparation increases their immunological capacity.[107] It is of interest to note that with some experimental designs such a recovery seems to be due to a reduced T-cell suppressor activity as if the treatment would have modified the ratios among different subsets of T-derived cells.[108] This interpretation is in agreement, on the other hand, with the finding that in autoimmune-prone strains of mice, the age-dependent decline of serum thymic factors activity occurs earlier than in nonsusceptible strains and that treatment with thymic hormone preparations may to a certain extent ameliorate the autoimmune phenomena in susceptible mice.[109]

In the context of the relevance of the thymus in aging processes, it should be mentioned that, according to recent studies, the thymus seems to be involved in the age-related deterioration of organs and apparatus other than the immune system. In particular, it has been demonstrated that some extra-immunological functions, such as the response of submandibular glands to synthetic catecholamines or the basal serum levels of triiodothyronine and insulin, which are altered in old age, can be corrected to young values by transplanting a neonatal thymus.[110] Although direct evidence is still lacking, it is conceivable that such an effect is mediated by humoral factors of thymic origin, rather than from the improved immunological efficiency.

With regard to the causes of the decline of thymic endocrine activity with advancing age, primary failure of the thymus, or secondary defect depending upon age-related modifications of the hormone-metabolic balance or upon progressive reduction of peripheral demand of thymic hormones themselves, are possibilities to be investigated. Preliminary data from our laboratory suggest that the deficient thymic hormone secretion in old age may be a secondary phenomenon during the first period of old age, while it depends on primary failure of the thymus in very old animals. Such an assumption is derived from the observation that with appropriate endocrinological manipulation, the thymus of a 20-month-old mouse can still be induced to increase the amount of thymic factor secreted, whereas in period of life over 24 months of age such an induction is impossible.[49]

Thyroid Hormones

It is generally accepted that with advancing age a decrease in thyroid-dependent body functions does occur although it is not obligatorily revealed by modified serum levels of thyroid hormones.[81] It has been recently proposed that such a defect might depend on a decreased peripheral sensitivity to thyroid hormones and that this phenomenon is due to the progressive increase with advancing age of a factor of the pituitary origin, which could antagonize the utilization of thyroid hormones by peripheral tissues.[83] This suggestion is further supported by the fact that removal of the hypophysis may increase thyroid hormone utilization and consequently recover a number of age-related immunodeficiencies.[84,111]

It is to be noted, however, that these findings can also be explained by qualitative alteration of pituitary hormones occurring in old age, which could give rise to prohormones competing at the periphery with thyroid hormone.[82]

The assumption that modification of thyroid hormone blood levels or their peripheral utilization may be responsible for some age-related immunodeficiencies is supported by another order of observations. Exogenous administration of thyroxine in old animals can increase both the plaque-forming-cell capacity and the PHA response of their spleen cells.[37-112]

These findings would agree with the observation that a progressive decline of peripheral conversion rate of T_4 to T_3 occurs with advancing age[113] and that exogenous injection of T_4 may activate such a conversion.[114] An alternative interpretation may be offered by data from preliminary experiments which have shown that the thyroxine-induced immunological recovery in old mice is accompanied by increased serum levels of thymic factors and that very old animals, which frequently do not respond to thyroxine treatment, do not show the serum increment of thymic factor activity.[49] Whether immunological recovery and resumption of thymic endocrine activity are concomitant phenomena or linked to each other remains to be established.

Glucocorticoids

With advancing age a progressive decline of the concentration of membrane receptor for glucocorticoids has been documented in the spleen cell population. Such an alteration may depend either on an age-related modification of the ratio among various subsets of lymphoid cells carrying different receptor densities or, more likely, on an intrinsic failure of old cells, which might be unable to maintain the proper turnover of receptor molecules.[115] The age-related defect in cell receptors may be responsible for the altered functional responsiveness of old cells to the glucocorticoid action: the ability of these hormones to inhibit the metabolism of lymphoid cells is greatly reduced in old age.[116]

Catecholamines

The concentration of membrane receptors for these low-molecular-weight hormones on lymphoid cells shows with advancing age alterations quite similar to that recorded for the glucocorticoid receptor.[117] Moreover, it has been shown that it is the number of receptor molecules which decreases with advancing age, whereas the affinity does not seem to change.[87] These findings, together with those obtained for glucocorticoid receptors in lymphoid cells and those documented in other systems of hormone-target cell receptor interaction, have suggested the idea that receptor loss is in general an age-related phenomenon, although the causes may be different according to the system under investigation.[87] In the case of catecholamines, the reduced receptor density may represent, in fact, a compensatory phenomenon directed to adjust cell responsiveness to the increased plasma hormone level.[118]

In this context it is worthwhile to note that the intracellular level of both cAMP and cGMP in spleen cells is also modified with advancing age: cAMP level is reduced while cGMP level increases with consequent decline of the cAMP/cGMP ratio.[51] Whether such an imbalance is due to the alteration in catecholamine receptor or to modification of other hormonal balances, which may also affect cyclic nucleotide pattern, is still an unsolved problem.

Finally, the important fact that a number of age-related and frequently hormone-dependent metabolic alterations influence the efficiency of the immune system should not be ignored. The increase in serum cholesterol level augments the viscosity of lymphocyte membranes and consequently alters their functionality.[119,120] In some cases the pharmacological correction of these metabolic disturbances brings a significant recovery from some age-related immunodeficiencies.[121]

From all these data the picture of the microenvironmental effects on immunological aging gains quite complex attributes, which only a coordinated and interdisciplinary investigation may hope to clarify.

Neuroendocrine-Immune System Interactions and Tumor Surveillance

It is generally accepted that tumor development is an age-related phenomenon since the frequency of spontaneous tumors is higher both in early periods of life and during aging than during maturity. A number of hypotheses have been developed in order to explain such a pattern and the majority of them are strictly linked to the mechanism which is believed to play a major role in tumor surveillance.

Since the immune system has been shown in many experimental designs to protect against tumor development, an age-dependent failure of such an immunological surveillance has been thought to be the main cause for the increased tumor incidence with advancing age.[122] Although this hypothesis has received a good amount of experimental evidence,[123] it does not seem at present that it can cover all clinical and experimental observations.

In particular, a strict connection between immunodeficiency states and tumor susceptibility is not documentable in all situations. The immunodeficient nude[124] and dwarf mice[112] do not show increased incidence of spontaneous tumor, nor is the "take" and growth of transplantable tumors augmented.[112] Also, newborn mice, which do not have a fully developed immune system, do not always represent better recipients for transplantable tumors than adult animals.[125]

An immunological explanation for these exceptions to the immunological surveillance theory may be offered by the lymphocyte-dependent enhancing effect on tumor development observed in defined experimental situations.[126]

Although most of these immunological mechanisms may certainly play a role in the development and growth of tumors, it is unlikely that the tumor-host relationships are strictly limited to this biological area.

Before the discovery of the immune system as a major defense mechanism against tumors, endocrinological implications connected with tumor surveillance[127] have been investigated. A number of endocrinological situations which could either favor or inhibit tumor growth have been identified and these findings have been documented not only for tumors derived from hormone-sensitive tissues, but also for tumors derived from parenchymal and connective tissues and from quite anaplastic tumors such as Sarcoma 180 or Erlich ascites tumor.[112]

The hormone dependency of many tumors has received renewed attention in recent years.[128] It has been shown that defined hormonal imbalances precede in some tumor-prone strains of mice the appearance of tumor themselves and in other situations may reduce their growth rate.[129] Moreover, it has also been demonstrated that even for the oncological virus-induced transformation of both human and animal cells, a number of hormones may play a role, either augmenting the expression of viral genome or enhancing the proliferation of transformed cells, the two effects not being correlated to each other.[130]

These findings, together with the observation that tumors may modify their hormone-sensitivity during serial transplant in syngeneic hosts, and that such a modification is directed more frequently toward an escape from hormone dependency than vice versa, have brought the postulation of a hormonal surveillance theory.[128] This hypothesis has also been investigated in relation to the age-related susceptibility of tumor development.[121-131] Although it is impressive that tumor susceptibility is doubtlessly higher both during development and aging when the neuroendocrine system is unbalanced and even during transitory periods of maturity, such as gestation,[132] which are characterized by hormonal alterations, direct evidence of this hypothesis is still lacking.

It is of interest to note, however, that both immunological and hormonal surveillance theories have been proposed, each neglecting the other. Such a procedure, according to the observations reported in the present paper, appears conceptually limited and suggests that a revision of the majority of the experiments supporting one or the other theory and in particular all conflicting or paradoxical findings is needed. A trial in this direction has been already fruitful.[112] The contradictory results obtained on the pituitary dependency of some transplantable tumors according to the fact that congenitally hypopituitary animals[133] or adult hypophysectomized animals[127] were used as hosts may be explained by taking into account that the former recipients suffer from both hypopituitarism and immunodeficiency, whereas the other animals show only the endocrinological disturbances, the immune system being unaffected shortly after hypophysectomy.[33] Moreover, the fact that, in spite of the immunodeficiency state, dwarf mice do not show an increased tumor take contradicts the theory that the immunodeficiency state does not fully justify tumor surveillance in these animals and that their endocrinological disturbances certainly represent factors interfering with tumor growth.[112] Whether these kinds of thoughts may be applied to the increased tumor incidence which occurs with advancing age, by hypothesizing that it depends more on the alterations of neuroendocrine-immune system interactions during aging[112-121] rather than on a pure immunological deficiency, remains the object of further investigations.

Conclusion and Perspectives

A large number of findings suggest that the progressive deterioration which occurs with advancing age in the neuroendocrine homeostasis is partially responsible for the age-related immunological deficiencies. The fragmentary and frequently contradictory findings clearly show that much more work is needed before we can attain the level of understanding necessary to hypothesize and speculate. Such a goal is certainly difficult to achieve, since homeostatic regulation mechanisms are quite complex and interact with each other, since their impact on the multifaceted immune system is presumably equally complex, and finally, since the target of such a neuroendocrine-immune system interaction is represented by the "old" cells, which remains to be discovered. This approach, although filled with the above-mentioned difficulties, may be quite fruitful since it may open the possibility to manipulate in a physiological, rather than in a pharmacological way, the immune disturbances and their consequences for body economy which occur with advancing age.

REFERENCES

1. **Gershon, R. K.**, T cell control of antibody production, in *Contemporary Topics in Immunobiology*, Cooper, M. D. and Warner, L. N., Eds., Plenum Press, New York, 1974, 1.
2. **Cantor H. and Boyse E. A.**, Regulation of cellular and humoral immune responses by T cell subclasses, *Cold Spring Harbor Symp. Quant. Biol.*, 41, 23, 1976.
3. **Walford, R. L., Meredith, P. J., and Cheney, K. E.**, Immunoengineering: prospects for correction of age-related immunodeficiency states, in *Immunology and Aging*, Makinodan, T. and Yunis, E., Eds., Plenum Press, New York, 1977, 183.
4. **Makinodan, T., Good, R. A., and Kay, M. M. B.**, Cellular basis of immunosenescence, in *Immunology and Aging*, Vol. 2, Makinodan, T. and Yunis, E., Eds., Plenum Press, New York, 1977, 9.
5. **Segre, D. and Segre, M.**, Humoral immunity in aged mice. II. Increased suppressor T cell activity in immunologically deficient old mice, *J. Immunol.*, 116, 735, 1976.
6. **Gerbase-DeLima, M., Meredith P., and Walford, R.**, Age-related changes, including synergy and suppression, in the mixed lymphocyte reaction in long-lived mice, *Fed. Proc. Fed. Am. Soc. Exp. Biol.*, 34, 159, 1975.
7. **Gershon, R. K. and Metzler, C. M.**, Suppressor cells in aging, in *Immunology and Aging*, Makinodan, T. and Yunis, E., Eds., Plenum Press, New York, 1977, 103.
8. **Davies, J. and Ryan, K. J.**, Comparative endocrinology of gestation, *Vitam. Horm. (N.Y.)*, 30, 223, 1972.
9. **Walford, R. L., Liu, R. K., Mathies, M., Gerbase-DeLima, M., and Smith, G. S.**, Long term dietary restriction and immune function in mice. Response to sheep red blood cells and to mitogens, *Mech. Ageing Dev.*, 2, 447, 1973/74.
10. **Liu, R. K. and Walford, R. L.**, The effect of lowered body temperature on life-span and immune and non-immune processes, *Gerontologia*, 18, 363, 1972.
11. **Stein, M., Schiavi, R. C., and Camerino, M.**, Influence of brain and behaviour on the immune system, *Science*, 191, 435, 1976.
12. **Solomon, G. F., Levine, S., and Kraft, J. K.**, Early experience and immunity, *Nature (London)*, 220, 821, 1968.
13. **Jankovic, B. D. and Isakovic, K.**, Neuro-endocrine correlates of immune response. I. Effects of brain lesions on antibody production, Arthus reactivity and delayed hypersensitivity in the rat, *Int. Arch. Allergy*, 45, 360, 1973.
14. **Isakovic, K. and Jankovic, B. D.**, Neuro-endocrine correlates of immune response. II. Changes in the lymphatic organs of brain lesioned rats, *Int. Arch. Allergy*, 45, 373, 1973.
15. **Brodie, B. B., Davies, J. I., Hynie, S., Krishna, G., and Weiss, B.**, Interrelationships of catecholamines with other endocrine systems, *Pharmacol. Rev.*, 18, 273, 1969.
16. **Fabris, N.**, Hormones and aging, in *Immunology and Aging*, Vol. 1, Makinodan, T. and Yunis, E., Eds., Plenum Press, New York, 1977, 72.
17. **Gavin, J. R., III.**, Polipeptide hormone receptor on lymphoid cells, in *Immunopharmacology*, Vol. 3, Hadden, J. W., Coffey, R. G., and Spreafico, F., Eds., Plenum Press, New York, 1977, 357.
18. **Lesniak, M. A.**, Binding of I^{125}-human growth hormone to specific receptors in human cultured lymphocytes: characterization of the interaction and sensitivity of radioreceptor assay, *J. Biol. Chem.*, 249, 1661, 1974.
19. **Archer, J. A., Gorden, P., Gavin, J. R., III, Lesniak, M. A., and Roth, J.**, Insulin receptors in human circulating lymphocytes: application to the study of insulin resistance in man, *J. Clin. Endocrinol. Metab.*, 36, 627, 1973.
20. **Lemarchand-Béraud, T., Holm, A. C., and Scazziga, B. R.**, Triiodothyronine and thyroxine nuclear receptors in lymphocytes from normal, hyper and hypothyroid patients, *Acta Endocrinol.*, 85, 44, 1977.
21. **Perper, R. J. and Davies, P.**, Modulation of the expression of the immune response by anti-inflammatory drugs, in *Immunopharmacology*, Vol. 3, Hadden, J. W., Coffey, R. G., and Spreafico, F., Eds., Plenum Press, New York, 1977, 227.
22. **Sorkin, E., Pierpaoli, W., Fabris, N., and Bianchi, E.**, Relation of growth hormone to the thymus and the immune response, in *Growth and Growth Hormone*, Pecile, E. and Muller, F., Eds., Excerpta Medica, Amsterdam, 1972, 132.
23. **Ernström, U. and Larsson, B.**, Thymic and thoracic duct contribution to blood lymphocytes in normal and thyroxin-treated guinea-pig, *Acta Physiol. Scand.*, 66, 189, 1966.
24. **Fabris, N.**, Immunodepression in thyroid-deprived animals, *Clin. Exp. Immunol.*, 15, 601, 1973.
25. **Fabris, N. and Piantanelli, L.**, Differential effect of pancreatectomy on humoral and cell-mediated immunity, *Clin. Exp. Immunol.*, 28, 315, 1977.
26. **Addock, E. W., III, Teasdale, F., Agust, C. S., Cox, S., Meschia, G., Battaglia, F. C., and Naughton, M. A.**, Human chorionic gonadotrophin: its possible role in maternal lymphocytes suppression, *Science*, 181, 835, 1973.

27. **Fabris, N., Piantanelli, L., and Muzzioli, M.,** Differential effect of pregnancy or gestagens on humoral and cell-mediated immunity, *Clin. Exp. Immunol.,* 28, 306, 1977.
28. **Munroe, J. S.,** Progesteroid as immunosuppressive agents, *J. Reticuloendothelial Soc.,* 9, 361, 1971.
29. **Eidinger, D. and Garrett, T. J.,** Studies on the regulatory effects of the sex hormones on antibody formation and stem cell differentiation, *J. Exp. Med.,* 136, 1098, 1972.
30. **Pierpaoli, W., Fabris, N., and Sorkin, E.,** Developmental hormones and immunological maturation, in *Hormones and the Immune Response,* Ciba Study Group No. 36, Wolstenholme, G. E. W. and Knight, J., Eds., Churchill, London, 1970, 126.
31. **Fabris, N., Pierpaoli, W., and Sorkin, E.,** Hormones and the immunological capacity. III. The immunodeficiency diseases of the hypopituitary Snell-Bagg dwarf mouse, *Clin. Exp. Immunol.,* 9, 209, 1971.
32. **Fabris, N., Pierpaoli, W., and Sorkin, E.,** Hormones and the immunological capacity. IV. Restorative effects of developmental hormones or of lymphocytes on the immunodeficiency syndrome of the dwarf mouse, *Clin. Exp. Immunol.,* 9, 227, 1971.
33. **Kalden, J. R., Evans, M., and Irvine, W. J.,** The effect of hypophysectomy on the immune response, *Immunology,* 18, 671, 1970.
34. **Basso, A. and Fabris, N.,** Recovery of age-dependent immunological decline by short-term treatment with L-thyroxine. II. Effect on antigen induced immune reactions, *Mech. Ageing Develop.,* to be submitted.
35. **Fabris, N., Pierpaoli, W., and Sorkin, E.,** Hormones and the immune response, in *Developmental Aspects of Antibody Formation and Structure,* Sterzl, J. and Riha, I., Eds., Czechoslovak Academy Press, Prague, 1970, 79.
36. **Dusquenoy, R. J., Mariani, T., and Good, R. A.,** Effect of hypophysectomy on the immunological recovery from X-irradiation, *Proc. Soc. Exp. Biol. Med.,* 132, 1176, 1969.
37. **Muzzioli, M., Mocchegiani, E., and Fabris, N.,** Recovery of age-dependent immunological decline in mice by short-term treatment with L-thyroxine. I. Effect on lymphoid cell subpopulations, *Mech. Ageing Develop.,* to be submitted.
38. **Upendra, S., and Owen, J. J. T.,** Studies on the maturation of thymus stem cells: the effects of catecholamines, histamine and peptide hormones on the expression of T cell alloantigens, *Eur. J. Immunol.,* 6, 59, 1976.
39. **Arrembrecht, S.,** Specific binding of growth hormone to thymocytes, *Nature (London),* 252, 255, 1974.
40. **Stavy, L.,** Stimulation of rat lymphocyte proliferation by hydrocortisone during the induction of cell-mediated immunity in vitro, *Transplantation,* 17, 173, 1974.
41. **Krug, U., Krug, F., and Cuatrecasas, P.,** Emergence of insulin receptors on human lymphocytes during in vitro transformation, *Proc. Nat. Acad. Sci. U.S.A.,* 9, 2604, 1972.
42. **Van Bekkum, D. V.,** *The Biological Activity of Thymic Hormones,* Kooyker Scientific Publications, The Netherlands, 1975.
43. **Goldstein, A. L., Low, T. L. K., McAdoo, M., McClure, J., Thurman, G. B., Rossio, J., Lai, C. Y., Chang, D., Wang, S. S., Harvey, C., Ramel, A. H., and Meienhofer, J.,** Thymosin: isolation and sequence analysis of an immunologically active thymic polypeptide, *Proc. Natl. Acad. Sci., U.S. A.,* 74, 725, 1977.
44. **Kook, A. I., Yakir, Y., and Trainin, N.,** Isolation and partial chemical characterization of THF, a thymus hormone involved in immune maturation of lymphoid cells, *Cell. Immunol.,* 19, 151, 1975.
45. **Goldstein, G.,** Isolation of bovine thymin: a polypeptide hormone of the thymus, *Nature (London),* 247, 11, 1974.
46. **Bach, J. F., Dardenne, M., Pleau, J. M., and Rosa, J.,** Biochemical characterization of a serum thymic factor, *Nature (London),* 226, 55, 1977.
47. **Bach, J. F. and Dardenne, M.,** Studies on thymus products. II. Demonstration and characterization of a circulating thymic hormone, *Immunology,* 25, 353, 1973.
48. **Pelletier, M., Montplaisir, S., Dardenne, M., and Bach, J. F.,** Thymic hormone activity and spontaneous autoimmunity in dwarf mice and their littermates, *Immunology,* 30, 783, 1976.
49. **Fabris, N., Mocchegiani, E., Spinaci, S., and Muzzioli, M.,** Endocrinological modulation of the serum level of thymic factor, *Eur. J. Immunol.,* submitted.
50. **Astaldi, A., Astaldi, G. C. B., Schellekens, P. Th. A., and Eijsvoogel, V. P.,** A thymic factor in human sera demonstrated by a cAMP assay, *Nature (London),* 260, 713, 1976.
51. **Tam, C. F. and Walford, R. L.,** Cyclic nucleotide levels in resting and mitogen-stimulated spleen cell suspensions from young and old mice, *Mech. Aging Develop.,* 7, 309, 1978.
52. **Melmon, K. L., Weinstein, J., Poon, T. C., Bourne, M. R.,** Shearer, G. M., Coffino, P., and Insel, P. A., Receptors for low-molecular-weight hormones on lymphocytes, in *Immunopharmacology,* Vol. 3, Hadden, J. W., Coffey, R. G., and Spreafico, F., Eds., Plenum Press, New York, 1977, 331.

53. **Hadden, J. W.,** Cyclic nucleotides in lymphocytes proliferation and differentiation, in *Immunopharmacology,* Vol. 3, Hadden, J. W., Coffey, R. G., and Spreafico, F., Eds., Plenum Press, New York, 1977, 1.
54. **Besedowski, H. O., del Rey, A., Sorkin, E., Da Prada, M., and Keller, M. H.,** Immunoregulation mediated by the sympathetic nervous system, *Cell. Immunol.,* in press.
55. **Wostmann, B. S.,** Defence mechanisms in germfree animals. I. Humoral defence mechanisms, in *The Germfree Animals in Research,* Coates, Marie E., Ed., Academic Press, New York, 1968, 197.
56. **Nomura, T., Ohsawa, N., Kageyama, K., Saito, M., and Tajima, Y.,** Testicular functions of germfree mice, in *Germfree Research,* Heneghan, J. B., Ed., Academic Press, New York, 1973, 515.
57. **Pierpaoli, W. and Sorkin, E.,** Alterations of adrenal cortex and thyroid in mice with congenital absence of the thymus, *Nature (London) New Biol.,* 238, 282, 1972.
58. **Webb, D. R., Nowowyeski, I., Dauphinée, M., and Talal, N.,** Antigen induced alterations in splenic prostaglandin and cyclic nucleotide levels in NZB mice, *J. Immunol.,* 118, 446, 1977.
59. **Besedovsky, H. O., Sorkin, E., Keller, M., and Muller, J.,** Changes in blood hormone levels during the immune response, *Proc. Soc. Exp. Biol. Med.,* 150, 466, 1975.
60. **Besedovsky, H. O. and Sorkin, E.,** Network of immune-neuroendocrine interactions, *Clin. Exp. Immunol.,* 27, 1, 1977.
61. **Sara, V. R. and Lazarus, L.,** A prenatal action of growth hormone on brain and behaviour, *Nature (London),* 250, 257, 1974.
62. **Jost, A., Vigier, B., Prepin, J., and Perchellet, J. P.,** Studies on sex differentiation in mammals, in *Recent Progress in Hormone Research,* Vol. 29, Greep, R. O., Ed., Academic Press, New York, 1973, 1.
63. **Bakke, J. L., Lawrence, N. L., Robinson, S., and Bennett, J.,** Endocrine studies in the untreated F1 and F2 progeny of rats treated neonatally with thyroxine, *Biol. Neonate,* 31, 71, 1977.
64. **Stuchlikova, E., Jurikova-Horakova, M., and Deyl, Z.,** New aspect of dietary effect on life prolongation in rodents. What is the role of obesity in aging?, *Exp. Gerontol.,* 10, 141, 1975.
65. **Foucherau-Péron, M., Duran Garcia, S., and Rosselin, G.,** Altération des recepteurs de l'hormone de croissance dans le nanisme genetique hypophysaire de la souris, *An. Endocrinol.,* 37, 83, 1976.
66. **Timiras, P. S. and Vernadakis, A.,** Structural, biochemical and functional aging of the nervous system, in *Developmental Physiology and Aging,* Timiras, P. S., Ed., Macmillan, New York, 1972, 502.
67. **Beck, C. H. M.,** Functional implications of changes in the senescent brain: a review, *Le J. Can. Sci. Neurol.,* 5, 417, 1978.
68. **Bondareff, W.,** Synaptic atrophy in the senescent hippocampus, *Mech. Ageing Develop.,* 9, 163, 1979.
69. **Brizzee, K. R. and Ordy, J. M.,** Age pigments, cell loss and hippocampal function, *Mech. Ageing Develop.,* 9, 143, 1979.
70. **Everitt, A. V.,** Conclusion: aging and its hypothalamic-pituitary control, in *Hypothalamus, Pituitary and Aging,* Everitt, A. V., and Burgess, J. A., Eds., Charles C Thomas, Springfield, Ill., 1976, 676.
71. **Timiras, P. S.,** Neurophysiological factors in aging: recent advances, in *10th Int. Cong. in Gerontol.,* Cong. Abstr., Vol. 1, 50, 1975.
72. **Frolkis, W., Bezrukov, V. V., and Sinitsky, V. N.,** Sensitivity of central nervous structures to humoral factors in aging, *Exp. Gerontol.,* 7, 185, 1972.
73. **Finch, C. E.,** Catecholamine metabolism in the brains of aging male mice, *Brain Res.,* 52, 261, 1973.
74. **Azizi, F., Vagenakis, A. G., Portnoy, G. F., Rapoport, B., Ingbar, S. H., and Braverman, L. E.,** Pituitary-thyroid responsiveness to intramuscular thyrotropin-releasing hormone based on an analysis of serum thyroxine, tri-iodothyronine and thyrotropin concentrations, *New Engl. J. Med.,* 292, 272, 1975.
75. **Landfield, P. W. and Lynch, G. S.,** Brain aging and plasma steroid levels: quantitative correlations, *Neurosci. Abstr.,* 3, 111, 1977.
76. **Dilman, V. M.,** Age-associated elevation of hypothalamic threshold to feed-back control, and its role in development, ageing, and disease, *Lancet,* 1, 1211, 1971.
77. **Kanugo, M. S., Patnaik, S. K., and Koul, O.,** Decrease in oestradiol receptor in brain of ageing rats, *Nature (London),* 253, 366, 1975.
78. **Baker, H. W. G., Burger, H. G., de Krester, D. M., Hudson, B., O'Connor, S., Wang, C., Mirovics, A., Court, J., Dunlop, M., and Rennie, G. C.,** Changes in the pituitary-testicular system with age, *Clin. Endocrinol.,* 5, 349, 1976.
79. **Furuhashi, N., Suzuki, M., Abe, T., Yamaya, Y., and Tukahashi, K.,** Changes in hypophysio-ovarian endocrinological function by aging in women, *Tohoku J. Exp. Med.,* 21, 231, 1977.
80. **Britton, G. W., Rotemberg, S., and Adelman, R. C.,** Impaired regulation of corticosterone levels during fasting in aging rats, *Biochem. Biophys. Res. Commun.,* 64, 184, 1975.
81. **Ingbar, S. H.,** Changes in thyroid hormone economy in aging man, in *10th Int. Cong. in Gerontol.,* Cong. Abstr., Vol. 1, 191, 1975.

82. **Segal, P. E.,** Interrelations of dietary and hormonal effects in aging, *Mech. Ageing Develop.*, 9, 511, 1979.
83. **Denckla, W. D.,** A time to die, *Life Sci.*, 16, 31, 1975.
84. **Bilder, G. E. and Denckla, W. D.,** Restoration of ability to reject xenografts and clear carbon after hypophysectomy of adult rats, *Mech. Ageing Develop.*, 6, 153, 1977.
85. **Everitt, A. V.,** The hypothalamic-pituitary control of ageing and age-related pathology, *Exp. Gerontol.*, 8, 265, 1973.
86. **Adelman, R. C., Stein, G., Roth, G. S., and Englander D.,** Age-dependent regulation of mammalian DNA synthesis and cell proliferation in vivo, *Mech. Ageing Develop.*, 1, 49, 1972.
87. **Roth, G. S.,** Hormone action during aging: alterations and mechanisms, *Mech. Ageing Develop.*, 9, 497, 1979.
88. **Andres, R. and Tobin, J. D.,** Endocrine systems, in *Handbook of the Biology of Aging,* Finch, C. E. and Hayflick, L., Eds., Van Nostrand-Reinhold, New York, 1977, 357.
89. **Roth, G. S. and Adelman, R. C.,** Age-related changes in hormone binding by target cells and tissues: possible role in altered adaptive responsiveness, *Exp. Gerontol.*, 10, 1, 1975.
90. **Holinka, C. F. Nelson, J. F., and Finch, C. E.,** Effect of estrogen treatment on estradiol binding capacity in uteri of aged rats, *Gerontologist,* 15, 30, 1975.
91. **Cooper, B. and Gregerman, R. I.,** Hormone-sensitivity fat cell adenylate cyclase in the rat, *J. Clin. Invest.*, 57, 161, 1976.
92. **Barnes, D. W. H., Ford, C. E., and Loutit, J. E.,** Grèffes en serie de moélle osseuse chez des souris irradiée, *Sang,* 30, 762, 1959.
93. **McCay, C. M.,** Chemical aspects of aging and the effect of diet upon aging, in *Cowdry's Problems of Ageing,* Lansing, L. I., Ed., Williams & Wilkins, Baltimore, 1952, 139.
94. **Fernandes, G., Good, R. A., and Yunis, E.,** Attempts to correct age-related immunodeficiency and auto-immunity by cellular and dietary manipulation in inbred mice, in *Immunology and Aging,* Vol. 1, Makinodan, T. and Yunis, E., Eds., Plenum Press, New York, 1977, 111.
95. **Price, G. B., and Makinodan, T.,** Immunologic deficiencies in senescence. II. Characterization of extrinsic deficiencies, *J. Immunol.*, 108, 413, 1972.
96. **Cherry, C. I., Einstein, R., and Glucksmann, A.,** Epithelial cords and tubules of rat thymus: effects of age, sex, castration, thyroid and other hormones on their incidence and secretory activity, *Br. J. Exp. Pathol.*, 48, 90, 1968.
97. **Sherman, J. D. and Dameshek, W.** "Wasting disease" following thymectomy in the hamster, *Nature (London),* 197, 469, 1963.
98. **Elders, M. J., Parham, B. A., and Hughes, E. R.,** Prevention of wasting disease by pregnancy associated with hypertrophy of the fetal thymus, *J. Exp. Med.*, 127, 649, 1968.
99. **Nossal, J. V., Bussard, A. E., Lewis, H., and Mazie, J. C.,** Formation of hemolitic plaques by peritoneal cells in vitro. I. A new technique enabling micromanipulation and yielding higher plaque numbers, in *Developmental Aspects of Antibody Formation and Structure,* Sterzel, J. and Riha, I., Eds., Czecoslovak Academic Press, Prague, 1970, 655.
100. **Fabris, N., Pierpaoli, W., and Sorkin, E.,** Lymphocytes, hormones and ageing, *Nature (London),* 240, 557, 1972.
101. **Fabris, N. and Piantanelli, L.,** Thymus, homeostatic regulation and aging, in *Proceedings of the Fifth European Symposium on Basic Research in Gerontology,* Schmidt, U. J., Ed., Springer-Verlag, Berlin, 1977, 151.
102. **Stutman, O., Yunis, E. J., and Good, R. A.,** Carcinogen-induced tumors of the thymus. IV. Humoral influence of normal thymus and functional thymomas and influence of postthymectomy period on restoration, *J. Exp. Med.*, 130, 809, 1969.
103. **Stutman, O.,** Intrathymic and extrathymic T cell maturation, *Immunol. Rev.*, 42, 138, 1978.
104. **Pierpaoli, W., Fabris, N., and Sorkin, E.,** The effects of hormones on the development of the immune capacity, in *Cellular Interactions in the Immune Response, 2nd Int. Convoc. Immunol.*, S. Karger, Basel, 1971, 25.
105. **Bartrop, R. W., Luckhurst, E., Lazarus, L., Kiloh, L. G., and Penny, R.,** Depressed lymphocyte function after bereavement, *Lancet,* 1, 8016, 1977.
106. **Bach, J. F., Dardenne, M., Papiernik, M., Barvis, A., Levasseur, P., and Lebrand, H.,** Evidence for a serum-factor secreted by the human thymus, *Lancet,* 2, 1056, 1972.
107. **Rovensky, J., Goldstein, P. J., Holt, L., Pekarek, J., and Mistina, T.,** Obnova funkcie T lymphocytor tymozinom u klinicky zdravych osob vyssiehoveku, *Cas. Cesk. Lek.*, 116, 1063, 1977.
108. **Doria, G.,** personal communication, June 1979.
109. **Bach, J. F., Bach, A. M., Charreire, J., Dardenne, M., Fourier, C., Papiernik, M., and Pleau, J. M.,** The circulating thymic factor (TF). Biochemistry, physiology, biological activities and clinical applications, in *The Biological Activity of Thymic Hormones,* Bekkum, D. W., Ed., Hooyker Scientific Publ., 1975, 145.

110. **Piantanelli, L., Basso, A., Muzzioli, M., and Fabris, N.,** "Thymus-dependent reversibility of physiological and isoproterenol-evoked age-related parameters in athymic (nude) and old normal mice," *Mech. Ageing Develop.*, 7, 171, 1978.
111. **Scott, M., Bolla, R., and Denckla, W. D.,** Age-related changes in immune function of rats and the effect of long-term hypophysectomy, *Mech. Ageing Develop.*, 11, 127, 1979.
112. **Piantanelli, L. and Fabris, N.,** Hypopituitary dwarf and athymic nude mice and the study of the relationships among thymus, hormones and aging, in *Genetic Effects on Aging*, Harrison, D. E. and Bergsma, D., Eds., Sinauer Associates, Sunderland, Mass, 1978, 315.
113. **Ooka, H.,** Changes in extrathyroidal conversion of thyroxine (T4) to 3,3′,5-triiodothyronine (T3) in vitro during development and aging of the rat, *Mech. Ageing Develop.*, 10, 151, 1979.
114. **Kaplan, M. M. and Utiger, R. D.,** Iodothyronine metabolism in liver and kidney homogenates from hyperthyroid and hypothyroid rats, *Endocrinology*, 103, 156, 1978.
115. **Roth, G. S.,** Age related changes in glucocorticoid binding by rat splenic leukocytes: possible cause of altered adaptive responsiveness, *Fed. Am. Soc. Exp. Biol.*, 34, 1975, 183.
116. **Roth, G. S.,** Reduced glucocorticoid responsiveness and receptor concentration in splenic leukocytes of senescent rats, *Biochim. Biophys. Acta*, 399, 145, 1975.
117. **Schocken, D. D. and Roth, G. S.,** Reduced beta adrenergic receptor concentrations in aging man, *Nature (London)*, 267, 856, 1977.
118. **Ziegler, M. G., Lake, C. R., and Kopin, I. J.,** Plasma noradrenaline increases with age, *Nature (London)*, 261, 333, 1976.
119. **Rivnay, B., Globerson, A., and Shinitzky, M.,** Viscosity of lymphocyte plasma membrane in aging mice and its possible relation to serum cholesterol, *Mech. Ageing Develop.*, 10, 71, 1979.
120. **Rivnay, B., Globerson, A., and Shinitzky, M.,** Perturbation of lymphocyte response to concanavalin A by exogenous cholesterol and lecithin, *Eur. J. Immunol.*, 8, 185, 1978.
121. **Dilman, V. M.,** Ageing, metabolic immunodepression and carcinogenesis, *Mech. Ageing Develop.*, 8, 153, 1978.
122. **Burnet, M. F.,** Immunological surveillance in neoplasia, *Transplant. Rev.*, 7, 3, 1971.
123. **Goodman, S. A. and Makinodan, T.,** Effect of age on cell-mediated immune responsiveness assessed in vivo by tumor resistance and in vitro by cytolytic activity, *Clin. Exp. Immunol.*, 19, 533, 1975.
124. **Rygaard, J. and Polvsen, C.,** The mouse mutant nude does not develop spontaneous tumours. An argument against immunological surveillance, *Acta Pathol. Microbiol. Scand. B*, 82, 99, 1974.
125. **Svetlana, N. Z., Svet-Moldavsky, J. G., and Karmanova, N. V.,** Nonimmune and immune surveillance. I. Growth of tumors and normal fetal tissues grafted into new born mice, *J. Natl. Cancer Inst.*, 57, 47, 1976.
126. **Prehn, R. T.,** Perspectives on oncogenesis: does immunity stimulate or inhibit neoplasia?, *J. Reticuloendothel. Soc.*, 10, 1, 1971.
127. **Gardner, W. U.,** Hormonal aspects of experimental tumorigenesis, in, *Advances in Cancer Research*, Vol. 1, Greenstein, J. P. and Haddow, A., Eds., Academic Press, New York, 1953, 173.
128. **Noble, R. L.,** Hormonal control of growth and progression in tumors of NB rats and theory of action, *Cancer Res.*, 37, 82, 1977.
129. **Pierpaoli, W., Haran-Ghera, N., Muller, J., Meshorer, A., and Bree, M.,** Endocrine disorders as a contributory factor to neoplasia in SJL/J mice, *J. Natl. Cancer Inst.*, 53, 731, 1974.
130. **Schaller, J. P., Milo, G. E., Blakeslee, J. R., and Olsen, R. G.,** Estrogen and androgen hormones on transformation of human cells in vitro by feline sarcoma virus, *Cancer Res.*, 36, 1980, 1976.
131. **Dilman, V. M.,** Changes in hypothalamic sensitivity in ageing and cancer, in *Mammary Cancer and Neuroendocrine Therapy*, Stoll, B. A., Ed., Butterworths, London, 1974, 197.
132. **Kallis, N. and Dagg, M. K.,** Immune response engendered in mice by multiparity, *Transplantation*, 2, 416, 1974.
133. **Bielschowsky, F. and Bielshowsky, M.,** Carcinogenesis in the pituitary dwarf mouse. The response of 2-aminofluorene, *Br. J. Cancer*, 14, 195, 1960.

BEHAVIOR AND AGING*

Richard L. Sprott

The study of the behavioral consequences of aging can be divided into two broad categories: age changes and age differences. Age changes are observed in longitudinal designs where it is possible to assess behavior in the same individuals on two or more occasions. Age differences are observed in cross-sectional designs where individuals of two or more ages are observed at the same time. Each method has its strengths and weaknesses and many investigators are now creating designs which combine both methods. See Schaie[1] for a complete discussion of this issue.

Another important distinction for behavioral aging research is that between performance and ability. Performance is the actual behavior observed in a test situation and is presumed to be influenced by many variables including health status, motivation, the condition of the central and peripheral nervous systems, and ability. Ability is usually used to mean "capacity", that is, some ideal level of performance which would be possible in the absence of any interference from other factors. A great deal of current behavioral-aging research is concerned with the performance-ability distinction, and an even greater proportion of current debate about the nature of age-dependent behavioral change revolves around the same issue. In general, behavioral development of simple behaviors is clear, and results from one laboratory to another are comparable. However, when more complex behaviors are examined, results are also more complex and data are often ambiguous. The tables which follow are not exhaustive, in that they do not include all behaviors for which some report of age effects exists. Rather these tables are an attempt to briefly summarize what is known with reasonable certainty about the effects of age upon major classes of behavior in mice (Table 1) and rats (Table 2). Table 3 contains a brief list of available reviews of human behavioral age changes and differences. Research findings in human studies tend to be more complex and diffuse, particularly for complex behavioral systems like learning, problem solving, personality, and sexuality.

Activity levels and psychomotor coordination decline with advancing age in almost all situations and species from early adulthood onward. Food intake stays constant or decreases slightly, while water intake usually increases in older individuals. Sexual behavior declines sharply in rodents and to a lesser degree in human subjects, and the decline in human sexual behavior appears to be due as much to loss of opportunity and to cultural expectations as to biological changes. Emotionality decreases in rodents, but increases in some situations in human subjects. However, the term is used very differently by different investigators and species comparisons are rarely possible. Rodent emotionality is measured by counting boluses in open-field tests, while human emotionality covers a broad spectrum of behaviors which interact independently with age.

The most controversial behavioral consequences of aging are losses of learning ability. Ability to learn simple tasks seems to be maintained by most healthy individuals (rodent or human), but decrements do occur in some situations. Performance declines in most complex tests. However, there is considerable debate about the meaning of these deficits since the performance decrements could reflect losses of ability, motivation, response speed, perceptual ability, or memory. Further, individual differences

* Preparation of this manuscript was supported by USPHS Grant AG 00250 from the National Institute on Aging.

Table 1
BEHAVIORAL AGE CHANGES IN MICE

Behavior	Strain	Sex	Nature of change	Oldest age at testing	Ref.
Activity (open-field)	C57BL/6J	♂	Decrease	18—30 months	2—4
	DBA/2J	♂	Decrease	18—30 months	2, 3
Activity (wheel running)	C57BL/6J	♂&♀	Decrease	26 months	4
	A/J	♂&♀	Decrease	23 months	4
Activity (home cage)	C57BL/6J	♂	Decrease	12—13 months	5
Aggression	C57BL/6J	♂	Increase	18 months	6
	DBA/2J	♂	Slight increase	18 months	6
Emotionality (defecation)	C57BL/6J	♂	No change	Up to 38 months	3
	DBA/2J	♂	No change	Up to 23 months	3
Feeding (alcohol preference)	C57BL/6J	♀	Decrease	26 months	7
	C57BL/6J	♂&♀	Decrease	26 months	4
	A/J	♂&♀	Decrease	23 months	4
Feeding (sucrose preference)	C57BL/6J	♀	Decrease	26 months	7
	C57BL/6J	♂&♀	Decrease	26 months	4
	A/J	♂&♀	No change	23 months	4
Feeding (water intake)	C57BL/6J	♂&♀	Increase	26 months	4
	A/J	♂&♀	Increase	23 months	4
Feeding (quinine discrimination)	C57BL/6J	♂&♀	Increase	26 months	4
	A/J	♂&♀	Decrease	23 months	4
Learning (maze)	C57BL/6J	♀	Decrease	26 months	7
Learning (shuttle avoidance)	C57BL/6J	♂	No change	15 months	8
Learning (passive avoidance)	C57BL/6J	♂	No change	30 months	9
	DBA/2J	♂	No change	30 months	9
	$B6D2F_1$	♂	Slight decrease	30 months	9
Learning (bar press-acquisition)	C57BL/6J	♂&♀	No change	26 months	4
	A/J	♂&♀	No change	23 months	4
Learning (bar press-extinction)	C57BL/6J	♂&♀	Fewer responses	26 months	4
	A/J	♂&♀	Fewer responses	23 months	4
Nest building	C57BL/6J	♂&♀	Poorer nests	26 months	4
	A/J	♂&♀	Poorer nests	23 months	4
Psychomotor coordination	C57BL/6J	♂	Decrease	18—24 months	6
	DBA/2J	♂	Decrease	18—24 months	6
	C57BL/6J	♂	Decrease	9.5—14.5 months	10

Table 2
BEHAVIORAL AGE CHANGES IN RATS

Behavior	Stock	Sex	Nature of change	Oldest age at testing	Ref.
Activity (open-field)	W[a]	♂	Increase	22 months	11
	S-D[b]	♂	Decrease	24 months	12
Activity (wheel running)	S-D	♂	Decrease	24 months	13
	S-D	♂	Decrease	25.8 months	14
	Various	♂&♀	Decrease	300 days	15 (review)
Emotionality (defecation)	S-D	♂&♀	Decrease	18 months	16
Feeding (food intake)	S-D	♂	No change	?	17
	?	♂	Decrease	?	18
Feeding (water intake)	?	♂	Increase	?	18
	S-D	♂	Increase	?	17
	W	♂	Increase	25 months	19
Feeding (alcohol preference)	S-D	♂	Decrease	24 months	20
Learning (maze)	W	♂&♀	Decrease	26 months	21
	W	♀	Decrease in complex maze	27 months	22
	U[c]	♀	Decrease	30 months	23
Learning (water avoidance)	S-D	♂&♀	Decrease	30 months	24
Learning (discrimination and reversal)	H[d]	♂	No change	18—23 months	25
Learning (active avoidance)	L-E H[e]	♂&♀	"Handled" — no change; unhandled — decrease	600 days	26
	L-E H	♂&♀	No change	650 days	27
	S-D	♂&♀	No enrichment effect	660 days	28
Learning (bar press)	S-D	♂	No change	24 months	29
	W	♂	No change	26 months	30
	W	♂	No senescent effect	800 days	31
Sexual behavior (copulation, ejaculation, mating)	Various	—	Decrease	Various	32 (review)

[a] Wistar.
[b] Sprague-Dawley.
[c] Unspecified.
[d] Hooded.
[e] Long-Evans hooded.

Table 3
LITERATURE REVIEWS OF HUMAN, AGE-DEPENDENT BEHAVIORS

Behavior	Nature of change	Ref.
Activity: sports and other exercise	Voluntary activity declines	33
Aggression	Decreases in men, increases in women	34
Emotionality	Increased response to stress and increased anxiety in some situations	32
Feeding: food, intake and nutrition	Intake declines, adequate nutrition often not achieved	35
Learning: verbal	Deficits for many, but not all individuals; learning speed decreases	36
Learning: perceptual and psychomotor	Decline in response speed, but not in rate of learning	37
Memory	Short-term memory declines for some types of material; long-term memory (recognition and recall) declines	38
Psychomotor coordination	Declines	35
Sexual behavior	Affected by marital status and social expectations; general decline in both sexes	32, 39

are large and are strongly influenced by health status, education level, occupation, age cohort, and social class. Most investigators agree that some deficits occur with advancing age, but little consensus exists for specific behaviors or causes.

REFERENCES

1. **Schaie, K. W.**, Quasi-experimental research designs in the psychology of aging, in *Handbook of the Psychology of Aging*, Birren, J. E. and Schaie, K. W., Eds., Van Nostrand Reinhold, New York, 1977, chap. 2.
2. **Sprott, R. L., and Eleftheriou, B. E.**, Open-field behavior in aging inbred mice, *Gerontologia*, 20, 155, 1974.
3. **Elias, P. K., Elias, M. F., and Eleftheriou, B. E.**, Emotionality, exploratory behavior, and locomotion in aging inbred strains of mice, *Gerontologia*, 21, 46, 1975.
4. **Goodrick, C. L.**, Behavioral differences in young and aged mice: strain differences for activity measures, operant learning, sensory discrimination, and alcohol preference, *Exp. Aging Res.*, 1, 191, 1975.
5. **Abel, E. L.**, Effects of ethanol and pentobarbital in mice of different ages, *Physiol. Psychol.*, 6, 366, 1978.
6. **Sprott, R. L.**, Behavioral characteristics of C57BL/6J, DBA/2J, and $B6D2F_1$ mice which are potentially useful for gerontological research, *Exp. Aging Res.*, 1, 313, 1975.
7. **Goodrick, C. L.**, Behavioral characteristics of young and senescent inbred female mice of the C57BL/6 strain, *J. Gerontol.*, 22, 459, 1967.
8. **Freund, G. and Walker, D. W.**, The effect of aging on acquisition and retention of shuttle box avoidance in mice, *Life Sci.* 10, 1343, 1971.
9. **Sprott, R. L.**, The interaction of genotype and environment in the determination of avoidance behavior of aging inbred mice, in *Genetic Effects on Aging*, Birth Defects Original Article Series, Vol. XIV-I, Bergsma, D., and Harrison, D. E., Eds., A. R. Liss, New York, 1978, chap. 6.
10. **Miquel, J., and Blasco, M.**, A simple technique for evaluation of vitality loss in aging mice, by testing their muscular coordination and vigor, *Exp. Gerontol.*, 13, 389, 1978.
11. **Goodrick, C. L.**, Activity and exploration as a function of age and exploration, *J. Genet. Psychol.*, 108, 239, 1966.
12. **Goodrick, C. L.**, Exploration of nondeprived male Sprague-Dawley rats as a function of age, *Psychol. Rep.*, 20, 159, 1967.
13. **Jakubczak, L. F.**, Age, food deprivation, and the temporal distribution of wheel running of rats, in *Proc. 78th Ann. Conv. Am. Psychol. Assoc.*, American Psychological Association, Washington, D.C., 1970, 689.
14. **Jakubczak, L. F.**, Age differences in the effects of water deprivation on activity, water loss and survival of rats, *Life Sci.*, 9, 771, 1970.
15. **Botwinick, J.**, Drives, expectancies and emotions, in *Handbook of Aging and the Individual*, Birren, J. E., Ed., University of Chicago Press, Chicago, 1959, chap. 21.
16. **Werboff, J., and Havlena, J.** Effects of aging on open field behavior, *Psychol. Rep.*, 10, 395, 1962.
17. **Osborn, G. K., Jones, D. C., and Kimeldorf, D. J.**, Water consumption of the ageing Sprague-Dawley male rat, *Gerontologia*, 6, 65, 1962.
18. **Everett, A. V.**, The change in food and water consumption and in faeces and urine production in ageing male rats, *Gerontologia*, 2, 21, 1958.
19. **Goodrick, C. L.**, Taste discrimination and fluid ingestion of male albino rats as a function of age, *J. Genet. Psychol.*, 115, 121, 1969.
20. **Goodrick, C. L.**, Alcohol preference of the male Sprague-Dawley albino rat as a function of age, *J. Gerontol.*, 22, 369, 1967.
21. **Goodrick, C. L.**, Learning, retention, and extinction of a complex maze habit for mature-young and senescent Wistar albino rats, *J. Gerontol.*, 23, 298, 1968.
22. **Goodrick, C. L.**, Learning by mature-young and aged Wistar albino rats as a function of test complexity, *J. Gerontol.*, 27, 353, 1972.
23. **Verzar-McDougall, E.**, Studies in learning and memory in ageing rats, *Gerontologia*, 19, 237, 1909.
24. **Birren, J. E. and Kay, H.**, Swimming speed of the albino rat. I. Age and sex differences, *J. Gerontol.*, 13, 374, 1958.

25. **Kay, H. and Sime, M.,** Discrimination learning with old and young rats, *J. Gerontol.,* 17, 75, 1962.
26. **Doty, B. A.,** Effects of handling on learning of young and aged rats, *J. Gerontol.,* 23, 142, 1968.
27. **Doty, B. A.,** Age and avoidance conditioning in rats, *J. Gerontol.,* 21, 287, 1966.
28. **Doty, B. A.,** The effects of cage environment upon avoidance responding of aged rats, *J. Gerontol.,* 27, 358, 1972.
29. **Goodrick, C. L.,** Operant responding of non-deprived young and senescent male albino rats, *J. Genet. Psychol.,* 114, 29, 1969.
30. **Goodrick, C. L.,** Light- and dark-contingent bar pressing in the rat as a function of age and motivation, *J. Comp. Physiol. Psychol.,* 73, 100, 1970.
31. **Goodrick, C. L.,** Adaptation to novel environments by the rat: effects of age, stimulus intensity, group testing, and temperature, *Develop. Psychobiol.,* 8, 287, 1975.
32. **Elias, M. F. and Elias, P. K.,** Motivation and activity, in *Handbook of the Psychology of Aging,* Birren, J. E. and Schaie, K. W., Eds., Van Nostrand Reinhold, New York, 1977, chap. 16.
33. **Shephard, R. J.,** Exercise and aging, in *The Biology of Aging,* Behnke, J. A., Finch, C. E., and Moment, G. B., Eds., Plenum Press, New York, 1978, chap. 8.
34. **Gutman, D.,** The cross-cultural perspective: notes toward a comparative psychology of aging, in *Handbook of the Psychology of Aging,* Birren, J. E. and Schaie, K. W., Eds., Van Nostrand Reinhold, New York, 1977, chap. 14.
35. **Young, V. R.,** Diet and nutrient needs in old age, in *The Biology of Aging,* Behnke, J. A., Finch, C. E., and Moment, G. B., Eds., Plenum Press, New York, 1978, chap. 9.
36. **Arenberg, D. and Robertson-Tchabo, E. A.** Learning and aging, in *Handbook of the Psychology of Aging,* Birren, J. E. and Schaie, K. W., Eds., Van Nostrand Reinhold, New York, 1977, chap. 18.
37. **Botwinick, J.,** Aids and types of learning, in *Aging and Behavior,* Springer-Verlag, New York, 1973, chap. 16.
38. **Craik, F. I.,** Age differences in human memory, in *Handbook of the Psychology of Aging,* Birren, J. E. and Schaie, K. W., Eds., Van Nostrand Reinhold, New York, 1977, chap. 17.
39. **Botwinick, J.,** Sexuality and sexual relations, in *Aging and Behavior,* Springer-Verlag, New York, 1973, chap. 4.

Development and Aging of the Immune System

MARROW STEM CELLS DURING DEVELOPMENT AND AGING*

Marvin L. Tyan

INTRODUCTION

Humoral and cell-mediated immune responses of mouse and man decrease with advancing age, and as a result, vulnerability to infectious, autoimmune, and neoplastic diseases may increase.[1] This decline in immune reactivity is the result of complex, incompletely understood changes in the immune system per se and in the environment in which it operates. The review which follows begins with descriptions of the origins and maturation of the immune system and other marrow stem cells in the hope that this knowledge will further an understanding of the manifold changes that occur with age in an organ which requires cellular renewal throughout life. Despite minor differences between mouse and man, the ontogeny and senescence of murine marrow stem cells will be described because this species has been studied most extensively.

Two classes of lymphocytes, B-cells and T-cells, and one representative of the reticuloendothelial system, the macrophage, have been shown to participate specifically in the induction and effectuation of immune responses in mice. In addition, mast cells, basophils, eosinophils, and polymorphonuclear cells are known to react specifically and nonspecifically as effector cells in antibody and cell-mediated immune reactions. Because of space and time considerations, the discussion which follows will be limited to lymphocytes and macrophages and to the marrow hematopoietic stem cells (colony-forming units, CFU) with which they interact.

MACROPHAGE

Origin of Monocyte-Macrophages

The blood islands of the yolk sac are the first sites of hematopoiesis in birds and mammals.[2] The precursors of cells capable of developing into functional macrophages are first detected in the mouse yolk sac on about the seventh or eighth day of gestation.[3] Although the early yolk sac contains the precursor of macrophage-monocytes, functional maturation of these cells does not appear to occur in that organ. Promonocytes and mature macrophages are found in the fetal liver by the 11th day of gestation, and the progenitors of these cells are found primarily if not exclusively in the marrow of neonatal and adult rodents and humans.[4-6]

Morphological Maturation of Monocyte-Macrophages

The precursors of monocyte-macrophages cannot be identified on the basis of morphological criteria, but their presence in tissues can be demonstrated by their ability to give rise in culture to typical mature cells which are characterized by abundant phase-dense granules, absence of peroxidase, avid phagocytosis, and a membrane receptor for the Fc portion of a subclass of IgG (FcR).[3] Adherent cells bearing these characteristic markers are first detected in small numbers in the fetal liver on the 11th day of gestation. By the 18th day they constitute 2 to 3% of all nucleated cells in the liver. Alloantigens controlled by the immune response region of the H-2 complex, Ia antigens which regulate interactions between macrophages and T-cells, can be demonstrated on the membranes of phagocytic cells taken from embryonic liver[7-10] (Table 1).

* This work was supported in part by VA Medical Research Funds and USPHS Grant AG-00990.

Table 1
ONTOGENY OF STEM CELLS

Day	
1	T/t membrane antigens
5	Implantation
6	H-2 and Fc receptor expressed and T/t suppressed
9	Precursors of T-cells, B-cells, macrophages, and other marrow constituents found in blood islands of yolk sac
10	Stem cells migrate to liver
12	Thymic rudiment appears and T-cell precursors migrate into area from the liver
18 to 20	Precursors begin to leave the liver and migrate to spleen and marrow
20	Birth
Adult	Bone marrow is the major source of stem cells of all types

Functional Maturation of Monocyte-Macrophages

The functions of the monocyte-macrophage are complex and protean. It would appear that early in embryonic life these cells are able to migrate normally, recognize and respond to antibody-coated and uncoated antigenic material, and to phagocytize and digest. Little, however, is known of the ontogenesis of macrophage antigen processing or of their ability to regulate the immune process through cell-to-cell contact with T-cells and B-cells or through the elaboration of soluble factors such as lymphocyte activating factor, B-cell activating factor, helper cell factors, colony-stimulating factor, and thymocyte-differentiating factor.[7] The few experiments that have been reported suggest that peritoneal macrophages from newborn mice cannot replace adult cells in macrophage dependent in vitro antibody responses.[11] However, it is not clear whether this is due to a functional deficiency of macrophages from neonatal mice or to suppressor activity commonly found in newborn mice (see below).

Functional Changes in Aged Mice

No studies have been reported on age-related quantitative or qualitative changes in the progenitors of monocyte-macrophages. However, the following is known with regard to the function of mature cells in old mice: (1) tenfold more antigen is required to produce a maximum immune response in vivo in old mice; however, in vitro, old and young spleen cells respond maximally to the same antigen dose; (2) the in vitro phagocytic activity of peritoneal macrophages is equal to, if not better than, that of young mice; (3) the activity of the lysosomal enzymes, cathepsin D, β-glucuronidase, and acid phosphatase increases gradually with age; (4) the ability of antigen-primed peritoneal macrophages from old mice to initiate primary and secondary antibody responses in vivo is comparable to that of young cells; and (5) the capacity of splenic accessory cells to cooperate with T- and B-cells in the initiation of in vitro responses to sheep red blood cells (SRBC) is unaffected by age.[12] These results have been accepted as evidence that the function of macrophages in processing antigen, initiation of immune responses, and in phagocytosis does not diminish appreciably with age. However, a recent report suggests that the ability of macrophages from old animals to promote in vitro responses to T-independent antigens may be significantly impaired.[13]

B-CELLS

Origin of B-Cells

Cells which secrete specific antibody in response to antigenic stimulation are known as B- or ''bursa-equivalent'' cells. The precursors of these cells appear in the yolk sac, liver, and caudal half of the embryo by the 9th day of a 20-day gestation.[14] Later in pregnancy they are concentrated in the embryonic liver but they also may be found in the lung, gut, blood, and marrow. Shortly after birth the bone marrow becomes the major if not sole source of these stem cells.[15] Immunoglobulin-producing cells and those that mediate cellular immune functions appear to arise as separate cell lines.[14,16-18] Although the bursa of Fabricius, a gut-associated lymphoepithelial structure, is essential for the maturation of B-cells in birds, an analogue of this organ has not been demonstrated in mammals.[19,20]

Ontogeny of B-Cell Membrane Markers

A number of membrane markers have been helpful in studies of the precursor-successor relationships in B-cell differentiation: (1) the receptor of the Fc portion of aggregated or antigen-complexed IgG (FcR);[21] (2) receptors for split products of the third and fourth components of complement (CR);[22] (3) membrane-bound immunoglobulin (sIg); (4) alloantigens controlled by the immune response region of the H-2 complex, Ia antigens;[23-25] (5) Ly-4;[26] (6) Pc.1;[27] and (7) membrane-bound IgD, sIgD.[28]

Fc receptors and CR can be demonstrated on cells from mouse embryos as early as the day after implantation (i.e., day six); after the ninth day of gestation these receptors are found only on cells taken from tissues which contain hematopoietic and lymphocytic precursors.[29] Although certain studies suggest that FcR and CR are expressed on the membranes of B-cells before the appearance of sIg,[21,30-33] this is not firmly established because they also are found on cell types, such as macrophages, which cannot be distinguished physically or morphologically from lymphoid stem cells with certainty.

No functional roles have been assigned as yet to FcR and CR. However, it has been suggested that FcR may be involved in B-cell/T-cell interactions[34] and/or in lymphocyte-mediated, antibody dependent cytotoxic reactions.[21] Two hypotheses of CR function have been advanced: (1) by binding antigen-antibody-complement complexes these receptors may focus antigen on B-cell membranes and increase the likelihood of interactions with antigen specific receptors,[35] and (2) the complex may serve as a ''second signal'' to the B-cell, leading to proliferation and terminal differentiation.[36] The time of appearance of CR in neonatal mice is under the control of at least two genetic loci, one of which (CRL-1) is associated with the major histocompatibility locus (H-2).[37] It also has been suggested that the expression of FcR may be partially under the control of H-2 associated genes.[38]

Cells synthesizing monomeric sIgM are first detected in the embryonic mouse on the tenth day of gestation.[39] Cells bearing monomeric sIgM, sIgG, or sIgA are readily demonstrated in fetal liver on the 15th or 16th day of pregnancy;[40,41] sIgD of the same idiotype and determinant specificity is expressed on splenic B-cells one to several weeks after birth.[42,43] It has been postulated that IgD facilitates the terminal stages of B-cell differentiation.[28]

Ia antigens are not found on bone marrow cells until about 4 weeks after birth; however, they have been demonstrated on splenic lymphocytes up to 2 weeks earlier.[44] This, together with the observation that sIg+, Ia− marrow cells can be induced to express Ia in vitro when stimulated with cAMP, lipopolysaccharide (LPS), or thymopoietin suggests that these glycoproteins normally are expressed after FcR, CR, and sIg. Ia antigens also can be demonstrated on T-cells, macrophages, and epidermal cells. More than 20 individual Ia specificities have been identified, and although no functional role has been assigned to them it is felt that they are involved in cell recognition and cell-to-cell interactions.[45] As noted above, at least three B-cell membrane markers (FcR, CR, and Ia) appear to be wholly or partially under the control of loci associated with the H-2 complex, a system that contains genes known to exert profound effects on immune responsiveness[46] and one that expresses its K and D products shortly after implantation.[47,48]

No data are available on the ontogeny of Ly-4, but what evidence does exist suggests that this alloantigen is expressed after sIg.[26] Pc.1 is an alloantigen found on terminally differentiated plasma cells.[27,44] No specific functions have been attributed to these two membrane proteins.

Ontogeny of B-Cell Function

Although fully mature B-cells are not found in the fetus until relatively late in pregnancy, from the tenth day of gestation onward small numbers of large cells which synthesize and release sIgM at a rapid rate are found in the fetal liver.[49] At about the same time antigen-binding cells (ABC) specific for a variety of antigenic determinants can be demonstrated in mouse liver. When these cells are cultured with antigen they respond with proliferation[51] and the appearance of cells bearing sIgM, sIgG, and sIgA[51-53] but little antibody is secreted.[51,54]

By the 15th day of pregnancy small cells bearing readily detectable sIgM, which turns over slowly, are found in the liver, and over the next few days cells with sIgG and sIgA can be demonstrated.[49,53] B-cells from fetal liver acquire the ability to respond to the mitogenic properties of dextran sulfate about day 16, LPS just prior to birth on day 19 or 20, and purified protein derivative (PPD) 3 or 4 days later.[39,49,55] The repertoire of ABC and antibody-secreting cells cultured in the presence of LPS does not change during development and is approximately 1:500 to 1000 for SRBC, 1:100 for horse red blood cells (RBC), 1:500 for TNP_3-SRBC, 1:50 for TNP_{30}-SRBC and 1:10 for NIP_{12} -SRBC.[49] B-cells obtained from fetal liver produce little specific antibody when cultured in vivo with thymus dependent and thymus independent antigens. When adult thymocytes are added, antibody production increases significantly although it is restricted in heterogenity and affinity; the secondary responses are comparable to those obtained with adult spleen cells.[55,56]

Spleen cells taken 1 day after birth produce few antibody secreting cells when cultured with thymus-independent antigens and even fewer when thymus-dependent antigens are added. Thereafter, the responses to thymus-independent antigens and to LPS mature rapidly reaching near adult levels by 2 or 3 weeks of age; however, responses to T-dependent antigens, and to the T-cell mitogens Con A and phytohemogglutinin (PHA) do not approach adult levels until 6 to 8 weeks after birth.[57,58] The response of neonatal spleen cells to thymus-dependent antigens can be enhanced by adding T-cells from adult mice only if endogenous T-cells are removed first.[57] These and other observations suggest that a small number of mature B-cells capable of producing specific antibody are present in the fetus just prior to birth but their ability to respond to antigenic stimulation is depressed by a relative or absolute excess of T-cell suppressor activity which gradually declines over the first 6 to 8 weeks of life (see Table 2).

Other studies have shown that the in vitro responses to SRBC by adult spleen cells but not those limited responses by B-cell precursors can be inhibited by masking Ia antigens with specific anisera or by blocking the FcR with aggregated IgG;[59-62] the cumulative evidence suggests that these agents act by impairing the induction of the primary antibody response at the stage of B-cell/T-cell interaction.

Table 2
ONTOGENY OF B-CELL FUNCTION

Day	
6	Cells with Fc and CR receptors first appear; significance not known
9	Cells which can be induced to express sIg and to proliferate when cultured with antigen appear in yolk sac
15 to 20	Cells expressing sIg appear "spontaneously" in liver and spleen
Birth	Rapid increase in ability to produce antibody to thymus-independent antigens; IgD expression begins
Birth to 6 weeks	Slow increase in ability to produce antibody to thymus-dependent antigens
2 to 5 weeks	Slow increase in CR positive lymphocytes in the spleen (strain variations)

When viewed together, these and other observations[63] suggest that B-cells mature in a step-wise manner advancing through several distinct differentiation compartments that can be characterized tentatively on the basis of what is known of the sequential appearance of certain cell-membrane and functional markers:

1. FcR±, CR±, sIg−, Ia−, sIgD−, Pc.1−, LPS− (precursor), (?) plus antigen
2. FcR+, CR±, sIg+, Ia−, sIgD−, Pc.1−, LPS− (ABC), (?) plus T-cells or T-factor
3. FcR+, CR+, sIg+, Ia+, sIgD+, Pc.1−, LPS+ (antibody secreting) to
4. FcR±, CR−, sIg−, Ia±, sIgD±, Pc.1+, LPS+ (plasma cell)

Age-Related Changes in B-Cell Precursors

Humoral immune responses decline dramatically with age as a result of changes in the immune system and its environment.[64,65] Old mice may generate 10- to 50-fold fewer antibody-forming cells in response to an optimal antigenic stimulus. Approximately 10% of this decline can be attributed to an altered environment that among other things may necessitate a tenfold increase in antigen to produce maximum stimulation.[65] Changes intrinsic to the immune system per se contribute the remainder of the defect: (1) there is decreased T-cell helper activity, altered T-cell: B-cell ratios, and increased/decreased suppressor activity, which result in major deficiencies in B-cell regulation,[65-72] (2) B-cell proliferation and/or differentiation is moderately impaired with the result that immunological burst size (i.e., the number of effector cells generated per immunocompetent unit) diminishes with age,[64,72] (3) the pattern of differentiation of B-cell precursor found in the marrow of aged mice may be altered,[72,73] and (4) there is a loss of IgG and high avidity antibody secreting cells.[74]

Although there is a paucity of knowledge regarding age-related changes in B-cell precursors, the following observations have been made. Marrow from old mice was found to contain more mature B-cells than did young marrow and the frequencies of B-cell progenitors appeared to be equal.[75] During culture with SRBC old marrow produced few new mature B-cells; this was due primarily to a maturation arrest at the stage of the ABC and, perhaps, to an impaired ability to generate new stem cells. Parallel experiments revealed that spleens from aging donors contained fewer mature sIgM+ and sIgG+ cells than did spleens from young mice. After culture with SRBC old spleen cells produced fewer mature antibody secreting cells due to the maturation arrest noted above; more striking, however, was the decline in B-cell progenitors. These findings suggest that aging mice may have a modest impairment of their ability to renew stem cell populations rapidly, and in addition, they have difficulty advancing beyond the ABC stage of development, perhaps due to defects in the T-cell regulating matrix noted above.

T-CELLS

Origin of T-Cells

T-cells are lymphocytes that differentiate within the thymus or perhaps under the influence of thymic hormones.[76] The progenitors of T-cells are first found in the placenta on the ninth day of gestation and somewhat later in the blood islands of the yolk sac.[16,77] They migrate into the fetal liver by the tenth day, and 2 days later they are found in the upper trunk where they have begun to invade the thymic rudiment. Thereafter, the pattern of migration is similar to that described for B-cells with the exception that they do not appear in the gut until after birth. During adult life the bone marrow serves as the major if not sole source of lymphoid stem cells.[15] Thymus lymphocytes increase greatly in number between the 14th and 18th days of gestation primarily due to proliferation of large cells in the thymic area destined to become cortex.[78]

Ontogeny of T-Cell Membrane Markers

T-cells express a variety of immunological functions. For example, they have helper and suppressor functions in antibody and cell-mediated responses, generate cytotoxic activity, and secrete soluble factors that induce inflammatory responses. It is not clear if this diversity of function reflects heterogeneity within T-cell progenitors or whether the responses are mediated by the descendants of one or a small number of stem cell lines. One approach being used to resolve this question and to follow the maturation of T-cells is to study the development and function of subsets of T-cells bearing the membrane antigens Thy-1(θ), Ly-1, Ly-2, and Ly-3.[78]

Thy-1 is first detected on the membranes of small and medium lymphocytes in the thymus on about the 14th or 15th day of gestation. At about the same time, these cells first become responsive to the T-cell mitogen, PHA.[57] At the end of pregnancy Thy-1+ cells are found in the spleen of the embryo, and after birth these cells appear to migrate from the thymus to lymph nodes first and somewhat later to the spleen.[79] The expression of Thy-1 is controlled by a gene on the ninth chromosome; the function of θ is unknown.

Ly antigens are found on thymocytes shortly after birth.[78] Each antigen is determined by a single genetic locus having two alleles. Ly-1 is located on chromosome 19, and Ly-2 and Ly-3 are closely associated on chromosome six. Virtually all Ly+ cells also express Thy-1; the function of these membrane antigens is not known. It has been shown that thymopoietin will induce T-cell precursors to express θ and Ly antigens on their cell-membranes without producing concomitant functional maturation of these cells.[80,81]

During the first week of life almost all Thy-1+ spleen cells are Ly-1,2,3+.[78] As the mouse grows older, the proportion of Ly-1,2,3+ cells declines while Ly-1+ and Ly-2,3+ cells increase. Cells bearing only Ly-2 or Ly-3 have not been detected.

Depletion of Ly-1+ cells from lymph node preparations abolishes T-cell mediated antibody helper activity, and removal of Ly-2,3+ cells impairs suppressor and killer activity.[78] These data suggest that lymphocytes undergoing thymus-dependent differentiation can be divided into subsets on the basis of the expression of particular Ly antigens, and that these subsets are associated with distinct functional qualities. These experiments, however, do not resolve the question as to whether T-cell subpopulations are descendant from one or several progenitors.

Table 3
ONTOGENY OF T-CELL FUNCTION

Day	
9	Stem cells in yolk sac
10	Stem cells in liver
12	Thymic rudiment appears
13 to 14	Antigen-binding cells found in thymus. Some proliferation in response to antigen in vitro
14 to 18	Theta expressed and PHA responsive cells in thymus
17 to 20	(a) Theta positive cells found in spleen, (b) acquisition of responsiveness to con A and foreign cells in vitro, (c) appearance of "suppressor effects" in fetal tissues
Birth	(a) Most cells are Ly 1, 2, 3 +, (b) GVH activity high in thymus and low in spleen
Birth to 6 weeks	(a) decreasing suppressor activity, (b) increasing helper activity, (c) Ly 1, 2, 3 + decreases as Ly 1 + and Ly 2, 3 + increase, (d) increasing GVH activity in the spleen

Ontogeny of T-Cell Function

The precursors of T-cells migrate from the liver and into the thymic rudiment on about the 12th day of gestation. There, under the influence of the thymic stroma and thymic macrophages, they acquire the ability to respond to the mitogen PHA by the 14th or 15th day.[57,82,83] Shortly thereafter, they are able to recognize and respond to allogeneic cells. By the end of pregnancy thymus lymphocytes respond less well to PHA but they now proliferate vigorously when exposed to Con A.

Thymocytes are able to produce severe *graft-vs.-host* disease at birth, but the peripheral lymphoid tissues are virtually devoid of this activity until several weeks after birth.[16] T-cells appear to mature more slowly in the peripheral lymphoid tissues than do B-cells. T-cell helper and killer activities do not approach adult levels until 6 to 8 weeks after birth, but it is possible that these functions are obscured by the readily demonstrable T-cell mediated suppressor activity present during this time. By the eighth week after birth, helper, suppressor, and effector activity has approached the equilibrium found in the adult mouse.

Thymic hormone activity is detected in the serum of the neonatal mouse shortly after birth and it reaches peak levels between 10 and 14 days later.[81] Thymopoietin levels in the serum begin to fall slowly at about 1 year of age and the values drop more rapidly during the final third of the normal life span (see Table 3).

Age-Related Changes in T-Cell Precursors

Humoral and cell-mediated immune responses decline dramatically with age. To a great degree this reduced immune responsiveness can be attributed to quantitative and qualitative changes in post-thymic T-cells: (1) the proportion of Thy-1 + cells in the spleen decreases after the age of 6 months and reaches 50% of peak adult values at about 2 years; this appears to be associated with a parallel decline in the density of θ antigen on the cell membrane;[84] (2) the number of lymph node-seeking lymphocytes is reduced in aged mice;[85] (3) the *graft-vs.-host* activity of old spleen cells is reduced but that of old bone marrow is unchanged;[86,87] (4) the cytolytic ability of terminally differentiated lymphocytes from old mice is undiminished; however, the capacity to generate these cells is significantly impaired;[88] and (5) there is decreased T-cell helper activity, altered T-cell:B-cell ratios, and variable but significant changes in T-cell suppressor activity.[65-72]

Table 4
MATURATION OF IMMUNE RESPONSIVENESS

Day 0 to 12	Normally unresponsive
12 to 20	Minimally responsive — ? actively suppressed
From birth	(a) Rapid increase in ability to produce antibody to T-independet antigens, (b) effector T cells in thymus, (c) slow increase in ability to produce antibody to T-dependent antigens, (d) slow increase in effector T-cells in spleen, and (e) slow decrease in suppressor activity and slow increase in helper activity
6 to 8 weeks	Adult levels of responsiveness reached

The following observations suggest that many of the deficiencies in T-cell function noted above can be attributed to changes in the central lymphoid organs, the marrow, and thymus: (1) old bone marrow has a decreased capacity to provide the thymus with T-cell progenitors. This is due to a reduction in the stem cell population and/or to a proliferative defect;[86,87,89] (2) the number of cortisone-resistant mature thymocytes declines with age;[90] (3) the thymus involutes progressively beginning just after sexual maturation[91] (4) the thymus of old mice has a reduced capacity to promote the maturation of stem cells;[92] (5) thymopoietin serum levels appear to decline in parallel with thymus involution;[80,81] and (6) the defect in T-cell antibody helper activity of old mice can be reversed by treatment with thymopoietin[93] (see Table 4).

NATURAL KILLER (NK) AND NATURAL CYTOTOXIC (NC) CELLS

The occurrence in nonimmune individuals of cells which are cytotoxic in vitro to transformed or normal allogeneic and syngeneic cells has been demonstrated in mice and other species.[93-96] Attention has been focused on these cells because of their possible roles as mediators of anti-tumor surveillance.[97] The first cell line to be described, the natural killer (NK) lymphocyte, has the following characteristics: (1) NK activity first appears during the third or fourth week of life, peaks at the third month, and declines continuously thereafter;[98] (2) NK cells are derived from bone marrow;[100] (3) the cells are found in spleen, peritoneum, blood, and lymph nodes but not in the thymus;[98] (4) NK activity is high in athymic nude mice;[98] (5) the cells are not macrophages, polymorphonuclear cells or B-cells;[93] (6) NK cells are not killed readily by anti-θ serum and complement, but low concentrations of FcR and θ have been demonstrated on their plasma membranes suggesting that they may be prethymic T-cells;[101,102] (7) NK activity is radio-resistant;[103] (8) NK activity is increased by interferon and by agents which increase interferon release or production;[93] (9) target cell susceptibility has specific and nonspecific components;[93] (10) levels of NK activity are controlled by dominant genes which are partially associated with H-2;[104] and (11) susceptibility to lysis by NK cells appears to be a dominant characteristic.[105]

NC cells share many of the characteristics of NK cells but differ in the following ways:[95,96] (1) NC activity is detected at birth and does not seem to decay with age; (2) NC cells are present in the thymus as well as spleen, blood, peritoneum, bone marrow, and lymph nodes; (3) strain variations in activity are not concordant; and (4) FcR and θ have not been demonstrated on the membranes of NC cells.

The NK cell also shares properties in common with two other systems: (1) the Hh (hemopoietic histocompatibility) system which determines resistance to parental or allogeneic marrow grafts by F_1 hybrids[103] and (2) the "M cell" which appears to mediate the genetically determined resistance of mice to the erythropoietic and immunosuppressive properties of the Friend virus complex.[106] Like NK activity, Hh and "M" cells (1) mature during the fourth week of life, (2) are derived from bone marrow, (3) are X-ray resistant, and (4) mature independent of the thymus. This suggests that NK, Hh and "M" cells (and, perhaps, NC cells) are subsets or developmental stages of prethymic T-cells.[102]

HEMATOPOETIC COLONY-FORMING CELLS (CFU)

Origin of CFU

The multipotential hematopoietic stem cell, the erythroid, myeloid, and megakargocytic colony-forming cell (CFU), is detected in the blood islands of the yolk sac on the seventh day of gestation, in the circulation by day nine or ten, and in the embryonic liver on day ten.[107] The liver remains the major hematopoietic organ of the fetus until day 16 when the stem cells begin to migrate to bone marrow. In the adult, the marrow is the primary source of CFU. Erythroid differentiation in the yolk sac and fetal liver is vigorous; in contrast, although myeloid stem cells are present in fetal liver in numbers approaching their frequency in marrow, differentiation into mature forms is absent.[107] Folowing grafting into an adult environmental fetal liver CFU form predominantly myeloid colonies and maturation proceeds normally. This suggests that the lack of myeloid differentiation in the fetus is due to inhibition, to the absence of a positive stimulus, or to a deficiency in the microenvironment.

Roles of Macrophages and Lymphocytes in the Regulation of Hematopoiesis

The mechanisms regulating the proliferation and differentiation of hematopoietic stem cells are complex and incompletely understood. It is known that both hormonal and cellular systems are involved in many of the pathways from precursor to functionally mature circulating cell. Macrophages and lymphocytes appear to be among the significant contributors to the regulation of CFU and some of what is known of their function is presented here:

1. Colony stimulating factor (CSF) is essential for the growth in vitro of mixed myeloid-macrophage colonies. Increasing CSF concentrations favor differentiation into myeloid cells and reduction in monocyte-macrophage production. E type prostaglandins (PGE) inhibit this effect. CSF and PGE are produced by mature macrophages, T-cells and B-cells, and/or by their interactions.[108]
2. In vitro, CSF suppresses erythropoietin-stimulated hemoglobin synthesis, and erythropoietin suppresses myeloid-macrophage colony formation induced by CSF.[109]
3. Thymocytes enhance the formation of spleen colonies by radiation-damaged marrow CFU and by parental CFU transplanted into F_1 recipients.[110,111]
4. Activated T-cells elaborate a factor which increases in vivo colony formation by marrow CFU.[112]
5. Lymphocytes have been shown to have both suppressor[113] and enhancing effects[114] on erythroid differentiation.
6. Bone marrow treated in vitro with anti-θ serum and complement and transplanted into anemic W/W^v mice produces normal numbers of spleen colonies, but the anemia is not corrected and the colonies are predominantly granulocytic with no potential to produce stem cells. The anemia is corrected when viable syngeneic thymocytes are added to the inoculum or the recipient is treated with thymosin after marrow transplantation.[115,116]

Age-Related Changes in Marrow CFU

It has been accepted generally that total marrow CFU do not decrease with age in healthy mice.[117,119] In an effort to reveal a latent proliferative defect in aged mice, marrow cells from 3- and 30-month-old mice were subject to severe recruitment pressure by serial transplantation every 12 days in lethally irradiated young hosts.[120] Contrary to expectation, the decline in colony formation noted with each transfer was slower when old marrow was tested. Further studies showed that (1) old marrow cells migrate normally and are not sequestered preferentially in the spleen, (2) marrow suppressor activity increases with age and old CFU are more sensitive to this activity, (3) treatment of young marrow with anti-θ serum and complement has no effect on spleen colony formation but similar treatment of old cells results in a significant reduction in spleen nodule formation which can be partially restored by the addition of young thymus cells to the inoculum, and (4) young marrow cells produce equal numbers of spleen colonies in normal and recently immunized hosts, but old marrow produces more colonies in sensitized recipients.

Taken together the data suggests that old marrow CFU are more sensitive than young to normal helper-suppressor stimuli, and that at the time of initial sampling (i.e., *in situ*) old marrow is responding predominantly, but not maximally, to T-cell helper activity. It is not clear from the results of these experiments whether the differences noted in old marrow are due to intrinsic changes in stem cells or to defects in one or several of the CFU regulatory mechanisms.

REGULATION OF MARROW ELEMENTS

As we have seen, a series of T-cell, B-cell, and monocyte helper and suppressor systems regulate virtually all immunological processes through the elaboration of soluble factors or by direct cell-cell interactions. The impact of these immunoregulatory systems on marrow elements during ontogeny and aging is great, but because of space and time limitations only a brief overview can be given here.

Ontogeny of Regulation

By the tenth day of gestation mouse amniotic fluid contains an agent, perhaps α-fetoprotein, which can suppress murine antibody and cell-mediated immune responses.[121-122] However, mouse amniotic fluid will not inhibit the responses of human cells to antigens or mitogens, and human amniotic fluid and cord sera do not inhibit immune responses by cells of either species.[122] By the 16th day of pregnancy, nonspecific suppressor cells which are resistant to anti-θ serum and complement are found in fetal liver; the level of suppressor activity is comparable to that of young adult bone marrow.[120]

After birth bone marrow contains (1) T-cell and macrophage helper activity which promotes T-cell, B-cell, and CFU maturation,[7,120] (2) monocytes which can inhibit early B-cell differentiation,[123,124] (3) B-cells which can nonspecifically inhibit T-cell and B-cell responses,[125] (4) prethymic T-cells which are able to suppress antibody responses,[126] and (5) mature suppressor T-cells which specifically affect immune responses.

As mentioned previously, T-cell suppressor activity predominates in the peripheral lymphoid tissues of the neonate until 6 to 8 weeks after birth by which time helper and suppressor activities reach the equilibrium found in adult mice (see Table 5).

Changes in Immunoregulation with Age

The following changes in immunoregulatory mechanisms have been described in old

Table 5
MANIFESTATIONS OF AGE-RELATED DECLINE IN IMMUNE RESPONSIVENESS

Delayed allograft rejection
Decreased intensity of preexisting delayed hypersensitivity reactions
Increased difficulty in inducing DHS
Decline in "natural" antibody titers
Decreased antibody production in response to new antigens

Table 6
ENVIRONMENTAL FACTORS IN AGE-RELATED DECLINE IN IMMUNE RESPONSIVENESS

A. 1. Antibody production by spleen cells from old mice is twice as great when cells are "cultured" in young mice
2. Antibody production by spleen cells from young mice is one-half as great when cells are "cultured" in old mice
3. Fewer CFU-S are detectable in old hosts, regardless of the age of the donor marrow
4. Above due to inhibitory factor or decline in normal growth factor

B. 1. In vivo, up to 10 × the normal optimal antigen load is required to maximally stimulate antibody-production in old mice
2. In vitro, the optimal antigen concentration for maximum stimulation is the same for cells from young and old mice

Table 7
AGE-RELATED CHANGES IN THYMUS DEPENDENT FUNCTION

Number of $\theta+$ cells decreased in spleen, but increased in marrow; density of θ decreased
GVH activity is decreased in spleen but increased in marrow
Helper function is impaired
Suppressor activity is increased in some strains, decreased in others
Responses to Con A, PHA and thymus-dependent antigens are decreased
Thymic stroma is defective in promoting the maturation of T-cells from young and old mice; thymopoietin levels decline
There are major defects in the ability of T-cells to regulate immune and hematopoietic responses
There is a decline in the number of marrow T-cell precursors and/or in their proliferative potential

Table 8
AGE-RELATED CHANGES IN B-CELLS

Maximum antibody responses may be decreased 50-fold
There is a slight decline in Ig + cells in old spleen but slight increase in marrow
There is a shift from IgM^+ to IgG^+
Responses to LPS and B-cell antigens are only slightly, if at all, decreased
T-cell:B-cell interactions are impaired; this is only partially corrected with young T-cells
There are decreased numbers of antigen-reactive units (T — A — B)
"Burst size" is decreased in response to antigen
There is a maturation arrest at stage of ABC
There is a decrease in the number of functionally normal stem cells

mice: (1) T-cell antibody helper activity declines;[70] (2) specific suppressor T-cell activity increases;[68] (3) nonspecific B-cell suppressor activity in bone marrow and spleen increases;[120,125] and (4) nonspecific T-cell suppressor activity decreases.[71,74] The particular defects encountered appear to be determined to a great degree by the genetic background and environmental experience of the animal tested (see Table 6).

Currently available evidence suggests that changes in regulatory mechanisms may be primarily responsible for the immunological defects noted in aged mice. Therefore, immunological rejuvenation may be more dependent upon restoration of these regulatory systems than on stem cell replacement (see Tables 7 and 8).

REFERENCES

1. **Makinodan, T. and Adler, W. H.,** Effects of aging on the differentiation and proliferation potentials of cells of the immune system, *Fed. Proc. Am. Soc. Exp. Biol.*, 34, 153, 1975.
2. **Bloom, W. and Bartlemaz, G. W.,** Hematopoiesis in young human embryos, *Am. J. Anat.*, 67, 21, 1940.
3. **Cline, M. J. and Moore, M. A. S.,** Embryonic origin of the mouse macrophage, *Blood,* 39, 842, 1972.
4. **Virolainen, M.,** Hematopoietic origin of macrophages as studied by chromosome markers in mice, *J. Exp. Med.*, 127, 943, 1968.
5. **Van Furth, R. and Cohn, Z. A.,** The origin and kinetics of mononuclear phagocytes, *J. Exper. Med.*, 128, 415, 1968.
6. **Thomas, E. D., Ramberg, R. E., Sale, G. E., Sparkes, R. S., and Golde, D. W.,** Direct evidence for a bone marrow origin of the alveolar macrophage in man, *Science,* 192, 1016, 1976.
7. **Beller, D. I., Farr, A. G., and Unanue, E. R.,** Regulation of lymphocyte proliferation and differentiation by macrophages, *Fed. Proc. Am. Soc. Exp. Biol.*, 37, 91, 1978.
8. **Hammerling, G. J., Mauve, G., Goldberg, E., and McDevitt, H. O.,** Tissue distribution of Ia antigens. Ia on spermatozoa, macrophages and epidermal cells, *Immunogenetics,* 1, 428, 1975.
9. **Delovitch, T. L. and McDevitt, H. O.,** Isolation and characterization of murine Ia antigens, *Immunogenetics,* 2, 39, 1975.
10. **David, C. S.,** Serologic and genetic aspects of murine Ia antigens, *Transplant. Rev.*, 30, 299, 1976.
11. **Hardy, B., Globerson, A., and Danon, D.,** Ontogenic development of the reactivity of macrophages to antigenic stimulation, *Cell. Immunol.*, 9, 282, 1973.
12. **Kay, M. M. B. and Makinodan, T.,** Immunobiology of aging: evaluation of current status, *Clin. Immunol. Immunopath,* 6, 394, 1976.
13. **Nordin, A. A. and Buchholtz, M.,** The effect of age on the *in vitro* immune response of C57BL/6 mice to a T-independent antigen, in *Immunological Aspects of Aging,* Sergre, D. and Smith, L., Eds., Alan R. Liss, New York, in press.
14. **Tyan, M. L. and Herzenberg, L. A.,** Studies on the ontogeny of the immune system. II, *J. Immunol.*, 101, 446, 1968.
15. **Tyan, M. L. and Cole, L. J.,** Bone marrow as the major source of potentially immunologically competent cells in adult mice, *Nature (London),* 208, 1223, 1965.
16. **Tyan, M. L.,** Studies on the ontogeny of the mouse immune system. I, *J. Immunol.*, 100, 535, 1967.
17. **Komuro, K. and Boyse, E. A.,** *In vitro* demonstration of thymic hormone in the mouse by conversion of precursor cells into lymphocytes, *Lancet,* 1, 740, 1973.
18. **Hammerling, U., Chin, A. F., and Abbott, J.,** Ontogeny of murine B lymphocytes: sequence of B cell differentiation from surface immunoglobulin negative precursors to plasma cells, *Proc. Nat. Acad. Sci. U.S.A.*, 73, 2008, 1976.
19. **Glick, B., Chang, T. S., and Jaap, R. A.,** The bursa of Fabricius and antibody production, *Poult. Sci.*, 35, 224, 1956.
20. **Warner, N. L. and Szenberg, A.,** Effect of neonatal thymectomy on the immune response in the chicken, *Nature (London),* 196, 784, 1962.
21. **Basten, A., Miller, J. A. F. P., Sprent, J., and Pye, J.,** A receptor for antibody on B lymphocytes. I. Method of detection and functional significance, *J. Exp. Med.*, 135, 610, 1972.
22. **Bianco, C., Patrick, R., and Nussenzweig, V.,** A population of lymphocytes bearing a membrane receptor for antigen-antibody-complement complexes. I. Separation and characterization, *J. Exp. Med.*, 132, 702, 1970.
23. **David, C. S., Shreffler, D. C., and Frelinger, J. A.,** New lymphocyte antigen system (Ina) controlled by the Ir region of the mouse H-2 complex, *Proc. Nat. Acad. Sci. U.S.A.*, 70, 2509, 1973.
24. **Hauptfeld, V., Klein, D., and Klein, J.,** Serological identification of an Ir-region product, *Science,* 181, 167, 1973.
25. **Hammerling, G., Deak, B. D., Mauve, G., Hammerling, U., and McDevitt, H. O.,** B lymphocyte alloantigens controlled by the I region of the major histocompatibility complex in mice, *Immunogenetics,* 1, 68, 1974.
26. **McKenzie, I. F. C. and Snell, G. D.,** Ly-4.2: a cell membrane alloantigen of murine B-lymphocytes. I. Population studies, *J. Immunol.*, 114, 848, 1975.
27. **Takahashi, T., Old, L. J., and Boyse, E. A.,** Surface alloantigens of plasma cells, *J. Exp. Med.*, 131, 1325, 1970.
28. **Vitteta, E. S. and Uhr, J. W.,** Immunoglobulin-receptors revisited. A model for the differentiation of bone marrow-derived lympohcytes is described, *Science,* 189, 964, 1975.
29. **Tyan, M. L.,** Ontogeny of Fc and complement receptors in mouse embryonic tissues, *Proc. Soc. Exp. Biol. Med.*, 150, 237, 1975.

30. **Ryser, J. E. and Vassalli, J.**, Mouse bone marrow lymphocytes and their differentiation, *J. Immunol.*, 113, 719, 1973.
31. **Dukor, P. and Hartmann, K. V.**, Bound C3 as the second signal for B cell activation, *Cell. Immunol.*, 7, 349, 1973.
32. **Werner, P., Siegel, F. P., Dickler, H., Fu, S., and Kunkel, H. G.**, Immunoglobulin synthesis *in vitro* by lymphocytes from patients with immune deficiency: requirement for a special serum factor, *Proc. Natl. Acad. Sci., U.S.A.*, 71, 531, 1974.
33. **Moller, G.** Effect of B-cell mitogens on lymphocyte subpopulations possessing C3 and Fc receptors, *J. Exp. Med.*, 139, 969, 1974.
34. **Tyan, M. L.**, Evidence for clustering of H-2K, H-2D and the Fc receptor on B cells, *Proc. Soc. Exp. Biol. Med.*, 151, 526, 1975.
35. **Bianco, C., Dukor, P., and Nussenzweig, V.**, Follicular localization of antigen: possible role of lymphocytes bearing a receptor for antigen-antibody-complement complexes, *Adv. Exp. Med. Biol.*, 12, 251, 1971.
36. **Dukor, P., and Hartmann, K. V.**, Bound C3 as the second signal for B-cell activation, *Cell. Immunol.*, 7, 349, 1973.
37. **Gelfand, M. C., Sachs, D. H., Lieberman, R., and Paul, W. E.**, Ontogeny of B lymphocytes. III. H-2 linkage of a gene controlling the rate of appearance of complement receptor lympohcytes, *J. Exp. Med.*, 139, 1142, 1974.
38. **Dickler, H. B., and Sachs, D. H.**, Evidence for identity or close association of the Fc receptor of B lymphocytes and alloantigens determined by the Ir region of the H-2 complex, *J. Exp. Med.*, 140, 779, 1974.
39. **Melchers, F., von Boehmer, H., and Phillips, R. A.**, B-lymphocyte subpopulations in the mouse, *Transplant. Rev.*, 25, 26, 1975.
40. **Gelfand, M. C., Elfenbein, G. G., Frank, M. M., and Paul, W. E.**, Ontogeny of B lymphocytes. II. Relative rates of appearance of lymphocytes bearing surface immunoglobulin and complement receptors, *J. Exp. Med.*, 139, 1125, 1974.
41. **Lawton, A. R. and Cooper, M. D.**, Modification of B lymphocyte differentiation by anti-immunoglobulins, *Contemp. Top. Immunobiol.*, 3, 193, 1974.
42. **Melcher, U., Vitteta, E. S., McWilliams, M., Philips-Quagliata, J., Lamm, F., and Uhr, J. W.**, Cell surface immunoglobulin. X. Identification of an IgD-like molecule on the surface of murine splenocytes, *J. Exp. Med.*, 140, 1427, 1974.
43. **Abney, E. and Parkhouse, R. M. E.**, Candidate for immunoglobulin D present on murine B lymphocytes, *Nature (London)*, 252, 600, 1974.
44. **Hammerling, U., Chin, A. F., Abbott, J., and Scheid, M. P.**, The ontogeny of murine B lymphocytes. I. Induction of phenotypic conversion of Ia^- to Ia^+ lymphocytes, *J. Immunol.*, 115, 1425, 1975.
45. **David, C. S.**, Serological and genetic aspects of murine Ia antigens, *Transpl. Rev.*, 30, 299, 1976.
46. **McDevitt, H. O. and Tyan, M. L.**, Genetic control of the antibody response in inbred mice, *J. Exp. Med.*, 128, 1, 1968.
47. **Heyner, S., Brinster, R. L., and Palm, J.**, Effect of iso-antibody on pre-implantation mouse embryos, *Nature (London)*, 222, 783, 1969.
48. **Palm, J., Heyner, S., and Brinster, R. L.**, Differential immunofluorescence of fertilized mouse eggs with H-2 and non-H-2 antibody, *J. Exp. Med.*, 133, 1282, 1971.
49. **Melchers, F., Andersson, J., and Phillips, R. A.**, Ontogeny of murine B lymphocytes: development of Ig synthesis and of reactivities to mitogens and to anti-Ig-antibodies, *Cold Spring Harbor Symp.*, 41, 147, 1976.
50. **Decker, J. M., Clarke, J., Bradley, L. M., Miller, A., and Sercarz, E. E.**, Presence of antigen-binding cells for five diverse antigens at the onset of lymphoid development: lack of evidence for somatic diversification during ontogeny, *J. Immunol.*, 113, 1823, 1974.
51. **Tyan, M. L., Ness, D. B., and Gibbs, P. R.**, Fetal lymphoid tissue; antibody production *in vitro*, *J. Immunol.*, 110, 1170, 1973.
52. **Owen, J. J. T., Cooper, M. D., and Raff, M. C.**, *In vitro* generation of B lymphocytes in mouse foetal liver, a mammalian "bursa equivalent", *Nature (London)*, 249, 361, 1974.
53. **Kearny, J. F. and Lawton, A. R.**, B lymphocyte differentiation induced by lipopolysaccharide. I. Generation of cells synthesizing four major immunoglobulin classes, *J. Immunol.*, 115, 671, 1975.
54. **Tyan, M. L.**, Fetal lymphoid tissues: increase in ABC induced by antigen, LPS and IgG, *Proc. Soc. Exp. Biol. Med.*, 152, 354, 1976.
55. **Siskind, G. W.**, Ontogeny of B-cell function, in *Immunological Aspects of Aging*, Segre, D. and Smith, L., Eds., Alan R. Liss, New York, in press.
56. **Szewczuk, M. R., Sherr, D. H., Cornacchia, A., Kim, Y. T., and Siskind, G. W.**, Ontogeny of B lymphocyte function. XI. The secondary response by neonatal and adult B cell populations to different T-dependent antigens, *J. Immunol.*, 122, 1294, 1979.

57. **Mosier, D. E. and Cohen, P. L.**, Ontogeny of mouse T-lymphocyte function, *Fed. Proc. Am. Soc. Exp. Biol.*, 34, 137, 1975.
58. **Spear, P. G. and Edelman, G. M.**, Maturation of the humoral immune response in mice, *J. Exp. Med.*, 139, 249, 1974.
59. **Tyan, M. L.**, Effects of masking lymphocyte membrane components, *Cell. Immunol.*, 10, 450, 1974.
60. **Tyan, M. L.**, Inhibition of *in vitro* immune responses by antisera to H-2 and Ir, *Proc. Soc. Exp. Biol. Med.*, 150, 847, 1975.
61. **Tyan, M. L.**, Effects of masking H-2 and Ir gene products *in vitro*, *Proc. Soc. Exp. Biol. Med.*, 151, 12, 1976.
62. **Pierce, C. W., Kapp, J. A., Solliday, S. M., Dorf, M. E., and Bennacerraf, B.**, Immune responses *in vitro*. XI. Suppression of primary IgM and IgG plaque-forming cell responses in vitro by alloantisera against leukocyte allo-antigens, *J. Exp. Med.*, 140, 921, 1974.
63. **Hammerling, U., Chin, A. F., and Abbott, J.**, Ontogeny of murine B lymphocytes: sequence of B-cell differentiation from surface-immunoglobulin-negative precursors to plasma cells, *Proc. Natl. Acad. Sci. U.S.A.*, 73, 2008, 1976.
64. **Heidrick, M. L. and Makinodan, T.**, Nature of deficiencies in age-related decline of the immune system, *Gerontologia*, 18, 305, 1972.
65. **Makinodan, T. and Adler, W. H.**, Effects of aging on the differentiation and proliferation potentials of cells of the immune system, *Fed. Proc. Am. Soc. Exp. Biol.*, 34, 153, 1975.
66. **Mathies, M., Lipps, L., Smith, G. S., and Walford, R. L.**, Age-related decline in sensitivity to PHA and pokeweed mitogens of spleen cells from hamsters and a long-lived mouse strain, *J. Gerontol.*, 28, 425, 1973.
67. **Gerbase-Delima, M., Wilkinson, J., Smith, G. S., and Walford, R. L.**, Age-related decline in thymic-independent immune function in a long-lived mouse strain, *J. Gerontol.*, 29, 261, 1974.
68. **Segre, D. and Segre, M.**, Humoral immunity in aged mice. II. Increased suppressor T cell activity in immunologically deficient old mice, *J. Immunol.*, 116, 735, 1976.
69. **Gerbase-Delima, M., Meredith, P., and Walford, R. L.**, Age-related changes, including synergy and suppression, in mixed lymphocyte reactions in long-lived mice, *Fed. Proc. Am. Soc. Exp. Biol.*, 34, 159, 1975.
70. **Doria, G.**, *In vitro* antibody response of spleen cells from aging mice, in *Immunological Aspects of Aging*, Segre, D. and Smith, L., Eds., in press.
71. **Meredith, P., Kristie, J. A., and Walford, R. L.**, Increased expression of LPS-induced autoantibody secreting B-cells and evidence for deregulation in aging mice, in *Immunological Aspects of Aging*, Segre, D. and Smith, L., Eds., in press.
72. **Price, G. B. and Makinodan, T.**, Immunologic deficiencies in senescence. I. Characterization of intrinsic deficiencies, *J. Immunol.*, 108, 403, 1972.
73. **Farrar, J. J., Loughman, B. E., and Nordin, A. A.**, Lymphopoietic potential of bone marrow cells from aged mice: comparison of the cellular constituents of bone marrow from young and aged mice, *J. Immunol.*, 112, 1244, 1974.
74. **Goidl, E. A., Innes, J. B., and Weksler, M. E.**, Immunological studies of aging, *J. Exp. Med.*, 144, 1037, 1976.
75. **Tyan, M. L.**, Studies on B-cell precursors in aging mice, *Fed. Proc. Am. Soc. Exp. Biol.*, 36, (Abstr.), 1289, 1977.
76. **Tyan, M. L.**, Thymus: role in maturation of fetal lymphoid precursors, *Science*, 145, 934, 1964.
77. **Tyan, M. L. and Cole, L. J.**, Mouse fetal liver and thymus: potential sources of immunologically active cells, *Transplant.*, 1, 347, 1963.
78. **Cantor, H. and Boyse, E. A.**, Development and function of subclasses of T cells, *J. Reticuloendo. Soc.*, 17, 115, 1975.
79. **Raff, M. C. and Owen, J. J. T.**, Thymus-derived lymphocytes: their distribution and role in the development of peripheral lymphoid tissues of the mouse, *Eur. J. Immunol.*, 1, 27, 1971.
80. **Stutman, O.**, The thymic hormones, in *Immunological Aspects of Aging*, Segre, D. and Smith, L., Eds., in press.
81. **Twomey, J. J. and Lewis, V. M.**, Aging, thymic involution, thymectomy and thymic hormone secretion, in *Immunological Aspects of Aging*, Segre, D. and Smith, L., Eds., in press.
82. **Van Den Twell, J. G. and Walker, W. S.**, Macrophage-induced thymic lymphocyte maturation, *Immunol.*, 33, 817, 1977.
83. **Beller, D. I. and Unanue, E. R.**, Thymic macrophages modulate one stage of T cell differentiation *in vitro*, *J. Immunol.*, 121, 1861, 1978.
84. **Brennan, P. C. and Jaroslow, B. N.**, Age-associated decline in theta antigen on spleen thymus-derived lymphocytes of $B6F_1$ mice, *Cell. Immunol.*, 15, 51, 1975.
85. **Gillette, R. W.**, Changes in the migration patterns of spleen and lymph node cells associated with thymectomy and aging, *J. Reticuloendo. Soc.*, 3, 204, 1975.

86. **Kismoto, S., Shigemoto, S., and Yamamura, Y.**, Immune response in aged mice, *Transplants,* 15, 455, 1973.
87. **Tyan, M. L.**, Impaired thymic regeneration in lethally irradiated mice given bone marrow from aged donors, *Proc. Soc. Exp. Biol. Med.,* 152, 33, 1976.
88. **Goodman, S. A., and Makinodan, T.**, Effect of age on cell-mediated immunity in long-lived mice, *Clin. Exp. Immunol.,* 19, 533, 1975.
89. **Tyan, M. L.**, Age-related decrease in mouse T cell progenitors, *J. Immunol.,* 118, 846, 1977.
90. **Gerbase-Delima, M. and Walford, R. L.**, Effect of cortisone in delineating thymus cell subsets in advanced age, *Proc. Soc. Exp. Biol. Med.,* 149, 562, 1975.
91. **Hirokawa, K.**, Age-related changes of thymus, *Acta Pathol. Jpn.,* 28, 843, 1978.
92. **Hirokawa, K. and Makinodan, T.**, Thymic involution: effect on T cell differentiation, *J. Immunol.,* 114, 1659, 1975.
93. **Welsh, R. M., Jr.**, Mouse natural killer cells: induction, specificity and function, *J. Immunol.,* 121, 1631, 1978.
94. **Pross H. F. and Baines, M. G.**, Spontaneous human lymphocyte-mediated cytotoxicity against tumor cells, *Cancer Immunol. Immunother.,* 3, 75, 1977.
95. **Stutman, O., Paige, C. J., and Figarella, E. F.**, Natural cytotoxic cells against solid tumors in mice. I. Strain and age distribution and target cell susceptibility, *J. Immunol.,* 121, 1819, 1978.
96. **Paige, C. J., Figarella, E. F., Cuttito, M. J., Cahan, A., and Stutman, O.**, Natural cytotoxic cells against solid tumors in mice. II. Some characteristics of the effector cells, *J. Immunol.,* 121, 1827, 1978.
97. **Baldwin, R. W.**, Immune surveillance revisited, *Nature, (London),* 270, 557, 1977.
98. **Heberman, R. B., Nunn, M. E., and Lavrin, D. H.**, Natural cytotoxic reactivity of mouse lymphoid cells against syngeneic and allogeneic tumors. I. Distribution of reactivity and specificity, *Int. J. Cancer,* 16, 216, 1975.
99. **Kiessling, R. E., Klein, E., Pross, H., and Wigzell, H.**, "Natural Killer" cells in the mouse. II. Cytotoxic cells with specificity for mouse Maloney leukemia cells. Characteristic of the killer cells, *Eur. J. Immunol.,* 5, 117, 1975.
100. **Haller, O. and Wigzell, H.**, Suppression of natural killer cell activity with radioactive strontium: effector cells are marrow dependent, *J. Immunol.,* 118, 1502, 1977.
101. **Heberman, R. B., Bartram, S., Haskill, J. S., Nunn, M., Holden, H. T., and West, W. H.**, Fc receptors on mouse effector cells mediating natural cytotoxicity against tumor cells, *J. Immunol.,* 119, 322, 1977.
102. **Heberman, R. B., Nunn, M. E., and Holden, H. T.**, Low density of Thy 1 antigen on mouse effector cells mediating natural cytotoxicity against tumor cells, *J. Immunol.,* 121, 304, 1978.
103. **Kiessling, R., Hochman, P. S., Haller, O., Shearer, G. M., Wigzell, H., and Cudkowicz, G.**, Evidence for a similar or common mechanism for natural killer cell activity and resistance to hemopoietic grafts, *Eur. J. Immunol.,* 7, 655, 1977.
104. **Petranyi, G. R., Kiessling, R., and Klein, G.**, Genetic control of "natural" killer lymphocytes in the mouse, *Immunogenetics,* 2, 53, 1975.
105. **Welsh, R. M., Zinkernagel, R. M., and Hallenbeck, L. A.**, Cytotoxic cells induced during lymphocytic choriomeningitis virus infection of mice. I. Specificities of the natural killer cells, *J. Immunol.,* in press.
106. **Kumar, V., Goldschmidt, L., Eastcott, J. W., and Bennett, M.**, Mechanisms of genetic resistance to Friend virus leukemia in mice, *J. Exp. Med.,* 147, 422, 1978.
107. **Moore, M. A. S. and Johnson, G. R.**, Hemopoietic stem cells during embryonic development and growth, in *Stem Cells of Renewing Populations,* Caisnie, A. B., Lala, P. K., and Osmond, D. G., Eds., Academic Press, New York, 1976, 323.
108. **Moore, M. A. S.**, Regulatory role of macrophages in hemopoiesis, *J. Reticuloendo. Soc.,* 20, 89, 1976.
109. **Van Zant, G. and Goldwasser, E.**, Simultaneous effects of erythropoeitin and colony-stimulating factor on bone marrow cells, *Science,* 198, 733, 1977.
110. **Lord, B. I. and Schofield, R.**, The influence of thymus cells in hemopoiesis: stimulation of hemopoietic stem cells in a syngeneic, *in vivo,* situation, *Blood,* 42, 395, 1973.
111. **Goodman, J. W. and Grubbs, C. G.**, The relationship of the thymus to erythropoiesis, in *Hemopoietic Cellular Proliferation,* Stohlman, F., Jr., Ed., Grune & Stratton, New York, 1970, 26.
112. **Cerny, J.**, Stimulation of bone marrow haemopoietic stem cells by a factor from activated T cells, *Nature (London),* 249, 63, 1974.
113. **Hoffman, R., Zanjani, E. D., Viva, J., Zalusky, R., Lutton, J. D., and Wasserman, L. R.**, Diamond-Blackfan syndrome. Lymphocyte mediated suppression of erythropoiesis, *Science,* 193, 899, 1976.
114. **Torok-Storb, B., Storb, R., and Weiden, P.**, The effects of lymphocytes from non-transfused dogs on the growth of erythroid colonies (EC) from DLA identical littermates, *Exp. Hematol.,* 5 (Suppl.), 97, 1977.

115. **Jedrzejczak, W. W., Sharkis, S. J., Ahmed, A., Sell, K. W., and Santos, G. W.,** Theta-sensitive cell and erythropoiesis: identification of a defect in W/W^v anemic mice, *Science,* 196, 313, 1977.
116. **Sharkis, S. J., Ahmed, A., Sensenbrenner, L. L., Jedrzejczak, W. W., Goldstein, A. L., and Sell, K. W.,** The regulation of hemopoiesis: effect of thymosin or thymocytes in a diffusion chamber, *Blood,* 52, 802, 1978.
117. **Coggle, J. E. and Proukakis, C.,** The effect of age on the bone marrow cellularity of the mouse, *Gerontologia,* 16, 25, 1970.
118. **Silini, G. and Andreozzi, U.,** Haematological changes in the aging mouse, *Exp. Gerontol.,* 9, 99, 1974.
119. **Chen, M. G.,** Age-related changes in hematopoietic stem-cell populations of a long-lived hybrid mouse, *J. Cell. Physiol.,* 78, 225, 1971.
120. **Tyan, M. L.,** Age-related changes in mouse CFU-S regulation, in *Immunological Aspects of Aging,* Segre, D. and Smith, L., Eds., in press.
121. **Murgita, R. A. and Tomasi, T. B., Jr.,** Suppression of the immune response by alpha-fetoprotein, *J. Exp. Med.,* 141, 269, 1975.
122. **Tyan, M. L.,** Immunosuppressive properties of mouse amniotic fluid, *Proc. Soc. Exp. Biol. Med.,* 151, 343, 1976.
123. **Unanue, E. R. and Calderon, J.,** Evaluation of the role of macrophages in immune induction, *Fed. Proc. Am. Soc. Exp. Biol.,* 34, 1737, 1975.
124. **Waldmann, T. A., Blaese, M., Broder, S., and Krakauer, R. A.,** Disorders of suppressor immunoregulatory cells in the pathogenesis of immunodeficiency and autoimmunity, *Ann. Int. Med.,* 88, 226, 1978.
125. **Singhal, S. K., Roder, J. C., and Duwe, A. K.,** Suppressor cells in immunosenescence, *Fed. Proc. Am. Soc. Exp. Biol.,* 37, 1245, 1978.
126. **Dauphinee, M. J. and Talal, N.,** Failure of NZB spleen to respond to prethymic bone marrow suppressor cells, *J. Immunol.,* 122, 936, 1979.

AGING OF THE IMMUNE SYSTEM

Robin E. Callard*

INTRODUCTION

The wealth of available data showing that immune function declines with age has been fully documented in several recent reviews.[1-3] Both humoral and cell mediated immunity are known to be decreased in old experimental animals and in man. Moreover, it is now clear that the major part of the defect lies within the cells of the immune system rather than the extracellular milieu of the senescent host.[4,5] In contrast, much less is known of either the mechanism of these changes or of their precise relationship to the diseases of old age.

This article emphasizes the effect of aging on cell-cell interactions in the immune system with particular reference to T-cell regulatory networks. In addition, an attempt has been made to determine some areas by which specific cellular defects may result in diminished responsiveness and the immunopathology of the aged.

STEM CELLS

Both lymphocytes and accessory cells required for immune function are derived from multipotent stem cells found predominantly in the bone marrow of adult mammals.[6-11] Defective stem cells or stem cell differentiation in the aged would, therefore, result in diminished immune responsiveness. For this reason, a lot of attention has been focused on stem cell function but, apart from some subtle defects which have been observed, the bulk of available data points towards an unimpaired stem cell pool in old animals (Figure 1).

Chen[12] found a decrease in the proportion of both splenic and in vitro colony-forming units (CFU_s and CFU_c) in bone marrow of aged BC3F1 mice, but this was accompanied by an increase in bone marrow cellularity and the total CFU per femur did not change. Plating efficiency of bone marrow stem cells from old mice was also determined and found to be similar to young controls. In contrast, it was much reduced for both old and young bone marrow transplanted into old irradiated recipients. These results suggest that the stem cell compartment in old mice was normal but that the local environment necessary for stem cell proliferation and/or differentiation was suboptimal. A slight decline with age in the number of bone marrow CFU_s was also reported by Albright and Makinodan.[13] In this case, however, a significant reduction in the proliferative capacity of each CFU_s occurred after seeding to the spleen of recipient mice. Although this result is consistent with a limit to stem cell division, other explanations such as defective regulation were not excluded.

From an immunological point of view, the most satisfactory way of assessing stem cells is not to measure CFU_s, which are granulocytic rather than lymphoid, but to determine their capacity to restore immune function in irradiated recipients. This type of experiment has been done by several groups with different results. For example, Harrison[14] obtained similar restoration of an antibody response to sheep red cells (SRC) in young irradiated recipients grafted 3 to 10 months earlier with bone marrow from young and old donors. In a further study, he showed that both phytohemagglutinin (PHA) and antibody responsiveness were fully restored in young irradiated recip-

* Address all correspondence to: Robin E. Callard, Immunology Unit, Department of Medicine, University of Sydney, New South Wales 2000, Australia.

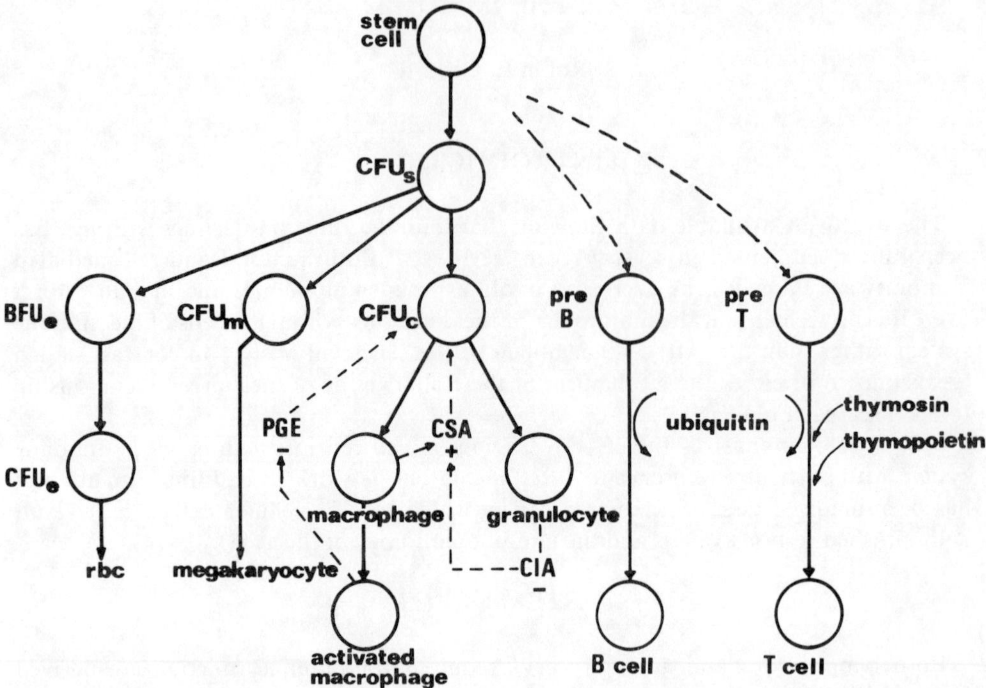

FIGURE 1. Stem cell differentiation — The simplified scheme here for stem cell differentiation is taken from References 6 to 11, 17 to 23, and 26 to 29. Note that the exact origin of lymphocyte cell lines is still uncertain. Abbreviations used are BFU, burst forming unit for erythrocytes; CFU_c, colony forming unit in culture; CFU_s, splenic colony forming unit; CFU_m, colony forming unit for megakaryocytes; CIA, colony inhibiting activity (lactoferrin); CSA, colony stimulating activity; PGE, prostaglandin E; --- = negative feedback; and --- + --- = positive feedback.

ients by bone marrow from aged donors even though the donors response to PHA and SRC was shown to be reduced.[15] In contrast, Farrar et al.[16] found that old bone marrow had a reduced capacity to generate B-cell functions in young irradiated recipients. In this study, spleen cells taken from recipient mice 4 weeks after reconstitution with bone marrow from donors pretreated with antilymphocyte serum (ALS) were combined with primed T-cells and tested for antibody production to SRC in vitro. The anti-SRC response obtained from donors grafted with old bone marrow was about one third that of donors grafted with young bone marrow. The different results obtained by Farrar[16] and Harrison[14,15] serve to illustrate a number of problems arising in this type of experiment.

First, it is now known that stem cell proliferation and differentiation is regulated by a variety of factors (see Figure 1 and References 8, 17-22). Perhaps most significant in the present context are T-cells which exert control over production of B-cells,[22] monocytes and granulocytes,[8] eosinophils,[20,21] erythrocytes,[21] and possibly CFU_s themselves.[23] As T-cell suppression is increased with age[24,25] it is imperative that this factor is taken into account when stem cell function in young and old mice is to be compared. For example, treatment of bone marrow preparations with anti-Thy.1 and complement should be done routinely in grafting experiments to remove contaminating T-cells. In this respect, it is interesting that in Harrison's experiments (see above) bone marrow stem cells from old and young donors were no longer comparable in restoration experiments if grafted into *thymectomized* irradiated recipients.[14] In this case, the diminished function of stem cells from old mice could be explained if functional T-cells needed first to be derived from stem cells in old marrow grafts before full reconstitution of the immune system could be achieved. Other factors are also required for differentiation of the many different lymphocyte subsets from committed pre B- and pre T-cells. Thymopoietin and ubiquitin, for example, induce human T-cell and B-cell differentiation in vitro, determined by the acquisition of FcR (Fc receptors) and surface membrane immunoglobulin (SMIg).[26] In addition, thymopoietin induces Thy.1, TL, and Lyl, 2, and 3 surface markers in murine T-cells.[27] Although thymopoietin acts on cells already committed to one line of differentiation rather than multipotent stem cells, it is clear that defective production of this hormone (or response to it) in old animals could result in an inability to maintain normal lymphocyte function. In this respect, it is relevant that thymosin, another thymic humoral factor which has been shown to induce T-cell surface markers in normal and nude mice,[28,29] has been reported to rejuvenate immune function in old mice.[30]

Second, full reconstitution of immune function in bone marrow-grafted irradiated mice may take longer than allowed in some experiments, especially since stem cells from old donors restore immune function more slowly that those from young controls. This difference is, however, lost after sufficient time has passed in the irradiated host[14,15] and could be the result of suboptimal regulation by T-cells or humoral factors rather than an intrinsic stem cell defect. Moreover, unless sufficient time is allowed to elapse after bone marrow transplantation, apparent defects in restoration by stem cells from old donors may be due to decreased function of mature lymphocytes already present in the transplanted bone marrow[16,31] rather than lymphocytes derived from stem cell differentiation in the host.

Third, it is always necessary to ensure that reconstitution of the irradiated recipient is by donor rather than host stem cells. This is usually accomplished by using the T_6 or other chromosome markers.[14]

Fourth, the use of serial transplantation procedures seems itself to impart a limit to the proliferative capacity of grafted stem cells.[32-34] This is true for bone marrow reconstitution of both irradiated recipients[32,34] and also *non*irradiated anemic W/W^v mice in which normal erythropoiesis can be restored with transplanted, normal, histocompatible stem cells.[35,36] These findings may be explained by a recent study in which evidence was provided for a limit to stem cell generation determined by the previous division history of each stem cell.[37] In this "generation-age" hypothesis a stem cell is lost to the stem cell compartment by forming two committed precursors to differentiated cell lines. Its place is then taken by the next oldest stem cell (age here is determined by its previous division history) and so on until ultimately the individual could run out of stem cells. The important question is whether such limits, if not simply an artifact of transplantation procedures, play any role in normal aging. There are several experiments which suggest not. For example, in Harrison's experiments with W/W^v anemic mice,[35] even though stem cell restoration of hemopoietic function was reduced by serial transplantation, there was no measurable difference between bone marrow from old and young donors. Moreover, by the fifth serial transplant, stem cells from old mice had produced erythrocytes normally for 77 to 84 months; that is, three to four times longer than the normal mouse life span. A quite different approach to this question was taken by Curtis and Tilley[38] who treated mice repeatedly with high doses of vinblastine over an extended period. This drug is cytotoxic for dividing cells and severely depletes peripheral and stem cell compartments. Recovery from the extended vinblastine treatment required a calculated 200 or more doublings of bone marrow stem cells in order to repopulate peripheral compartments, yet no loss of chromosomal integrity or any decrease in the ability of these cells to divide was detected. More recently, a definitive answer to the relative effects of serial transplantation and aging *in situ* has been provided by Ogden and Micklem[39] and Harrison.[34] In these experiments, chromosomally marked stem cells from old and young donors were mixed in equal proportions and infused into young irradiated recipients. The overriding advantage of this approach is that the environment, including regulatory soluble factors and T-cells, is the same for both old and young stem cells. In both primary and secondary hosts, reconstitution of T-cell and B-cell function (determined by response to PHA and lipopolysaccharide [LPS]) was equally distributed between stem cells from old and young donors, neither having an advantage over the other. This remained true even after four to five serial transfers when both donor populations ceased to replicate. Thus, whatever the reason for the decline following serial transplantation, stem cells from aged donors do not seem to be defective and can function normally in a suitable environment. They are, therefore, similar to other rapidly dividing cells such as intestinal crypt cells[40] and, of course, germinal cells, which can maintain normal populations in the aged presumably by selection for fully functional self-replicating units. This being so, the selective effect of aging on lymphocytes as compared, for example, with myelomonocytic lines, which are apparently unaffected by age, still needs to be explained. In this respect, it is worth considering the relative life spans of these cells. T-cells are longer lived than B-cells[41] which in turn are longer lived than monocytes,[42] and this is the order in which activity of these cells is lost with age.[43-45] It seems as if cells with a short half life which are continually replaced from normal bone marrow stem cells can maintain normal function throughout life. This hypothesis is testable and, if true, may provide a means for rejuvenation of immune function in the aged.

T-CELLS

Ever since T lymphocytes were shown to be a separate lineage from B lymphocytes it has become increasingly apparent that they are functionally extremely heterogeneous. It is only over the past few years, however, that the different T-cell subsets, in the mouse,with their highly specialized but quite separate functions have been identified by antisera specific for differentiation antigens. In particular, the Ly series, especially Lyl, 2, and 3, have played a major role, although in man, T-cell subsets have been identified by FcR (Fc receptors) for different classes of immunoglobulin (IgG, IgM and IgA),[46,47] by heteroantisera, for example TH_1 and TH_2,[48,49] and by autoantibodies present in some human diseases such as juvenile rheumatoid arthritis (JRA),[50] but these are much less well-defined than those characterized with Ly antisera in the mouse*. It is likely, however, that the many laboratories currently working with antibody-forming hybridomas will soon have monoclonal antibodies specific for human T-cell subsets. For further information on T-cell subsets the reader is referred to References 51—57.

Because of the functional and phenotypic heterogenity of T-cells, it is not sensible to talk of an overall loss of "T-cell function" with age when only one T-cell response has been measured. Furthermore, since most T-cell responses involve complex cell interactions, the observed loss of function with age may not always indicate a defect in a single defined T-cell subset. For this reason, the different T-cell functions, their interacting cell subpopulations and the changes which occur with age are discussed separately. Quantitative changes in T-cell subsets defined by surface phenotypes are discussed later in the section entitled "Mechanisms".

* Since this review was written, a number of monoclonal antibodies defining subsets of human T lymphocytes have been described. Two major categories of T-cell subsets have been identified; T helper/amplifier and T suppresor cytotoxic cells, characterized by OKT4/Leu 3A and OKT8/Leu 2A antibodies, respectively. (Beverly, P. C. L., Linch, D., and Callard, R. E., *Modern Trends in Leukemia*, Vol. 4, Springer-Verlag, Basel, 1980.)

T-Cell Mitogens

Diminished responsiveness to PHA has been described in aged mice,[58] rats,[59] hamsters,[60] and humans.[61] It does not appear to be due to either suppression or faulty presentation by accessory cells required for this response.[45] The defect, therefore, probably resides in the responding population of T-cells. It is now known, however, that only a subset of T-cells is activated by PHA in both mice and humans. In mice, the reactive cell is a T-cell with the surface phenotype Lyl* 2^+,[62] Ia^-,[63] Qal^+,[57] and is therefore distinct from both helper T-cells which are Lyl^+2^-,[64] and suppressor T-cells which are Lyl^-2^+, Ia^+.[65] They are also functionally distinct from both helper and suppressor T-cells.[66] Although the normal function of PHA reactive cells is unknown, a clue may be found in the recent finding of a role for Lyl^+2^+ cells as amplifiers for both helper and suppressor T-cells.[67-68] Similarly, an Lyl^+2^+ Qal^+ T-cell subset has been identified which, when activated by Lyl^+ Qal^+ cells, can participate in specific suppression as part of an immunoregulatory T-cell circuit.[69] Moreover, loss of this Lyl^+2^+ Qal^+ subset in NZB mice is associated with the loss of immune competence and autoimmune disease characteristic of this strain.[109] Although it is uncertain which, if any, of these subsets are identifiable with PHA reactive cells, it is clear that disturbances in them could profoundly affect normal immune function in aged mice.

In man, T-cell subsets and, therefore, PHA reactive cells are less well-defined. T-cells with FcR for IgM ($T\mu$) respond more readily to PHA than $T\gamma$ (T-cells with FcR for IgG) suggesting that they may be identifiable with helper T-cells required for polyclonal antibody synthesis in response to pokeweed mitogen (PWM).[47] Distinguishing T-cell subsets by FcR is not, however, totally satisfactory since these markers have been shown to be unstable by the transition of $T\gamma$ to $T\mu$ in vitro.[70] Human PHA reactive T-cells have also been shown to be JRA^+, in contrast to concanavalin A (Con A) reactive cells which are JRA^-.[50] Thus, in man also, PHA acts only on a T-cell subset. However, since the normal in vivo function of this subset is unknown, the effect of diminished responsiveness to PHA on general immune competence in aged humans is unclear.

Responsiveness to another T-cell mitogen, Con A, is also decreased with age in both mice[71] and humans.[72] Con A, also, acts on a T-cell subpopulation albeit a different one to PHA. In mice, the responding cell has the surface phenotype Lyl^+2^-[62] Ia^+.[63] Anti-Qal serum and complement reduces the Con A response by only 40% suggesting that the majority of responding cells are Qal^-.[57] Evidence in humans for Con A activation of a T-cell subset comes from experiments in which PBL (peripheral blood lymphocytes) were treated with JRA serum and complement. The Con A response was not affected and the subset can therefore be distinguished from PHA responding T-cells which are JRA^+.[50] The Con A reactive subset is itself probably heterogeneous including suppressor cells in both mice[73] and man.[74] Suppressor cells generated by Con A from murine spleen cells carry the expected phenotype Lyl^-2^+, Ia^+.[75] On the other hand, Con A induced suppressors in humans are derived from the $T\mu$ "helper" population rather than the expected $T\gamma$ cells.[76,77] Although the exact relationship between these suppresor cells, and T-cells concerned with immune regulation in vivo is uncertain, changes in Con A reactivity with age may reflect alterations in immunoregulation which could have a profound effect on immune competence and autoimmunity in old animals. The relationship between suppressor cells and immune function in the aged is discussed in more detail below.

Cell Mediated Cytotoxicity and Graft-vs.-Host Response

The ability to make normal lymphocytotoxic responses to both alloantigens and virus infected targets is diminished with age.[43,78,79] This response requires an interaction between helper T-cells (T_h) and killer cells (T_k) which can be distinguished with anti-Ly sera as Lyl^+2^- and Lyl^-2^+, respectively.[53] * Moreover T_h are clonally activated by Ia antigens whereas T_k recognize K, D antigens alone, in an allogeneic response, or in association with foreign (e.g., viral) antigens. It is the activity of the T_h cell, which proliferates but does not itself form T_k cells, which has been shown in allogeneic mixed lymphocyte responses to decline with age in both mice and humans.[81-83] As this cell is necessary for the generation of lymphocytotoxic responses, it will be necessary to do reconstitution experiments with cells from old and young mice depleted of Lyl^+ and $Ly2^+$ cells before the loss of cytotoxic activity can be attributed to diminished T helper function or defective T_k lymphocytes themselves.

Alloreactivity in graft-vs.-host responses (GvH) is also decreased with age.[84] GvH is a complex and poorly understood phenomenon although recent work has indicated that the response is regulated by suppressor cells in mouse[85] and man.[86] It is interesting that GvH T_s (T suppressor cells) have the same surface phenotype (Lyl^+2^+, Ia^+)[85] as the nonspecific T_s found to be increased in old mice,[24] both of which are different from T_s regulating antibody responses which are Lyl 1, 2^+, Ia^+.[65] Whether or not they have a role in the loss of alloreactivity in aged mice has yet to be determined.

Delayed Type Hypersensitivity

In delayed type hypersensitivity (DTH), Lyl^+ T-cells recognize antigen in association with Ia on antigen presenting cells.[87] The ensuing response results in the release of a variety of soluble factors responsible for monocyte infiltration and the typical inflammatory response of DTH. This response has obvious in vivo significance and, unlike PHA and alloreactivity, its age related decline in humans[88,89] is immediately relevant to the increased susceptibility to infection which occurs with age.[90]

In theory, the loss of DTH activity with age could be due to defective T-cells, antigen presenting cells, or monocyte function; although the latter two are considered unlikely since no defect in antigen presentation or monocyte function with age has yet been reported.[45] In addition, Lyl^+2^- Ia^- suppressor T-cells have been described in DTH.[91,92] Enhanced activity of this T-cell subset could inhibit DTH reponses in the aged.

The investigation of declining DTH with age has several advantages over studies of other T-cell functions. First, it has clear relevance to the main role of the immune system; to protect against infection. Second, DTH can be readily tested in vivo in both experimental animals and man. Third, in mice, the interacting cell populations are relatively well-defined and can be easily manipulated in in vivo experiments to determine where the defect lies. With these advantages, it is surprising that so little attention has been paid to DTH in aging populations.

Helper T-Cells

Recent findings have shown that T-cell help required for thymus dependent antibody-formation is mediated by a complex of interacting helper, amplifier, and suppressor T-cell subsets.[69,93] Thus, the loss of T helper function which occurs with age[94-96] is not necessarily synonomous with the existence of a defect in the T_h subset. Indeed, the age related loss of T-cell help in thymus dependent primary and secondary antibody production[94] is quite clearly not just due to defective helper cells since highly active nonspecific T suppressor cells are also present in T-cell preparations from old mice.[24,25,94,97] Whether or not a defect also exists in Lyl^+ T helper cells per se is not known. This question could be answered by transfer experiments in which T-cell preparations from old mice are depleted of T suppressor cells by treatment with anti-Ly2 or anti-Ia serum and complement. Future work should also take into account the two,

* Recent evidence suggests that T_k concerned with killing syngeneic tumors may be $Ly1^+2^+$.[80]

recently described interacting Lyl⁺2⁻ T_h subsets which can be distinguished with anti-Qal sera[57] or by adherence to nylon wool.[93]

Loss of helper function with age may also result from a failure of Ia associated antigen presentation or, at the effector stage, from an inability to interact with B-cells via, for example, soluble factors.[98] Finally, recent work has demonstrated a requirement for idiotype as well as antigen specific T helper cells in antibody responses.[99] No attempt has yet been made to determine the role of T helper cells concerned with idiotype networks in the loss of helper function with age.

In man, T helper function necessary for polyclonal antibody formation in response to pokeweed mitogen (PWM) has been shown to be increased rather than decreased with age.[100] The significance of this finding is unclear. It is unlikely to be due to decreased suppressor activity by $T\gamma$ cells since this T-cell subset was shown to be increased both in this study and by others.[101] This could, however, be tested directly by irradiation, which abrogates suppressor activity, leaving helper function intact.[102] Monocytes are also known to modulate PWM responses[103] but possible changes in this cell population were not taken into account.

The major advantage in using PWM induced antibody-formation for determining helper function in aged humans is that histocompatibility between cooperating T(E+) and B(E−) cell populations is not required[104] thereby permitting reconstitution experiments with old and young donors. However, this property also raises doubts about the validity of this approach since genetic restriction in lymphocyte interactions is well established. A recently developed in vitro system for specific T-dependent antibody-formation by human blood lymphocytes which does show genetic restriction[105] should provide a method for future investigation of specific helper function in man.

Suppressor T-Cells

Disturbances in suppressor cell function in the aged could have two distinct results. On the one hand, increased suppressor activity with age would lead to diminished immune function. Alternatively, decreased suppressor function and/or disturbances in regulatory networks might be responsible for the increased incidence of autoimmunity in the aged. In fact, an increase rather than a decrease in nonspecific suppressor activity has been described in old mice by several workers.[24,25,97] Moreover, the appearance of suppressor function is associated with an increase in the proportion of I-J⁺ T-cells in the spleens of old mice (Table 1). Characterization of the cells mediating suppression has shown them to be T-cells found in spleen, lymph nodes and bone marrow, which nonspecifically suppress primary and secondary antibody responses to thymus dependent and thymus independent antigens. Treatment with anti-Ia, Lyl, or Ly2 sera and complement completely abrogates their activity which was shown, by reconstitution experiments, to be dependent on interacting Lyl⁺ and Ly2⁺ subsets.[24] This latter finding is somewhat reminiscent of the work of Eardley et al.[69] and Cantor et al.[56] who have described suppression generated from Lyl⁺2⁺, Qal⁺ cells by Lyl⁺2⁻, Qal⁺ helper cells. Unfortunately, the Qal phenotype of the nonspecific suppressor cells in old mice has not yet been determined.

The apparent lack of antigen specificity of old suppressor cells may be due to each cell being nonspecific in its action as has been described for some T suppressor cell hybridomas[106] or, alternatively, to polyclonal expansion of antigen specific T supressor cells. There is also the possibility that these cells are specific for idiotypic[99] or allotypic[107] determinants rather than antigen thereby representing disturbances in regulatory networks.

In contrast to the appearance of nonspecific T-cell suppression in old mice, generation of antigen specific T suppressor cells to deaggreagated human gamma globulin

Table 1
COMPARISON OF T-CELL SUBSETS IN SPLEENS OF OLD AND YOUNG MICE[a]

Surface phenotype	Donor CBA mice	Number of mice analyzed	Proportion of spleen cells ± 1SE	(range)
Thy.1⁺	Old	9	29 ± 3	(18—39)
	Young	10	39 ± 1	(35—43)
Lyl⁺	Old	8	17 ± 3	(4—26)
	Young	6	24 ± 1	(23—27)
Ly2/3⁺	Old	4	18 ± 4	(7—25)
	Young	8	11 ± 2	(7—26)
I-J⁺	Old	9	5.3 ± 1.5	(2.0—16.3)
	Young	6	2.0 ± 0.1	(1.8—2.2)
Ig⁺ (B-cells)	Old	7	57 ± 5	(43—75)
	Young	10	46 ± 1	(41—52)

[a] The proportion of each T-cell subset was determined by radioautographical analysis of spleen cells labelled with specific antisera (kindly supplied by Dr. I. F. C. McKenzie), followed by ^{125}I-protein A. I-J⁺ cells were assayed by Dr. C. R. Parish. The slight decrease in proportion of Thy.1⁺ and Lyl⁺ cells in old mice could be accounted for by the increase in Ig+ (B) cells. The increase in Ly2/3⁺ cells is consistent with the two- to threefold increase of I-J⁺ suppressor T-cells and is probably real. In general, the relationship between T-cell subsets breaks down with age as indicated by the increase in the range of values obtained from old mice.

(HGG), which have the surface phenotype, Lyl⁻2⁺, Ia⁺, is apparently unaffected.[24] Although the importance of suppression for the maintenance of self-tolerance is strongly supported by the finding that reconstitution of T-cell deprived mice with T-cells depleted of Ly2⁺ cells results in the spontaneous production of divers autoantibodies,[108] the absence of any evidence for decreased suppressor activity in the aged argues against the notion that this is responsible for the observed high incidence of autoimmunity. Apparently, the relationship between depletion of Lyl⁺2⁺, Qal⁺ cells and loss of suppression with autoimmune disease in NZB mice[109] may not be typical of more normal strains.

In man, suppressor function is not as well-defined. T-cells with Fc receptors for IgG (Tγ) have been shown to be inhibitory in PWM induced antibody responses but well-defined antigen specific T suppressor cells analagous to those found in the mouse have yet to be described. Nonetheless, Tγ suppressor cells are altered with age. For example, the proportion of Tγ is significantly increased with age[100] especially in females.[101] The question of how this increase in Tγ cells might affect immune function in the aged is more difficult to answer. In one study[100] PHA responsiveness was negatively correlated with the increased proportion of Tγ cells. However, T helper activity in PWM induced antibody formation, which is mediated by Tμ cells and suppressed by Tγ cells, was enhanced rather than diminished. Conflicting results have also appeared from comparisons of Con A induced T-cell suppression in young and old humans. Hallgren and Yunis[110] reported a decrease in Con A induced suppression of Con A induced mitogen responses with age, whereas Antel et al.[111] reported an increase. Contrary to expectations, Con A induced suppressor cells are derived from the putative helper (Tμ) rather than the Tγ suppressor population.[77] It is, therefore, uncertain how or if changes in suppression induced by Con A are related to the increase in Tγ cells. Although the significance for immune function in the aged of altered suppression measured in these

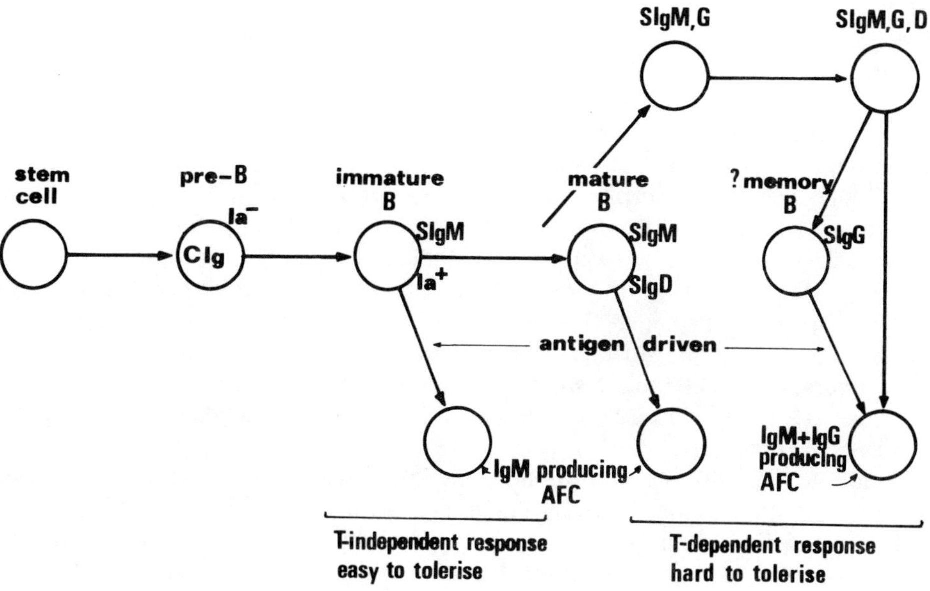

FIGURE 2. B-cell ontogeny — This scheme of B-cell differentiation has been simplified from the data given in References 118—122. Abbreviations used are AFC, antibody-forming cell; CIg, cytoplasmic immunoglobulin; and SIg, surface immunoglobulin.

artificial systems may be questionable, disturbances in T-cell suppression are associated with some forms of agammaglobulinemia[112] and changes in the proportion of Tγ cells have been found in a variety of immunologically related diseases.[113-114]

Increased suppressor activity with age may be an important factor in the loss of immune function but it is unlikely to be the only one. For example, diminished PHA reactivity in old mice could not be explained in this way.[45] Nonetheless, the appearance of nonspecific suppression with age may have profound in vivo effects. For example, recent work has shown that in vivo abrogation of suppressor cells with an anti-I-J alloantiserum enhances tumor rejection suggesting that resistance to syngeneic tumor growth may be regulated by T suppressor cells.[115,117] The possibility that the increased incidence of tumors in the aged may result from enhanced suppressor activity, should therefore be considered.

B-CELLS

B-cells do not constitute a homogeneous population. Several subsets can be identified by surface markers which either represent stages of maturity or commitment to making a particular Ig class. A simplified version of the B-cell lineage in mice is shown in Figure 2 and is essentially the same in man.[118] It is important to keep in mind that different techniques for determining B-cell function actually relate to different B-cell subsets. For example, changes in B-cell responses with age to different thymus independent antigens (e.g., SIII and LPS) probably indicate defects in B-cell subsets at different maturational states.[122] Similarly, reports of increased resistance to induction of B-cell tolerance in aged mice[123] may be due to a shift in B-cell subsets from immature, easily tolerized cells to those more mature and less easily tolerized.[120] These points need to be considered in the following discussion on changes in B-cell function with age.

Most B-cell responses, including antibody-formation to T independent antigens, are subject to a variety of T-cell regulatory controls. For this reason, it is important that comparisons between B-cells from old and young donors are made in a "neutral" environment. That is, either in the absence of T-cells, or following reconstitution of T-cell depleted B-cells with a single source of functional (young) T-cells. Without this precaution, it is difficult to determine whether the observed age changes are due to B-cell defects per se or to disturbances in T-cell regulation. With this in mind, there are three ways in which B-cell responses have been shown to decline with age.

First, old mice respond less well to the T independent antigen pneumococcal polysaccharide type III (SIII).[124,125] Moreover, neither treatment with ALS[125] or adoptive transfer of spleen cells treated with anti-Thy-1 and complement into young irradiated recipients,[124] reduced the difference in responsiveness between cells from old and young donors. From this experiment, a defect in B-cells per se can be concluded. Moreover, since SIII elicits only IgM antibody, the defect can probably be attributed to an immature B-cell subset (see above).

Second, old mice also do not respond as well to T dependent antigens. In this case, it is imperative that comparisons are made by reconstituting purified B-cells (i.e., T-cell depleted) from old and young animals with purified T-cells from young donors. Both primary and secondary (memory) B-cell responses have been studied in this way and have been shown to decline with age.[94,126] Thus, anti-Thy.1 treated spleen cells from old mice combined with activated thymocytes responded less well than young B-cells in a primary in vitro response to trinitrophenyl-sheep red cells (TNP-SRC).[126] Similarly, when B-cells prepared by treatment with anti-Thy.1 serum and complement were taken from naive old and young donors, transferred with equal numbers of purified young T-cells into young irradiated recipients, and immunized with dinitrophenyl-keyhole limpet hemocyanin (DNP-KLH), B-cells from old donors made much less anti-DNP antibody than those from young donors.[94] A similar approach was taken to determine memory B-cell function in old mice, only the procedure was more complex because of the necessity for priming both old and young B-cells in the presence of normal young T-cells. Purified B-cells from old and young donors were first primed with DNP-KLH in the presence of nylon wool purified young T-cells in young irradiated recipients. Three weeks later, primed B-cells from these animals were combined with HGG primed young T-cells, transferred into a secondary irradiated recipient, and immunized with DNP-HGG. Anti-DNP antibody was determined after 7 days. In this way, primed B-cells from old mice were shown to be less functional than those from young mice.[94] The poor B memory response could, however, have been due to either defective generation of memory B-cells on primary exposure to antigen (DNP-KLH), or to a failure of B memory cells to become antibody-forming cells on exposure to the second antigen (DNP-HGG), or both. Although this experiment does not distinguish between these two possibilities it may be possible to do so by quantifying antigen binding B-cells following primary exposure to antigen.[127] In either case, the experiment demonstrates a true B-cell defect since in both phases of the response, B-cells were only exposed to normal young T-cells.

Third, B-cell function in old mice has been studied with polyclonal B-cell activators such as LPS. In some cases, a considerable loss of activity has been reported[124,128] albeit slightly less so, or later than, observed for T-cell responses.[128] On the other hand, some workers failed to find any significant change with age at all.[43,44] But, in none of these examples, were B-cells depleted of T-cells, and so the possibility of inhibition by regulatory T-cells could not be excluded. In another study, however, suppression was not detected in mixing experiments with old cells responding to LPS.[45] Thus, for this mitogen at least, the decreased response of old cells was probably due to a real decline in B-cell function.

In man, the study of B-cell function has been hindered by several factors including both the necessity of relying almost exclusively on in vitro techniques and the absence of a true B-cell mitogen. Those which are known to activate human B-cells such as PWM, protein A from *Staphylococcus aureus* and water soluble extract from Nocardium all require T-cell help. Kishimoto et al.[100] found an increase in Ig production and no change in the proliferative response to PWM in aged humans. By contrast Weksler and Hutteroth[83] have described a decreased proliferative response to PWM with age. In neither case, however, could the changed responsiveness be attributed specifically to B-cells. To do so, reconstitution of purified B-cells from old and young donors with young, albeit allogeneic, T-cells is required. The response to PWM should then be measured by polyclonal antibody formation, rather than proliferation.

Human B-cell function determined by specific antibody-formation is even more difficult to measure. Natural antibody to flagellin[168] and natural isoagglutinins[129] are both decreased with age in man. Moreover, following in vivo immunization with flagellin, less specific IgG antibody was produced in aged people although total antibody was the same in both old and young.[168] Neither of these observations, however, give any direct information on B-cell function in specific antibody responses. To do so, it will be necessary to go to the recently developed methods for specific in vitro antibody production using human blood lymphocytes.[105,130]

MACROPHAGES AND ANTIGEN PRESENTING CELLS

Typical macrophage functions such as phagocytosis and enzyme degradation have been measured in old animals. In each case, macrophages from old donors functioned as well as or even better than those from young donors.[131-133] Macrophages from old mice prepared by adherence to plastic have also been shown to be normal in their capacity to support in vitro collaborative antibody responses.[134,135] Moreover, diminished responsiveness of old mice to PHA was shown to reside entirely in the nonadherent T-cell population. Both the presentation and supportive roles played by accessory cells in this response were normal.[45]

Recent work, however, has suggested that antigen presenting cells may not be typical macrophages. Thus, accessory cells in in vitro collaborative antibody responses express I-A and I-E/C Ia antigens which are found on a subpopulation only of peritoneal exudate adherent cells (PEC).[136,137] A further step in the identification of antigen presenting cells has come from work with Ia$^+$ splenic dendritic cells which are adherent but nonphagocytic,[11,138] and the similar Ia$^+$ skin Langerhans cell.[139] Both these cells are bone marrow derived and are extremely potent stimulators of mixed lymphocyte response (MLR): splenic dendritic cells are 300× more potent than B-cells.[11] Antigen pulsed Langerhans cells are also able to induce T-cell proliferative responses.[139] These findings suggest that nonphagocytic dendritic cells rather than macrophages may be the true antigen presenting (accessory) cell. With this in mind, the reported changes in MLR stimulating activity of PEC from old mice[45] may suggest a defect in antigen presentation. In addition, follicular localization of antigen in spleens and lymph nodes of old mice is diminished.[140] Taken together, these findings suggest that accessory cell function in old animals should be re-evaluated.

MECHANISMS

The past phenomenological approach to the aging immune system is currently being replaced by attempts to understand the underlying mechanisms. There are two types of explanation for the loss of immune competence with age: (1) quantitative; in which the lack of response is due to depletion of immunocompetent cells and (2) qualitative; in which intracellular defects prevent the relevant cells from responding to appropriate antigenic, mitogenic, or intercellular signals. These are discussed separately below.

Cell Depletion: A Quantitative Defect

Cell depletion was proposed as a possible mechanism for the waning of immune function with age as a consequence of two observations. First, was Hayflick's finding that cultured fibroblasts had a limited in vitro proliferative capacity which led to the notion of a finite life span for regenerating cell lines.[141] Second, Albright and Makinodan[142] and later Price and Makinodan[4] obtained evidence from limiting dilution assays for depletion of "immunocompetent units"[1] in old mice. These two basic observations have led to the idea that involution of the thymus acts as a biological clock by which a "Hayflick limit" to the proliferative capacity of thymocytes and thymus-derived cell lines would result in depletion of the T-cell pool and a concomitant decline in cell mediated immunity and antibody production to thymus-dependent antigens.[143] A similar argument has also been proposed for bone marrow procursors of B-cell lines. There are, however, a number of arguments against this hypothesis.

1. The bulk of available evidence does not support the notion of diminished proliferative capacity of bone marrow stem cells in old mice (see section entitled "Stem Cells").
2. The evidence for cell depletion is based primarily on limiting dilution experiments[4,144] and supported by blocking experiments using colchicine.[124,144,145] Taken together with other work, in which the defect was shown not to be due to changes in cell cycle time or diminished capacity for cell division,[146] these studies clearly show that fewer cells in old animals respond to the mitogenic or antigenic signal. They do not, however, distinguish between depletion of these cells and some other intracellular defect preventing those present from responding. To do this, a more direct method for quantifying precursor cells must be used.
3. Quantitative studies of T-cells in mice and humans have shown either no change or, at best, a slight decrease in proportion with age which could only account for a small part of the observed loss in function.[101,145-149] Similarly, B-cell numbers are either unchanged or slightly increased with age.[100,124] Indeed, in some instances, the increase in B-cell numbers completely accounted for the slight decrease in T-cell proportions.[124] A more direct test for cell depletion has been done by comparing antigen and mitogen responses of a known number of cells with the proportion of specific precursor cells in old and young mice.[94,124] In these experiments similar numbers of specific antigen binding B-cells (which are antibody-forming cell precursors) were found in old and young mice yet the antibody response to each antigen was very much reduced in old mice. Similarly, the subset of T-cells which responds to PHA[66] was not depleted in old mice despite a greatly diminished PHA response.[145] Quantitation of lymphocyte subsets using specific Ly antisera in mice (Table 1) and FcR markers in humans has supported the above findings. No consistent depletion of any lymphocyte subset was noted but disturbances in the balance of subsets was seen in some individual mice suggesting a breakdown in homeostatic control. A consistent *increase* in one lymphocyte subset has, however, been reported. These are I-J bearing T-cells in mice (Table 1) and Tγ cells in humans[100,101] both of which probably represent suppressor T-cells.[76,169] This finding is consistent with the observed increase in suppressor activity with age (see section entitled "Suppressor T-Cells").
4. Involution of the thymus is often presented as circumstantial evidence for deple-

tion of T-cells with age and has been invoked as a biological clock for senescence. Recent work by Kay[151] has suggested that thymic processing of bone marrow stem or pre-T-cells may cease, under normal circumstances, as early as 6 to 10 weeks of age in the mouse; although its ability to restore a normal T-cell pool following, for example, irradiation, remains for much longer. This observation, taken together with the known capacity for T-cell renewal in the periphery[152] suggests that peripheral T-cell numbers can be maintained long after any proposed decrease in thymic function. Complete removal of the thymus does, however, have an early effect on some T-cell subsets, although most T-cell functions are not noticeably diminished for many months.[109,153]

Membrane Abnormalities: An Example of a Qualitative Defect

The lack of experimental support for the cell depletion hypothesis has stimulated investigations into possible qualitative defects. Since most cell interactions in immune responses are mediated via the cell surface, it is appropriate to look at this organelle in lymphocytes from aged animals. Several abnormalities have been reported.

1. Evidence for new antigenic determinants arising in old cells has been obtained in MLR with syngeneic young responder cells, and confirmed by raising cytotoxic antisera, specific for old cells, in young mice immunized with lymphoid cells from syngeneic old donors.[154] In each case, mice of the same sex were used in order to avoid responses to H-Y antigens. In agreement with these findings, Gozes et al.[155] obtained a syngeneic GvH response in popliteal lymph nodes of young C57BL/6 mice given footpad injections of syngeneic cells from old donors. These observations have considerable implications for the immunopathology of aging. In particular, chronic lymphostimulation arising from autoreactivity to these changes in membrane antigens could result, as is known for chronic GvH, in an increased incidence of lymphoid tumors (especially reticular cell sarcoma) and autoimmunity,[156] both of which are characteristic of aging. Moreover, interference in surface interactions necessary for lymphocyte responses to antigens and mitogens may contribute to loss of immune function in the aged.
2. Cap formation and endocytosis of B-cell surface Ig following cross-linking with anti-Ig is slower on lymphocytes from old compared with young Lewis rats.[157] Although this may have been due to the slightly lower proportion of B-cells with a high density of SMIg detected in these animals, alternative explanations such as changes in membrane fluidity or in the microfilaments and microtubules of the cytoskeleton required for capping[158] were not excluded. Membrane fluidity of lymphocytes from old mice has, however, been studied by other investigators. In electron spin resonance (ESR) experiments, fluidity at the surface and deep in the membrane, determined with different spin labels, was shown to be similar in spleen and lymph node preparations from old and young mice (Raison and Callard, unpublished observations). By contrast, recent work by Rivnay et al.[159] has shown a 20% increase in microviscosity of the lymphocyte plasmalemma in old animals due to an increase in the cholesterol/phospholipid ratio. Similar preliminary findings have been reported by Woda[157] who measured microviscosity by antisotropy of the fluorophore 1,6-diphenylhexatriene. Such pertubations in lymphocyte surface membranes have been shown to decrease responsiveness to Con A[160] and may also result in autoimmune responses from the exposure of naturally hidden determinants.[159] The different results obtained from ESR and microviscosity experiments are probably due to the different techniques used. Nonetheless, it would be worth measuring, for example, lateral diffusion rates of surface components tagged with fluorescein as has been done with Con A and Fc receptors.[161]

3. Perturbations in cyclic nucleotide synthesis measured by increases in CAMP and CGMP following surface binding of mitogens has been reported recently.[162] Similarly, in recent work from our laboratory, lymphocytes from old donors were shown to respond less well to PHA, LPS, and prostaglandin E as measured by increasing CAMP levels (Callard and Ellis, manuscript in preparation). Moreover, much higher basal levels of CAMP, which may itself be a switch off signal,[163] were found in unstimulated lymphoid cells from old mice. Since adenyl and guanyl cyclases are membrane-bound enzymes which are activated by modulation of surface receptors[150] these findings provide further evidence for the presence of membrane abnormalities in old animals.

There are a variety of ways in which membrane changes could occur with age including; the appearance of new differentiation antigens, modification of the cell membrane by continued exposure to environmental chemical haptens, quantitative differences in the expression of normal cell surface antigens (for example Ig idiotype, perhaps as a result of monoclonal expansion of a B-cell line), changes in cholesterol/phospholipid ratio as already described,[159] expression of viral antigens or, finally, by insertion into the cell membrane of altered proteins arising from somatic mutation or from errors in protein synthesis, both of which have been postulated as causes of cellular aging.[165,166] At the present time, no distinction between these possibilities can be made. However, the technology is now available for raising monoclonal antibodies to the altered membrane components[167] which will permit isolation and characterization of these determinants. Whatever the explanation, it is clear that age related changes in lymphocyte membranes are to be found, and by interfering with cell interactions may result both in loss of immunological activity and in chronic lymphostimulation, thereby leading to autoimmune disease and neoplasia.[156]

ACKNOWLEDGMENTS

The author wishes to express his thanks to Dr. Ian Addison for his useful comments and to Anna Murchie for her patience in typing the manuscript.

REFERENCES

1. **Kay, M. M. B.,** An overview of immune ageing, *Mech. Ageing Dev.*, 9, 39, 1979.
2. **Meredith, P. J. and Walford, R. L.,** Autoimmunity, histocompatibility and ageing, *Mech. Ageing Dev.*, 9, 61 1979.
3. **Makinodan, T. and Yunis, E., Eds.,** *Immunology of Aging*, Vol. 1, Plenum Press, London, 1977.
4. **Price, G. B. and Makinodan, T.,** Immunologic deficiencies in senescence. I. Characterization of intrinsic deficiencies, *J. Immunol.*, 108, 403, 1972.
5. **Price, G. B. and Makinodan, T.,** Immunologic deficiencies in senescence. II. Characterization of extrinsic deficiencies, *J. Immunol.*, 108, 413, 1972.
6. **Abramson, S., Miller, R. G., and Phillips, R. A.,** The identification in adult bone marrow of pluripotent and restricted stem cells of the myeloid and lymphoid systems, *J. Exp. Med.*, 145, 1567, 1977.
7. **Till, J. E. and McCulloch, E. A.,** A direct measurement of the radiation sensitivity of normal mouse bone marrow cells, *Radiat. Res.*, 14, 213, 1961.
8. **Cline, M. J. and Golde, D. W.,** Cellular interactions in hematopoiesis, *Nature (London)*, 277, 177, 1979.
9. **Greaves, M. and Janossy, G.,** Patterns of gene expression and the cellular origins of human leukemias, *Bichem. Biophys. Acta*, 516, 193, 1978.

10. **Golde, D. W., Burgaleta, C., Sparkes, R. S., and Cline, M. J.,** The philadelphia chromosome in human macrophages, *Blood,* 49, 367, 1977.
11. **Steinman, R. M.,** Dendritic cells: a new population of mouse adherent cells active in MHC-linked functions, *Proc. 13th Int. Leuc. Cult. Conf.,* Toronto, in press.
12. **Chen, M. G.,** Age related changes in hemopoietic stem cell populations of a long lived hybrid mouse, *J. Cell. Physiol.,* 78, 225, 1971.
13. **Albright, J. W. and Makinodan, T.,** Decline in the growth potential of spleen-colonizing bone marrow stem cells of long lived ageing mice, *J. Exp. Med.,* 144, 1204, 1976.
14. **Harrison, D. E. and Doubleday, J. W.,** Normal function of immunologic stem cells from aged mice, *J. Immunol.,* 114, 1314, 1975.
15. **Harrison, D. E., Astle, C. M., and Doubleday, J. W.,** Stem cell lines from old immunodeficient donors give normal responses in young recipients, *J. Immunol.,* 118, 1223, 1977.
16. **Farrar, J. J., Loughman, B. E., and Nordin, A. A.,** Lymphopoietic potential of bone marrow stem cells from aged mice: comparison of the cellular constituents of bone marow from young and aged mice, *J. Immunol.,* 112, 1244, 1974.
17. **Burgess, A. W., Wilson, E. M. A., and Metcalf, D.,** Stimulation by human placental conditioned medium of hemopoietic colony formation by human marrow cells, *Blood,* 49, 573, 1977.
18. **Ruscetti, F. W. and Chervenick, P. A.,** Regulation of the release of colony-stimulating activity from mitogen stimulated lymphocytes, *J. Immunol.,* 114, 1513, 1975.
19. **Basten, A., Boyer, M. H., and Beeson, P. B.,** Mechanism of Eosinophilia 1. Factors affecting the eosinophil response of rats to trichinella spiralis, *J. Exp. Med.,* 131, 1271, 1970.
20. **Basten, A. and Beeson, P. B.** Mechanism of Eosinophilia. II. Role of the lymphocyte, *J. Exp. Med.,* 131, 1288, 1970.
21. **Nathan, D. G., Chess, L., Hillman, D. G., Clarke, B., Breard, J., Merler, E., and Housman, D. E.,** Human erythroid burst-forming unit: T-cell requirement for proliferation in vitro, *J. Exp. Med.,* 147, 324, 1978.
22. **Sherr, D. H., Szewczuk, M. R., and Sisking, G. W.,** Ontogeny of B-lymphocyte function. V. Thymus cell involvement in the functional maturation of B lympohcytes from fetal mice transferred into adult irradiated hosts, *J. Exp. Med.,* 147, 196, 1978.
23. **Cerny, J.,** Stimulation of bone marrow hemopoietic stem cells by a factor from activated T-cells, *Nature (London),* 249, 63, 1974.
24. **Callard, R. E., Fazekas, De St., Groth, B., Basten, A., and McKenzie, I. F. C.,** Immune function in aged mice v. role of suppressor cells, *J. Immunol.,* 124, 52, 1980.
25. **Segre, D. and Segre, M.,** Humoral immunity in aged mice II. Increased suppressor T-cell activity in immunologically deficient old mice, *J. Immunol.,* 116, 735, 1976.
26. **Kagan, W. A., Siegal, F. P., Gupta, S., Goldstein, G., and Good, R. A.,** Early stages of human marrow lymphocyte differentiation: induction in vitro by thymopoietin and ubiquitin, *J. Immunol.,* 122, 686, 1979.
27. **Scheid, M. P., Goldstein, G., Hammerling, G., and Boyse, E. A.,** Lymphocyte differentiation from precursor cells in vitro, *Ann. N.Y. Acad. Sci.,* 249, 531, 1975.
28. **Scheid, M. P., Hoffman, M. K., Komuro, K., Hammerling, U., Abbott, J., Boyse, E. A., Cohen, G. H., Hooper, J. A., Schulaf, R. S., and Goldstein, A. L.,** Differentiation of T-cells induced by preparations from thymus and by non-thymic agents. The determined state of the precursor cell, *J. Exp. Med.,* 138, 1027, 1973.
29. **Komuro, K. and Boyse, E. A.,** Induction of T lymphocytes from precursor cells in vitro by a product of the Thymus, *J. Exp. Med.,* 138, 479, 1973.
30. **Goldstein, A. L.,** Thymosin: the endocrine thymus and its role in the ageing process, *XIth International Congress of Gerontology Symposia,* Scimed, Tokyo, 1978, 22.
31. **Osmond, D. G. and Norsal, G. J. V.,** Differentiation of lympohcytes in mouse bone marrow. I. Quantitative radioautographic studies of antiglobulin — binding by lymphocytes in bone marrow and lymphoid tissues, *Cell. Immunol.,* 13, 117, 1974.
32. **Cudkowicz, G., Upton, A. C., and Shearer, G. M.,** Lymphocyte content and proliferative capacity of serially transplanted mouse bone marrow *Nature (London),* 201, 165, 1964.
33. **Lajtha, L. G. and Schofield, R.,** Regulation of stem cell renewal and differentiation: possible significance in ageing, *Adv. Gerontol. Res.,* 3 131, 1971.
34. **Harrison, D. E., Astle, C. M., and Delaittre, J. A.,** Loss of proliferative capacity in immunohemopoietic stem cells caused by serial transplantation rather than ageing, *J. Exp. Med.,* 147, 1526, 1978.
35. **Harrison, D. E.** Normal function of transplanted marrow cell lines from aged mice, *J. Gerontol.,* 30, 279, 1975.
36. **Harrison, D. E.,** Defective erythropoietic responses of aged mice not improved by young marrow, *J. Gerontol.,* 30, 286, 1975.
37. **Rosendaal, M., Hodgson, G. S., and Bradley, T. R.,** Organization of hemopoietic stem cells: the generation: age hypothesis, *Cell Tissue Kinet.,* 12, 17, 1979.

38. **Curtis, H. J., and Tilley, J.**, The life span of dividing mammalian cells in vivo, *J. Gerontol.*, 26, 1, 1971.
39. **Ogden, D. A. and Micklem, H. S.**, The fate of serially transplanted bone marrow cell populations from young and old donors, *Transplantation*, 22, 287, 1976.
40. **Lesher, S., Sacher, G. A.**, Effects of age on cell proliferation in mouse duodenal crypts, *Exp. Gerontol.*, 3, 211, 1968.
41. **Sprent, J. and Basten A.**, Circulating T and B lymphocytes of the mouse, II. Lifespan, *Cell. Immunol.*, 7, 40, 1973.
42. **Volkman, A.**, Monocyte kinetics and their changes in infection, in *Immunobiology of the Macrophage*, Nelson, D., Ed., Academic Press, New York, 1976, 291.
43. **Adler, W. H., Jones, K. H., and Nariuchi, H.**, Ageing and immune function, recent advances in, *Clin. Immunol.*, 1, 77, 1978.
44. **Makinodan, T., Good, R. A., Kay, M. M. B.**, Cellular basis of immunosenescence, in *Immunology and Aging*, Vol. 1, Good, R. A. and Day, S. B., Eds., Plenum Medical Book, London, 1977, 9.
45. **Callard, R. E.**, Immune function in aged mice. III. Role of macrophages and effect of 2-mercaptoethanol in the response of spleen cells from old mice to phytohaemagglutinin, lipopolysaccharide and allogeneic cells, *Eur. J. Immunol.*, 8, 697, 1978.
46. **Lum, L. G., Muchmore, A. V., Keren, D., Decker, J., Koski, I., Stober, W., and Blaese, R. M.**, A receptor for IgA on human T lympohcytes, *J. Immunol.*, 122, 65, 1979.
47. **Moretta, L., Ferrarini, M., Mingari, M. C., Moretta, A., and Webb, S. E.**, Subpopulations of human T cells identified by receptors for immunoglobulins and mitogen responsiveness, *J. Immunol.*, 177, 2171, 1976.
48. **Evans, R. L., Breard, J. M., Lazarus, H., Schlossman, S. F., and Chess, L.**, Detection, isolation and functional characterization of two human T-cell subclasses bearing unique differentiation antigens, *J. Exp. Med.*, 145, 221, 1977.
49. **Evans, R. L., Lazarus, H., Penta, A. C., and Schlossman, S. F.**, Two functionally distinct subpopulations of human T-cells that collaborate in the generation of cytotoxic cells responsible for cell-mediated lympholysis, *J. Immunol.*, 120, 1423, 1978.
50. **Strelkauskas, A. J., Schauf, V., Wilson, B. S., Chess, L., and Schlossman, S. F.**, Isolation and characterization of naturally occurring subclasses of human peripheral blood T-cells with regulatory functions, *J. Immunol.*, 120, 1278, 1978.
51. **Beverly, P. C. L.**, Functional subsets of lympohcytes, *J. Clin. Path.*, 32, (Suppl.), in press.
52. **Chess, L. and Schlossman, S. F.**, Human lympohcyte subpopulations, *Adv. Immunol.*, 25, 213, 1977.
53. **Cantor, H. and Boyse, E. A.**, Lympohcytes as models for the study of mammalian cellular differentiation, *Immunol. Rev.*, 33, 105, 1977.
54. **Boyse, E. A. and Cantor, H.**, Immunogenetic aspects of biologic communication: a hypothesis of evolution by program duplication, *Birth Defects Orig. Artic. Ser.*, 14, 249, 1978.
55. **Simpson, E. and Beverley, P. C. L.**, T-cell subpopulations, in *Progress in Immunology*, Vol. 3, Mandel, T. E., Cheers, C., McKenzie, I. F. C., and Nossal, G. J. V., Eds., Australian Academy of Sciences, Canberra, 1977, 206.
56. **Cantor, H., Hugenberger, J. Boudreau, L. McV., Eardley, D. D., Kemp, J., Shen, F. W., and Gershon, R. K.**, Immunoregulatory circuits among T-cell sets. III. Identification of a subpopulation of T-helper cells that induces feedback inhibition, *J. Exp. Med.*, 148, 871, 1978.
57. Stanton, T. H., Calkins, C. E., Jandinski, J., Schendel, D. J., Stutman, O., Cantor, H., and Boyse, E. A., The Qa-1 antigenic system. Relation of Qa-1 phenotypes to lymphocyte sets, mitogen responses and immune functions, *J. Exp. Med.*, 148, 963, 1978.
58. **Hori, Y., Perkins, E. H., and Halsall, M. E.**, Decline in phyto hemagglutinin responsiveness of spleen cells from ageing mice, *Proc. Soc. Exp. Biol. Med.*, 144, 48, 1973.
59. **Nielson, H. E.**, The effect of age on the response of rat lymphocytes in mixed leucocyte culture, to PHA and graft-versus-host reaction, *J. Immunol.*, 112, 1194, 1974.
60. **Mathies, M., Lipps, L., Smith, G. S., and Walford, R. L.**, Age related decline in response to phytohemagglutinin and pokeweed mitogen by spleen cells from hamsters and a long lived mouse strain, *J. Gerontol.*, 28, 425, 1973.
61. **Pisciotta, A. V., Westring, D. W., de Prey, C., and Walsh, B.**, Mitogenic effect of phytohemagglutinin at different ages, *Nature*, 215, 193, 1967.
62. **Hirst, J. A., Beverley, P. C. L., Kisielow, P., Hoffman, M. K., and Oettgen, H. F.**, Ly antigens: markers of T cell function on mouse spleen cells, *J. Immunol.*, 115, 1555, 1975.
63. **Neiderhuber, J. E., Frelinger, J. A., Dine, M. S., Schoffner, P., Dugan, E., and Shreffler, D. C.**, Effects of anti-Ia sera on mitogenic responses II. Differential expression of the Ia marker on phytohemagglutinin and concanavalin A — reactive T-cells, *J. Exp. Med.*, 143, 372, 1976.
64. **Cantor, H., Shen, F-W., and Boyse, E. A.**, Separation of helper T-cells from suppressor T-cells expressing different Ly components. II. Activation by antigen: after immunization, antigen-specific suppressor and helper activities are mediated by distinct T-cell subclasses, *J. Exp. Med.*, 143, 1391, 1976.

65. **Basten, A., Miller, J. F. A. P., Loblay, R., Johnson, P., Gamble, J., Chia, E., Pritchard-Briscoe, H., Callard, R. E., and McKenzie, I. F. C.,** T-cell dependent suppression of antibody production. I. Characteristics of suppressor T-cells following tolerance induction, *Eur. J. Immunol.,* 8, 360, 1978.
66. **Callard, R. E. and Basten, A.,** Identification of T-cell subpopulations binding phytohaemagglutinin: functional characteristics, *Eur. J. Immunol.,* 8, 247, 1978.
67. **Tada, T., Taniguchi, M., and Okumura, K.,** Regulation of antibody response by antigen-specific T-cell factors bearing I region determinants, in *Progress in Immunology,* Vol. 3, Elsevier/North Holland, Amsterdam, 1977, 369.
68. **Feldmann, M., Beverley, P., Erb, P., Howie, S., Kontiainen, S., Maoz, A. Mathies, M., McKenzie, I., and Woody, J.,** Current concepts of the antibody response: heterogeneity of lymphoid cells, interactions and factors, *Cold Spring Harbor Symp. Quant. Biol.,* 41, 113, 1977.
69. **Eardley, D. D., Hugenberger, J., McVay-Boudreau, L., Shen, F-W., Gershon, R. K., and Cantor, H.,** Immunoregulatory circuits among T-cell sets. I. T-helper cells induce other T-cell sets to exert feedback inhibition, *J. Exp. Med.,* 147, 1106, 1978.
70. **Pichler, W. J., Lum, L., and Broder, S.,** Fc-receptors on human T lymphocytes. 1. Transition of $T\gamma$ to $T\mu$ cells, *J. Immunol.,* 1540, 1978.
71. **Heidrick, M. and Makinodan, T.,** Nature of cellular deficiencies in age-related decline of the immune system, *Gerontologia,* 18, 305, 1972.
72. **Hallgren, H. M., Kersey, J. H., Dubey, D. P., and Yunis, E. J.,** Lymphocyte subsets and integrated immune function in ageing humans, *Clin. Immunol. Immunopathol.,* 10, 65, 1978.
73. **Dutton, R. W.,** Suppressor T-cells, *Transplant. Rev.,* 26, 39, 1975.
74. **Haynes, B. F. and Fauci, A. S.,** Activation of human B lymphocytes. III. Concanavalin A induced generation of suppressor cells of the plaque-forming cell response of normal human B lymphocytes, *J. Immunol.,* 118, 2281, 1977.
75. **Jandinski, J., Cantor, H., Tadakuma, T., Peavy, D. L., and Pierce, C. W.,** Separation of helper T-cells from suppressor T-cells expressing different Ly components. I. Polyclonal activation: suppressor and helper activities are inherent properties of distinct T-cell subclasses, *J. Exp. Med.,* 143, 1382, 1976.
76. **Moretta, L., Webb, S. R., Grossi, C. E., Lydyard, P. M., and Cooper, M. D.,** Functional analysis of two human T-cell subpopulations: help and suppression of B-cell responses by T-cells bearing receptors for IgM and IgG, *J. Exp. Med.,* 146, 184, 1977.
77. **Hayward, A. R., Layward, L., Lydyard, P. M., Moretta, L., Dagg, M., and Lawton, A. R.,** Fc-receptor heterogeneity of human suppressor T-cells, *J. Immunol.,* 121, 1, 1978.
78. **Goodman, S. A. and Makinodan, T.,** Effect of age on cell-mediated immune responsiveness assessed in vivo by tumor resistance and in vitro by cytolytic activity, *Clin. Exp. Immunol.,* 19, 533, 1975.
79. **Doherty, P. C.,** Diminished T-cell surveillance function in old mice infected with lymphocyte choriomeningitis virus, *Immunology,* 32, 751, 1977.
80. **Shimizu, K. and Shen, F-W.,** Role of different T-cell sets in the rejection of syngeneic chemically induced tumors, *J. Immunol.,* 122, 1162, 1979.
81. **Konen, T. G., Smith, G. S., and Walford, R. L.,** Decline in mixed lymphocyte reactivity of spleen cells from aged mice of a long lived strain, *J. Immunol.,* 110, 1216, 1973.
82. **Gerbase, De Lima, M., Meredith, P., and Walford, R. L.,** Age related changes, including synergy and suppression in the mixed lymphocyte reaction in long lived mice, *Fed. Proc. Fed. Am. Soc. Exp. Biol.,* 34, 159, 1975.
83. **Weksler, M. E. and Hutteroth, T. H.,** Impaired lymphocyte function in aged humans, *J. Clin. Invest.,* 53, 99, 1974.
84. **Kishimoto, S., Shigemoto, S., and Yamamura, Y.,** Immune response in aged mice. Change of cell mediated immunity with ageing, *Transplantation,* 15, 455, 1973.
85. **Shand, F. L.,** Ly and Ia phenotype of suppressor T-cells induced by graft-vs-host reaction, *Eur. J. Immunol.,* 7, 746, 1977.
86. **Reinherz, E. L., Parkman, R., Rappeport, J., Rosen, F. S., and Schlossman, S. F.,** Aberrations of suppressor T-cells in human graft-versus-host disease, *N. Engl. J. Med.,* 300, 1061, 1979.
87. **Vadas, M. A., Miller, J. F. A. P., McKenzie, I. F. C., Chism, S. E., Shen, F-W., Boyse, E. A., Gamble, J. R., and Whitelaw, A. M.,** Ly and Ia antigen phenotypes of T-cells involved in delayed-type hypersensitivity and suppression, *J. Exp. Med.,* 144, 10, 1976.
88. **Toh, B. H., Roberts-Thomson, I. C., Mathews, J. D., Whittingham, S., and MacKay, I. R.,** Depression of cell mediated immunity in old age and the immunopathic diseases, lupus erythermatosus, chronic hepatitis and rheumatoid arthritis, *Clin. Exp. Immunol.,* 14, 193, 1973.
89. **Mackay, I. R.,** Ageing and immunological function in man, *Gerontologia,* 18, 285, 1972.
90. **Gardiner, I. D. and Remington, J. S.,** Age-related decline in resistance of mice to infection with intracellular phathogens, *Infect. Immunol.,* 16, 593, 1977.
91. **Moorhead, J. W.,** Tolerance and contact sensitivity to DNFB in mice. VI. Inhibition of afferent sensitivity by suppressor T-cells in adoptive tolerance, *J. Immunol.,* 117, 802, 1976.

92. **Ramshaw, I. A., McKenzie, I. F. C., Bretscher, P. A., and Parish, C. R.,** Discrimination of suppressor T-cells of humoral and cell-mediated immunity by anti-Ly and anti-Ia sera, *Cell. Immunol.*, 31, 346, 1977.
93. **Tada, T., Takemori, T., Okumura, K., Nonaka, M., and Tokuhisa, T.,** Two distinct types of helper cells involved in the secondary antibody response: independent and synergistic effects of Ia^- and Ia^+ helper T-cells, *J. Exp. Med.*, 147, 446, 1978.
94. **Callard, R. E. and Basten, A.,** Immune function in aged mice. IV. Loss of T-cell and B-cell function in thymus dependent antibody responses, *Eur. J. Immunol.*, 8, 552, 1978.
95. **Krogsrud, R. L. and Perkins, E. H.,** Age related changes in T-cell function, *J. Immunol.*, 118, 1607, 1977.
96. **Segre, M. and Segre, D.,** Humoral immunity in aged mice. 1. Age-related decline in the secondary response to DNP of spleen cells propagated in diffusion chambers, *J. Immunol.*, 116, 731, 1976.
97. **Goidl, E. A., Innes, J. B., and Weksler, M. E.,** Immunolgical studies of ageing. II. Loss of gG and high avidity plaque-forming cells and increased suppressor activity in ageing mice, *J. Exp. Med.*, 144, 1037, 1976.
98. **Feldmann, M., Cecka, J. M., Cosenza, H., David, C. S., Erb, P., James, R., Howie, S., Kontiainen, S., Maurer, P., McKenzie, I. F. C., Parish, C., Rees, A., Todd, I., Torano, A., Winger, L., and Woody, J.,** On the nature of specific factors and the integration of their signals by macrophages, ICN-UCLA Conference on T and B Lymphocytes, Academic Press.
99. **Herzenberg, L. A., Black, S. T., and Herzenberg, L. A.,** Regulatory circuits and antibody responses, *Eur. J. Immunol.*, 10, 1, 1980.
100. **Kishimoto, S., Tomino, S., Inomata, K., Kotegawa, S., Sacto, T., Kuroki, M., Mitsuya, H., and Hisamitsu, S.,** Age related changes in the subsets and functions of human T lympohcytes, *J. Immunol.*, 121, 1773, 1978.
101. **Gupta, S. and Good, R. A.,** Subpopulations of human T lymphocytes. X. Atlerations in T,B, Third population cells and T-cells with receptors for immunoglobulin M ($T\mu$) or G ($T\gamma$) in ageing humans, *J. Immunol.*, 122, 1214, 1979.
102. **Haynes, B. F. and Fauci, A. S.,** Activation of human B lymphocytes. VI. Immunoregulation of antibody production by mitogen-induced and naturally occurring suppressor cells in normal individuals, *Cell. Immunol.*, 36, 294, 1978.
103. **Dimitriu, A. and Fauci, A. S.,** Activation of human B lymphocytes. IX. Modulation of antibody production by products of activated macrophages, *J. Immunol.*, 120, 1818, 1978.
104. **Hirano, T., Kuritani, T., Kishimoto, T., and Yamamura, Y.,** In vitro immune response of human peripheral lymphocytes. I. The mechanism(s) involved in T-cell helper functions in the pokeweed mitogen-induced differentiation and proliferation of B-cells, *J. Immunol.*, 119, 1235, 1977.
105. **Callard, R. E.,** Specific in vitro antibody response to influenza virus by human blood lympohcytes, *Nature (London)*, 282, 734, 1979.
106. **Taniguchi, M. and Miller, J. F. A. P.,** Specific suppressor factors produced by hybridomas derived from the fusion of enriched suppressor T-cells and a T lymphoma cell line, *J. Exp. Med.*, 148, 373, 1978.
107. **Herzenberg, L. A., Chan, E. L., Ravitch, M. M., Riblet, R. J., and Herzenberg, L. A.,** Active suppression of immunoglobulin allotype synthesis. III. Identification of T-cells as responsible for suppression by cells from spleen, thymus, lymphnode and bone marrow, *J. Exp. Med.*, 137, 1311, 1973.
108. **Cantor, H. and Gershon, R. K.,** Immunological circuits: cellular composition, *Fed. Proc.*, in press.
109. **Cantor, H., McVay-Boudreau, L., Hugenberger, J., Naidorf, K., Shen, F-W., and Gershon, R. K.,** Immunoregulatory circuits among T-cell sets. II. Physiological role of feedback inhibition in vivo: absence in NZB mice, *J. Exp. Med.*, 147, 1116, 1978.
110. **Hallgren, H. M. and Yunis, E. J.,** Suppressor lymphocytes in young and aged humans, *J. Immunol.*, 118, 2004, 1977.
111. **Antel, J. P., Weinrich, M., and Arnason, B. G. W.,** Circulating suppressor cells in man as a function of age, *Clin. Immunol. Immunopathol.*, 9, 134, 1978.
112. **Waldmann, T. A., Broder, S., Krakauer, R., MacDermott, R. P., Durm, M., Goldman, C., and Meade, B.,** The role of suppressor cells in the pathogenesis of common variable hypogammaglobulinemia and the immunodeficiency associated with myeloma, *Fed. Proc.*, 35, 2067, 1976.
113. **Moretta, L., Christina Migari, M., Webb, S. R., Pearl, E. R., Lydyard, P. M., Grossi, C. E., Lawton, A. R., and Cooper, M. D.,** Imbalance in T-cell subpopulations associated with immunodeficiency and autoimmune syndromes, *Eur. J. Immunol.*, 7, 696, 1977.
114. **Santoli, D., Moretta, L., Lisak, R., Gilden, D., Koprowski, H.,** Imbalances in T-cell subpopulations in multiple sclerosis patients, *J. Immunol.*, 120, 1369, 1978.
115. **Fujimoto, S., Greene, M. I., and Sehon, A. H.,** Regulation of the immune response to tumor antigens. I. Immunosuppressor cells in tumor bearing hosts, *J. Immunol.*, 116, 791, 1976.

116. **Greene, M. I., Dorf, M. E., Pierres, M., and Benacerraf, B.,** Reduction of syngeneic tumor growth by an anti-I-J alloantiserum, *Proc. Natl. Acad. Sci., U.S.A.,* 74, 5118, 1977.
117. **Perry, L. L., McClusky, R. T., Benacerraf, B., and Greene, M. I.,** Enhanced syngeneic tumor destruction by in vivo inhibition of suppressor cells using anti-I-J alloantiserum, *Am. J. Pathol.,* 92, 491, 1978.
118. **Gathings, W. E., Lawton, A. R., and Copper, M. D.,** Immunofluorescent studies of the developments of pre-B cells, B lympohcytes and immunoglobulin diversity in humans, *Eur. J. Immunol.,* 7, 804, 1977.
119. **Abney, E. R., Cooper, M. D., Kearney, J. F., Lawton, A. R., and Parkhouse, R. M. E.,** Sequential expression of immunoglobulin on developing mouse B lymphocytes: a systematic survey that suggests a model for the generation of immunoglobulin isotype diversity, *J. Immunol.,* 120, 2041, 1978.
120. **Norsal, G. J. V. and Pike, B. L.,** Mechanisms of clonal abortion tolerogenism. I. Response of immature hapten specific B lympohcytes, *J. Exp. Med.,* 148, 1161, 1978.
121. **Vitetta, E. S., Cambier, J. C., Kettman, J. R., Strober, S., Yuan, D., Zan-Bar, I., and Uhr, J. W.,** B-cell differentiation and murine IgD, in *Progress in Immunology,* Vol. 3, Mandel, T. E., Ed., 1977, 65.
122. **Mosier, D. E., Mond, J. T., and Goldings, E. A.,** The ontogeny of thymic independent antibody responses in vitro in normal mice and mice with an x-linked B-cell defect, *J. Immunol.,* 119, 1874, 1977.
123. **McIntosh, K. R. and Segre, D.,** B- and T-cell tolerance induction in young-adult and old mice, *Cell. Immunol.,* 27, 230, 1976.
124. **Callard, R. E., Basten, A., and Waters, L. K.,** Immune function in aged mice. II. B-cell function, *Cell. Immunol.,* 31, 26, 1977.
125. **Mason Smith, A.,** The effects of age on the immune response to type III pneumococcal polysaccharide (SIII) and bacterial lipopolysaccharide (LPS) in BALB/c, SJL/J and C3H mice, *J. Immunol.,* 116, 469, 1976.
126. **Kishimoto, S., Takahama, T., and Mizumachi, H.,** In vitro immune response to the 2,4,6-trinitrophenyl determinant in aged C57BL/6 mice: changes in the humoral immune response to avidity for the TNP determinant and responsiveness to LPS effect; with aging, *J. Immunol.,* 116, 294, 1976.
127. **Ada, G. L.,** Antigen binding cells in tolerance and immunity, *Transplant. Rev.,* 5, 105, 1970.
128. **Gerbase-De Lima, M., Wilkinson, J., Smith, G. S., and Walford, R. L.,** Age related decline in thymic independent immune function in a long lived mouse strain, *J. Gerontol.,* 29, 261, 1974.
129. **Somers, H. and Kuhns, W. J.,** Blood group antibodies in old age, *Proc. Soc. Exp. Biol. Med.,* 141, 1104, 1972.
130. **Ballieux, R. E., Heijnen, C. J., Uytdehaag, F., and Zegers, B. J. M.,** Regulation of B cell activity in man: role of T-cells, *Immunol. Rev.,* 45, 1, 1979.
131. **Perkins, E. M.,** Phagocytic activity of aged mice, *J. Reticuloendothel. Soc.,* 9, 642, 1971.
132. **Cantrell, W. and Elko, E. E.,** Effect of age on phagocytosis of carbon in the rat, *Exp. Paristolol.,* 34, 337, 1973.
133. **Heidrick, M. L.,** Age related changes in hydrolase activity of peritoneal macrophages, *Gerontolgist,* 12, 28, 1972.
134. **Heidrick, M. L. and Makinodan, T.,** Presence of impairment of humoral immunity in nonadherent spleen cells of old mice, *J. Immunol.,* 3, 1502, 1973.
135. **Perkins, E. H. and Makinodan, T.,** Nature of humoral immunologic deficiencies of the aged, in *Proc. 1st Rocky Mt. Symp. Ageing,* Colorado State University, Fort Collins, 1971, 80.
136. **Cowing, C., Schwartz, B. D., and Dickler, H. B,.** Macrophage Ia antigens. I. Macrophage populations differ in their expression of Ia antigens, *J. Immunol.,* 120, 378, 1978.
137. **Hodes, R. J., Ahmann, G. B., Hathcock, K. S., Dickler, H. B., and Singer, A.,** Cellular and genetic control of antibody responses in vitro. IV. Expression of Ia antigens on accessory cells required for responses to soluble antigens including a response under Ir gene control, *J. Immunol.,* 121, 1501, 1978.
138. **Steinman, R. M., Kaplan, G., Witmer, M. D., and Cohn, Z. A.,** Identification of a novel cell type in peripheral lymphoid organs of mice. V. Purification of spleen dendritic cells, new surface markers, and maintenance in vitro, *J. Exp. Med.,* 149, 1, 1979.
139. **Stingl, G., Katz, S. I., Clement, L., Green, I. and Schevach, E. M.,** Immunologic functions of Ia bearing epidermal langerhans cells, *J. Immunol.,* 121, 2005, 1978.
140. **Legge, J. S. and Austin, C. M,.** Antigen localization and the immune response as a function of age, *Aust. J. Exp. Biol. Med. Sci.,* 46, 361, 1968.
141. **Hayflick, L.,** The limited in vitro lifetime of human diploid cell strains, *Exp. Cell. Res.,* 37, 614, 1965.
142. **Albright, J. F. and Makinodan, T.,** Growth and senescence of antibody-forming cells, *J. Cell. Physiol.,* 67 (Suppl. 1), 185, 1966.

143. **Burnet, F. M.,** An immunological approach to ageing, *Lancet,* 2, 358, 1970.
144. **Weksler, M. E., Innes, J., Kuntz, M. M., and Inkeles, B.,** Cytokinetic basis of the impaired responses of lymphocytes from aged humans to plant lectins, *XIth International Congress Gerontology Symposia,* 1978, 120.
145. **Callard, R. E. and Basten, A.,** Immune function in aged mice. I. T-cell responsiveness using phytohemagglutinin as functional probe, *Cell. Immmunol.,* 31, 13, 1977.
146. **Gershon, H., Merhav, S., and Abraham, C.,** T-cell division and ageing, *Mech. Ageing Dev.,* 9, 27, 1979.
147. **Ben-zuri, A., Galili, U., Russell, A., and Schlessinger M.,** Age associated changes in subpopulations of human lympohcytes, *Clin. Immunol. Immunopathol.,* 7, 139, 1977.
148. **Hallgren, H. M., Kersey, J. H., Dubey, D. P., and Yunis, E. J.,** Lymphocyte subsets and integrated immune function in ageing humans, *Clin. Immunol. Immunopathol.,* 10, 65, 1978.
149. **Clot, J., Charmasson, E., and Brochier, J.,** Age dependent changes of human blood lympohcyte subpopulations, *Clin. Exp. Immunol.,* 32, 346, 1978.
150. **Shelton Earp, H., Utsinger, P. D., Yount, W. J., Logue, M., and Steiner, A. L.** Lymphocyte surface modulation and cyclic mycleotides. I. Topographic correlation of cyclic adenosine 3′:5′ monophosphate and Immunoglobulin immunofluorescence during lymphocyte capping, *J. Exp. Med,* 145, 1087, 1977.
151. **Kay, M. M. B.,** Effect of age on T-cell differentiation, *Fed. Proc.,* 37, 1241, 1978.
152. **Sprent, J.,** Recirculating Lymphocytes, in *The Lymphocyte, Structure and Function,* Marchelonis, J. J., Ed., Marcel Dekker, New York, 1977, 43.
153. **Miller, J. F. A. P.,** Effect of thymectomy in adult mice on immunological responsiveness, *Nature (London),* 208, 1337, 1965.
154. **Callard, R. E., Basten, A., and Blanden, R. B.,** Loss of immune competence with age: a qualitative abnormality in lympohcyte membranes, *Nature (London),* 281, 218, 1979.
155. **Gozes, Y., Umiel, T., Meshover, A., and Trainin, N.,** Syngeneic GvH induced in popliteal lymph nodes by spleen cells of old C57BL/6 mice, *J. Immunol.,* 121, 2199, 1978.
156. Gleichmann, E., Gleichmann, H., and Wilke, W., Autoimmunization and lymphomagensis in parent to F_1 combinations differing at the major histocompatibility complex: model for spontaneous disease caused by altered self antigens, *Trans. Rev.,* 31, 156, 1976.
157. **Woda, B. A. and Feldman, J. D.,** Density of surface immunoglobulin and capping on rat B lymphocytes. I. changes with ageing, *J. Exp. Med.,* 149, 416, 1979.
158. **Gabbioni, G., Chaponnier, C. Zumbe, A., and Vassali, P.,** Actin and tubulin co-cap with surface immunoglobilins in mouse B lymphocytes, *Nature (London),* 269, 697, 1977.
159. **Rivnay, B., Globerson, A., and Shinitzky, M.,** Viscosity of lymphocyte plasma-membrane in ageing mice and its possible relation to serum cholesterol, *Mech. Ageing Dev.,* 10, 71, 1979.
160. **Rivnay, B., Globerson, A., and Shinitzky, M.,** Perturbation of lympohcyte response to Concanavalin A by exogenous cholesterol and lecithin, *Eur. J. Immunol.,* 8, 185, 1978.
161. **Edinin, M.,** Lateral diffusion and the function of cell plasma membranes, *Progress in Immunology,* Vol. 3, Mandel, T. E., Cheers, T. E., Cheers, C., Mckenzie, I. F. C., and Nossal, G. J. V., Australian Academy Sciences, Canberra, 1979, 17.
162. **Heidrick, M. L.,** Imbalanced cyclic-AMP and cyclic-GMP levels in concanavalin-A stimulated spleen cells from aged mice, *J. Cell. Biol.,* 57, 139a, 1973.
163. **Smith, J. W., Steiner, A. L., Newberry, W. M., and Parker, C. W.,** Cyclic adenosine 3′5′ monophosphate in human lympohcytes. Alterations after phytohaemagglutinin stimulation, *J. Clin. Invest.,* 50, 432, 1971.
164. **Schramm, M., Orly, J., and Eimerl, S.,** Coupling of hormone receptors to adenylate cyclase of different cells by cell fusion *Nature (London),* 268, 310, 1977.
165. **Burnet, F. M.,** *Intrinsic Mutogenesis: A Genetic Approach to Ageing,* Medical and Technical Publ. St. Leonardgate, Lancaster, England, 1974.
166. **Orgel, L. E.,** Ageing of clones of mammalian cells, *Nature (London),* 243, 441, 1973.
167. **Melchers, F., Potter, M., and Warner, N. L., Eds.,** *Lympohcyte hybridomas. Current Topics in Microbiology and Immunology,* Springer-Verlag, New York, 1978, 81.
168. **Roberts-Thomson, I. C., Whittingham, S., Youngchaiyud, U., and Mackay, I. R.,** Ageing, immune response and mortality, *Lancet,* 2, 368, 1974.
169. **Murphy, D. B., Herzenberg, L. A., Okumura, K., Herzenberg, L. A., and McDevitt, H. O.,** A new I subregion (I-J) marked by a locus (Ia-4) controlling surface determinants on suppressor T lymphocytes, *J. Exp. Med.,* 144, 699, 1976.

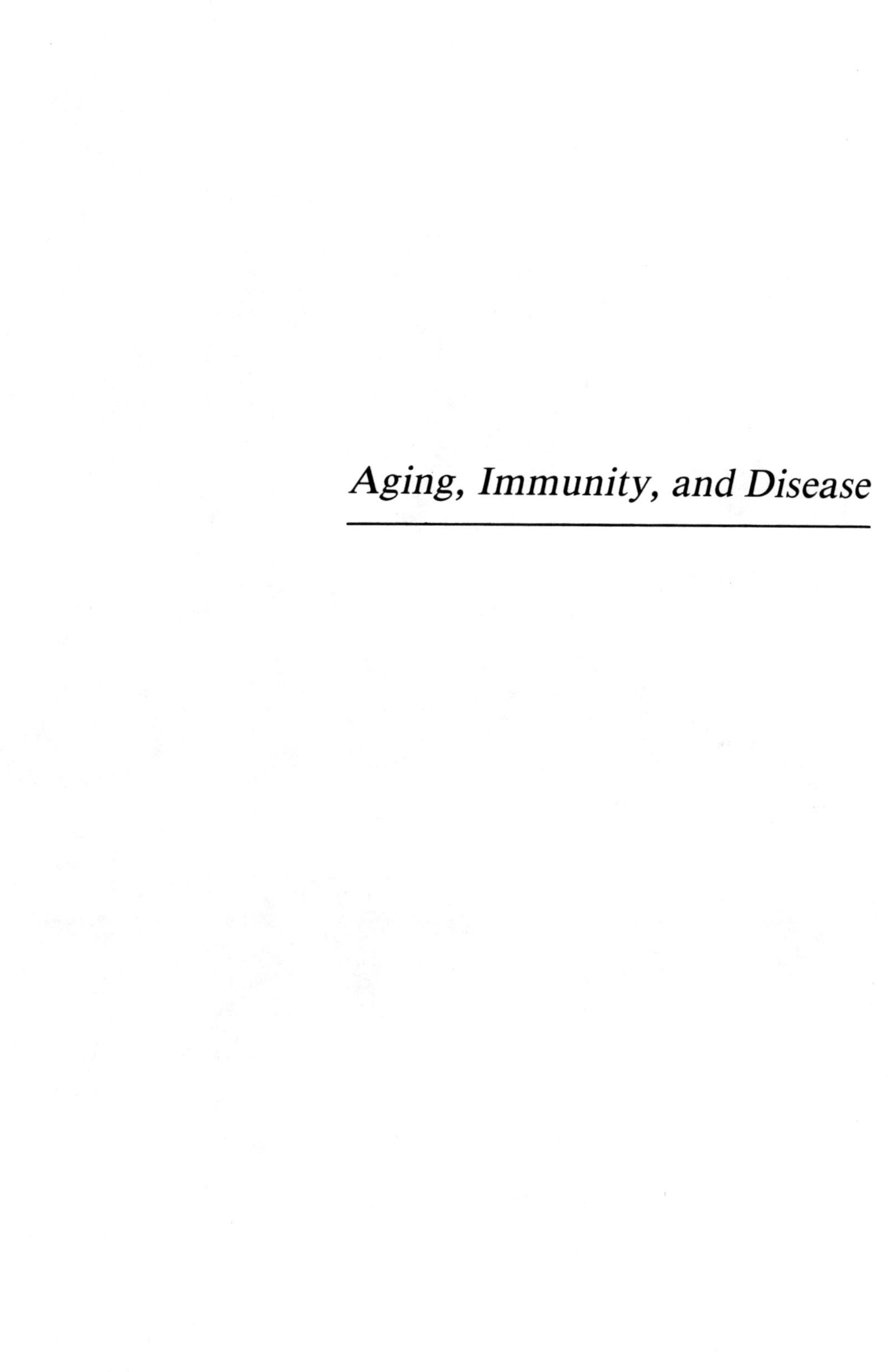

Aging, Immunity, and Disease

DIETARY RESTRICTIONS AND IMMUNE RESPONSES IN THE AGED

Ronald Ross Watson and David V. Safranski*

INTRODUCTION

For centuries man has recognized the association between malnutrition and disease. One compelling hypothesis that might explain, in part, the increased morbidity and mortality suffered by malnourished populations, is that nutritional deficiencies impair immune responsiveness, thus reducing antimicrobial protection in the nutritionally deprived.[1] On the other hand, nutritional intakes can be reduced in animals to enhance longevity by, in part, changing development of immune responses.[2] A major impediment to experimental approaches to test these hypotheses lies in the complexity of the nutritional and immunological aspects of the problem. Human malnutrition in different populations is most often both quantitatively and qualitatively distinct. It may include deficiencies in protein, calories, vitamins, and trace minerals, usually in a large variety of permuted combinations.[3] This fact makes direct comparisons difficult between different populations. Aging populations also have changes in their various immune systems which require that individuals be well aged-matched. The techniques commonly used to define nutritional status are often subjective and imprecise, and in many cases appropriate control values are unavailable. One related difficulty which prevents a critical evaluation of some of the human studies is the failure to distinguish between the various forms or degrees of malnutrition.

Worldwide protein-calorie malnutrition is the most common form of acquired immunodeficiency.[1,4] Most of the human studies to date have focused on severe protein-calorie malnutrition in hospitalized children.[1] While such children represent most dramatically the effects of nutritional deficiency on disease susceptibility, they comprise only a small percentage (3 to 5%) of malnourished children in most developing countries.[4,5] In contrast, up to 60% of all preschool children in many preindustrial societies may suffer from the milder forms of malnutrition.[5,6] Many aged humans in the U.S. who are undernourished have major contributing complications or causes of the nutritional stress including cancer, alcoholism, prolonged hospitalization, major illness, etc. A recent review shows that most studies of uncomplicated malnutrition and immunity involve young animals or children with maturing immune systems.[1] General conclusions and observations respecting the effects of various nutritional deficiencies on young immune systems are often instructive as similar data on aged animals and humans are sometimes lacking.[1] Key host defenses systems briefly reviewed are complement, secretory (mucosal) immunity, and cellular immunity.

IMMUNE SYSTEMS AFFECTED BY SHORT-TERM NUTRITIONAL STRESSES IN ADULT OR AGED INDIVIDUALS

Complement

The key role of the complement system in host resistance is amplification of other arms of the immune system; opsonization, phagocytosis, immune adherence, chemotaxis, and viral neutralization. Increased incidence and severity of disease has been associated with genetic deficiencies of complement components. Children with kwa-

* All correspondence for David V. Safranski should be sent to: Southern Illinois University, School of Dental Medicine, Carbondale, IL.

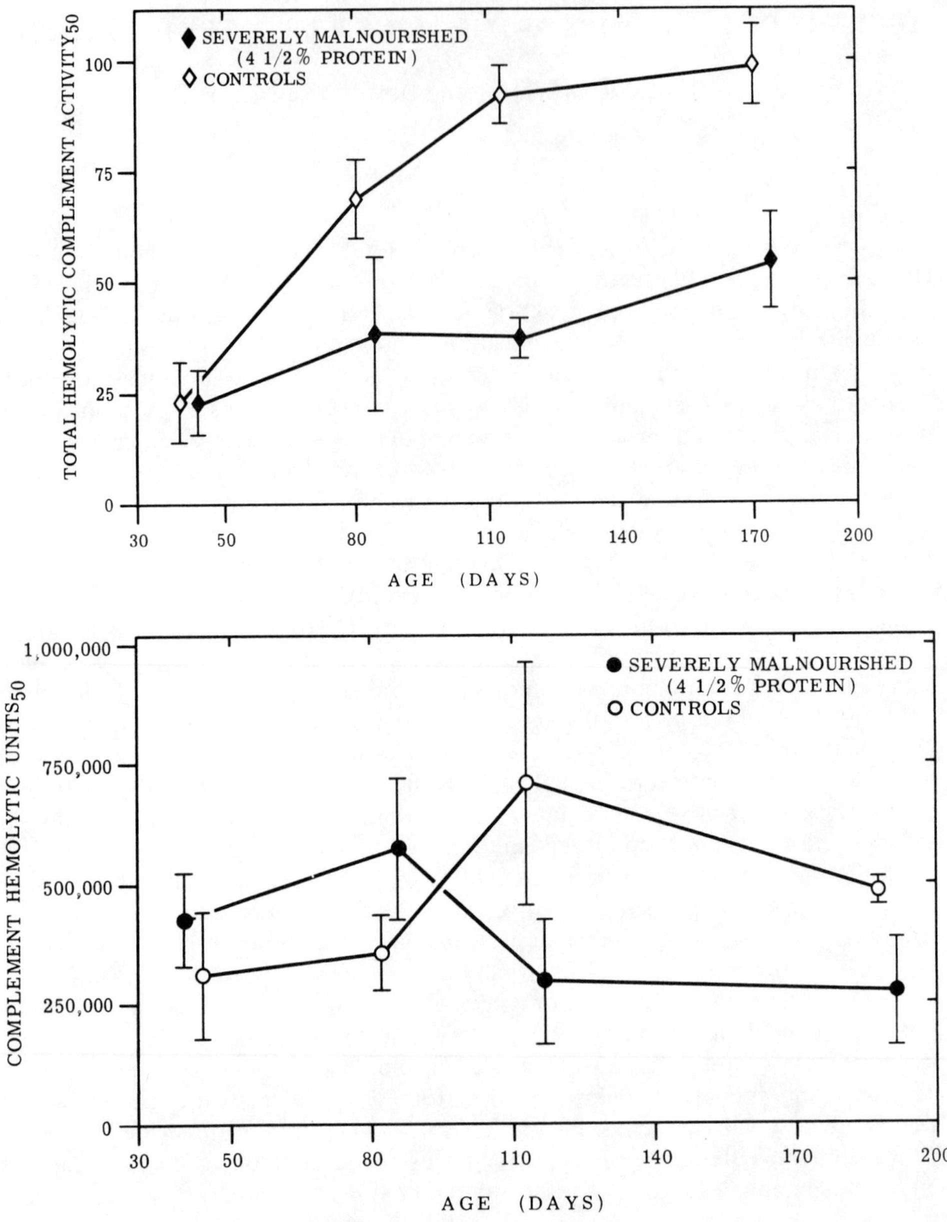

FIGURE 1. Changes in total hemolytic complement activity and C4 complement hemolytic units in normal and adult guinea pigs on a very low (4½%) protein diet. (From Peterson, B. H., Watson, R. R., and Holmes, D. H., © *J. Nutr.*, 110, 2159, 1980, American Institute of Nutrition. With permission.)

shiorkor and marasmus have increased incidence of infection and decreased complement levels.[1] Almost all studies of severely malnourished children or animals show a significant decrease in total hemolytic complement. For example, studies with protein-calorie malnourished Columbian children[6] and Thai[7] children showed a decrease in C_3, but not C_4. In mature adult guinea pigs a 4½% protein diet caused a suppression of total hemolytic complement (Figure 1) and C_2 (Figure 2), but not C_4 or C_8.[8] These results are similar to young rats fed a low protein diet beginning at weaning.[8] C_3 levels in aged (26 months) BALB/C mice fed either 4% or 0% protein diet were not significantly suppressed (Watson, Safranski, and Putt — unpublished data).[77]

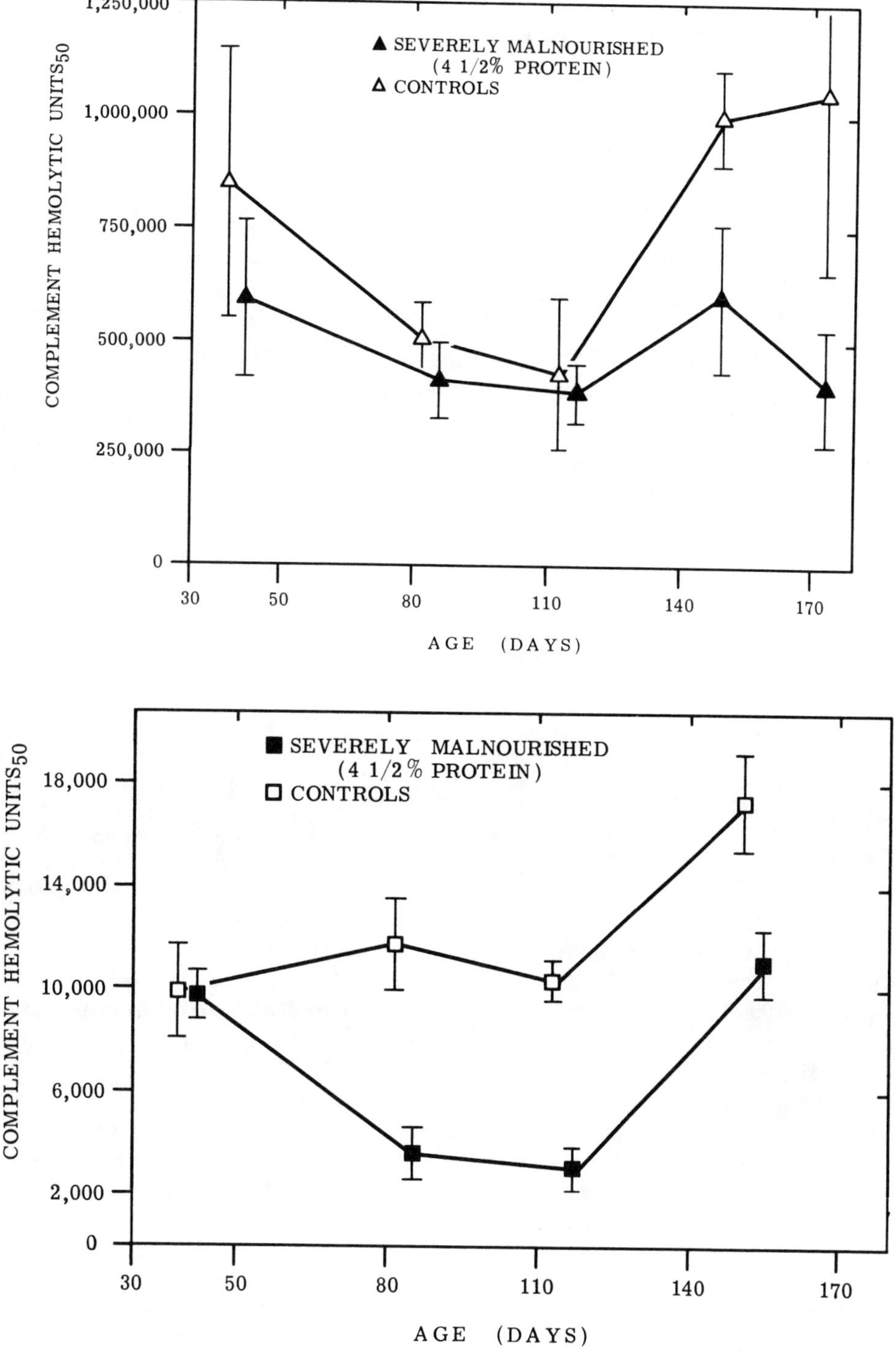

FIGURE 2. Changes in total hemolytic complement (C8 and C2) units in normal and adult guinea pigs on a very low (4½%) protein diet. (From Peterson, B. H., Watson, R. R., and Holmes, D. H.,© *J, Nutr.*, 110, 2159, 1980, American Institute of Nutrition. With permission.)

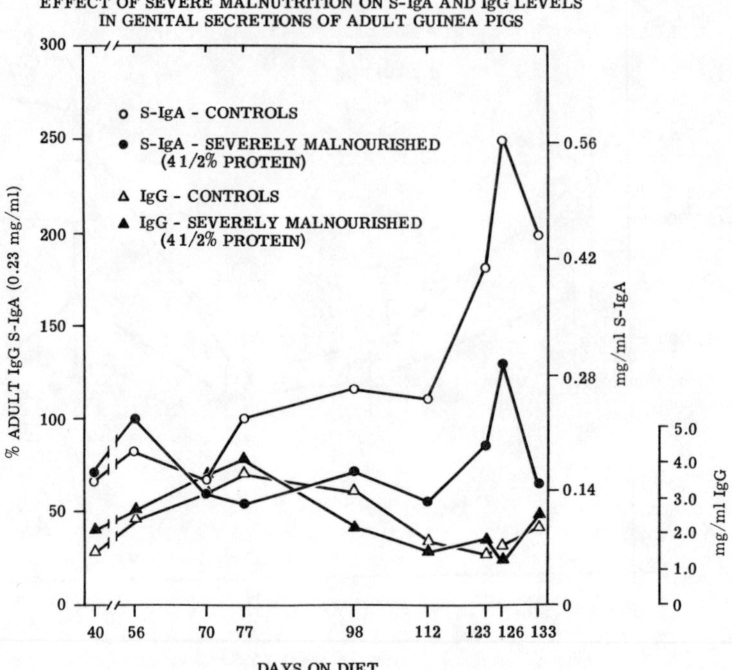

FIGURE 3. Effect of severe malnutrition on IgA and IgG levels in genital secretions of adult guinea pigs.

Secretory Immunity

Secretory immunity includes secretion flow, S-IgA (secretory immunoglobulin A), IgG, lysozyme, mucosal cellular immunity, and lactoperoxidase.[9] Very little is known about the effects of various types of nutritional stress on secretory host defense.[9,10] Recently, protein undernutrition has been shown to suppress significantly the secretion of lysozyme into tears of children.[9-11] The synthesis and secretion into tears of other locally produced proteins, S-IgA and amylase, was also impaired.[11] In severely protein undernourished Thai,[12] Indian,[13] and Colombian[14] children, the levels of S-IgA in secretions was found to be significantly reduced (35 to 50%) while IgG levels were unaffected.

Nasopharyngeal S-IgA antibodies to live attenuated polio virus vaccine and measles virus vaccine were very low or undetectable[13] in some malnourished Indian children with severe protein-calorie malnutrition. The reduced anti-measles S-IgA response could be due to decreased transportation of S-IgA antibodies into the secretions or a poorer response to the viral antigens by reduced production of the IgA antibodies. A current review[1] of the literature revealed no publication relating to secretory immunity in undernourished, aged humans, and only one publication in mature animals. Vaginal S-IgA, tear S-IgA but not vaginal IgG were suppressed by moderate (9%) as well as severe (4¼%) protein malnutrition (Figure 3) in mature guinea pigs.[15]

Cell-Mediated Immune Responses

Severe malnutrition in young animals and children is associated with profound impairment of cell-mediated immune functions.[1] Both the number and functional capability of T lymphocytes are markedly reduced, as is the delayed hypersensitivity response to antigens and sensitizing chemicals.[16,17] In general, the severity of immunological impairment parallels the severity of the nutritional deficiency.[16-27] Preliminary evidence supports the hypothesis that severe nutritional deficiencies interfere with lymphokine production by T lymphocytes and may alter the T lymphocyte subpopulations which have a suppressor function.[1] In addition, the efficacy of vaccines which stimulate primarily a cell-mediated immunity (e.g., BCG — an attenuated strain of microbacteria tuberculosae) may be impaired in severely malnourished vacinees.

In adults or aged humans the studies which have been done are usually complicated by surgery, cancer, and/or disease, in addition to malnutrition.[1] In contrast to malnourished children, protein malnutrition in adults hospitalized following surgery caused no significant changes in numbers of blood lymphocytes.[1,27] However the number of T-cells was higher than in well-nourished controls. Others have not observed a change in T-cell numbers.[25] In 12 adult patients with less than 85% of standard weight-height ratio and normal serum albumin (adult marasmus), in vitro measures of cellular immunity were not affected, while in vivo ones were.[25] The expression of intradermal skin test to candidin and streptokinase-streptodornase was suppressed. This may be caused by changes in expression of the inflammatory response which is inferred to occur in children[18] since lymphocyte transformation by B-cell and T-cell mitogens was normal.[25] Similar experiments in mature animals show a suppression in cellular immune responses. However, like the studies in adult humans, the mature cellular immune systems are more resistant to nutritional stress.[1] For example, female BALB/c mice at 5 or 6 (immature), and 35 weeks of age (mature) have been placed on isocaloric nonrestricted (20% protein) control or restricted (4% protein) experimental diets.[24] A significant decline in percentages of cell-mediated immune responses (θ-bearing cell percentages, phytohemagglutinin [PHA], induced mitogenesis, mixed lymphocyte reaction [MLR]) occurred as early as 2 weeks for the immature mice on the restricted diet. Suppression continued for up to 8 weeks before returning to near control values.

In mature, protein restricted mice, there were no significant changes in θ-cell numbers or spleen per body weight ratios. Protein restriction also did not influence θ-bearing cell percentages, but did suppress PHA and MLR responses after 6 weeks (Figure 4). A significant suppression of antibody-dependent cellular cytotoxic (ADCC) responses was also noted after 16 weeks on the diet.[24]

The mature mice were much more resistant to changes in the parameters tested. The transient reductions that occurred in PHA and MLR responses were not due to declines in θ cell numbers, but to some suppressive effect induced by the diet. The decrease in ADCC responses at 16 and 17 weeks can also be attributed to diet induced suppression. Developing cellular immune systems of immature mice are more sensitive to moderate protein restriction (i.e., immunosuppression occurs after a shorter interval) than those of mature mice.

ENHANCEMENT OF CELLULAR IMMUNITY AND/OR LONGEVITY BY DIETARY RESTRICTION

Undernutrition is often associated with increased incidence and/or severity of many bacterial, viral, and parasitic diseases.[3] It is well-documented[3,21] that the life span of children, young animals, as well as adults are *decreased* when severely stressed by low protein or severe vitamin deficiencies. This appears to be caused, in large part, by immunosuppression induced by diet. Much less is known about the effects of marginal undernutrition, which is extremely prevalent worldwide. Several studies have recently shown an *enhancement* of cellular immunity in mature animals fed *ad libitum* a low protein (8%) diet.[22,23] In one study alveolar macrophages but not the polymorphonuclear leukocytes (PMN) from marginally malnourished adult guinea pigs and rats had more superoxide dismutase activity.[22] An explanation for the increase in superoxide

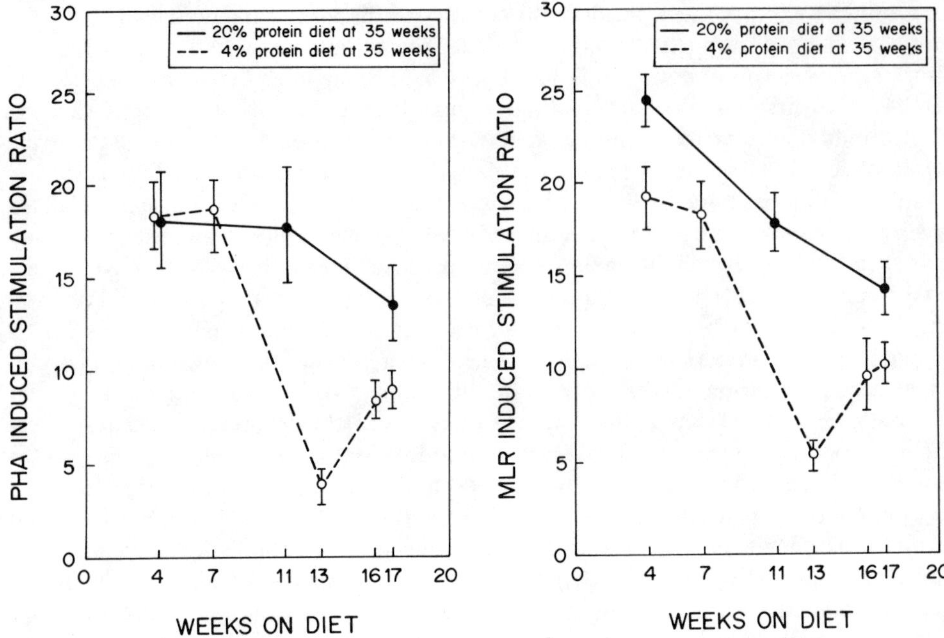

FIGURE 4. Changes by low protein diet in phytohemagglutinin (PHA) responses of mature BALB/c mice. (left panel) Changes caused by a low protein diet in the mixed lymphocyte reaction (MLR) reponses of mature BALB/C mice. (From Watson, R. R. and Haffer, K., *Mech. Ageing Dev.*, 12, 269, 1980. With permission.)

dismutase activity of the alveolar macrophages in chronic protein insufficiency, may be due to an activation by lymphocytes. It has also been shown that marginally malnourished mice fed an 8% protein diet from weaning had increased cellular immunity as measured by graft-vs.-host reaction, lymphocyte transformation, and skin graft rejection.[23] In addition, peritoneal marcophages from mice suffering from chronic protein insufficiency engulfed *Listeria monocytogenes* at a significantly greater rate than controls.[23] It is assumed that the macrophages of these mice were activated due to an absolute increase in T-cell population and increased immunocompetence of effector T-cells stimulated by the increased numbers of other pathogens found in the malnourished animals.[22,23] Dietary protein fed to weaning guinea pigs must be below 3% for a prolonged period of time to reduce T-cell function measured by skin test response in mycobacterium immunized guinea pigs.[22] Others have shown that early or lifelong moderate dietary restrictions often increases longevity in laboratory animals. The fact that the life span of experimental animals can be extended is also well-documented.[29-43] Dietary regimes of restricted intakes of total food,[29-32] protein,[33-36] amino acids,[37] calories,[38-40] as well as variations in the proportion and level of protein and carbohydrate[41-43]intake beginning at weaning, have been shown to reduce age-specific morbidity and mortality rates. Following the discovery of this phenomenon, current research has been directed toward elucidating possible mechanisms and completely understanding the full potential of dietary manipulations of longevity.

The addition of the aging parameter to the long-term interactions between undernutrition, disease, and immunity has been studied with difficulty. As the organism ages, there occurs an overall decline in immune capabilties, accompanied by an increased incidence of inappropriate responses directed toward the self.[44-46] Mouse strains genetically predetermined to develop autoimmune diseases provide an ideal subject as their life span is severely reduced and can be more conveniently studied. For example, Fernandes and co-workers[53] have used nutritionally stressed female C3H/UMC mice and reduced the incidence of spontaneous mammary carcinomas from 70% in the controls to 0%. The undernourished mice were aliquoted food, that if shared equally, would yield a 40% caloric reduction as compared to *ad libitum* fed controls. B-cell response to lipopolysaccharides (LPS) and the number of plaque forming cells (PFC) in the spleen were the same in both groups, while T-cell proliferative responses to PHA, concanavalin A (Con A), and LPS were increased in the undernourished group. The caloric restrictions in this case did not significantly lengthen life span, although the longest surviving mice were on the restricted diet. Visscher and co-workers[54] also found a significant reduction in tumors from 63% in the controls to 0% in C_3H mice fed about 50% of the calories of controls. Body weight was reduced and the percent survival at 16 months was increased in the undernourished animals. NZB mice which are genetically predisposed to autoimmune hemolytic anemia were also benefited by a low protein (6% casein), isocaloric diet.[55] On the low protein diet (5 g/day), total body and spleen weights of 7- to 10-months-old animals were considerably lower, while the thymus glands were over two times larger than controls. The undernourished mice had improved cellular immunologic capabilities in the form of an increased ability to mediate graft-vs.-host reactions and more vigorous cell-mediated killer cell immunity after immunization against DBA/2 mastocytoma cells. The normal decline with age of PHA and Con A responsiveness was abrogated by the low protein. Certain humoral immunologic conditions also improved with a more vigorous antibody production to sheep red blood cells. However this low protein diet did not extend life span of the NZB mice. On the other hand, a diet relatively low in fat and high in protein[56] showed increases in life span and immune competence when fed to NZB mice.

However, Fernandes et al.[57] have also shown NZB mice fed *ad libitum* a diet relatively high in fat and low in protein suffer an increased incidence of autoimmune hemolytic anemia and corresponding decline in longevity. Surprisingly, males on the high fat/low protein diet had a significantly shorter life span than males on the low fat/high protein diet. Females showed no difference.

In another related study, an increase in life span of (NZB × NZW) F1 hybrid mice (which develop a systemic lupus erythematosis-like immune complex nephropathy) was obtained by restricting caloric intake.[58] Controls were given 5 g per mouse per day and 50% caloric restriction was accomplished by feeding 2.5 g per mouse per day. A similar phenomenon was found by restricting dietary phenylalanine and tyrosine.[59] Gardner, et al.[60] did experiments to show that the improvement in longevity of the "diet-cured" (NZB × NZW) F1 mouse was apparently unrelated to the production of endogenous type C virus (implicated as the disease causing agent) or a reduction in host response (measured as antibody titer to the virus).

Jose et al.[61] and Walford et al.,[62] working with C57BL/6J female mice, provide some tangible evidence supporting the theory that dietary restriction causes a delay in maturation of the immune system and hence enhances longevity. Walford et al.[62] fed 3.5 g of food (21.5% casein, 14.5 calories) 4 days a week followed by a triple portion, while the restricted mice were fed 3.5 g of the same diet (enriched in vitamins and salts) twice a week with a double proportion on the weekend. Body weights and spleen indexes for mice restricted 18 weeks and 55-weeks-old were significantly lower than controls. In a comparison of the number of IgM and IgG plaque forming cells produced in response to SRBC, 17- to 18-week-old mice on the restricted diet were similar but the antibody responses were diminished. However at 52-weeks-old, while still showing a similar response curve and peak response at the same day, the malnourished mice had the greater number of PFCs. Response of spleen cells by 17-week-old and 52-week-old mice to PHA and PWM was similar in pattern to above, while the Con

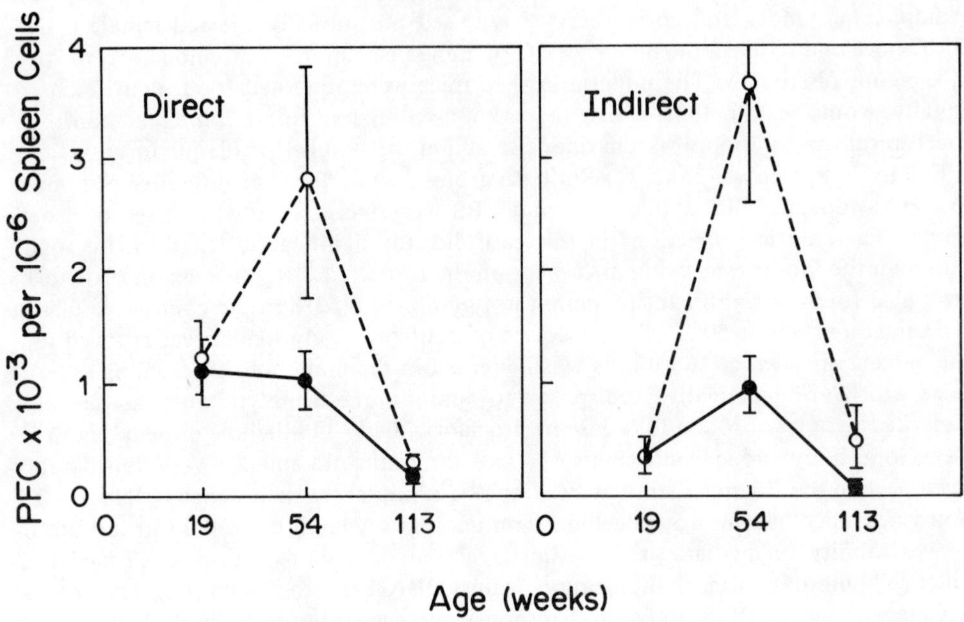

FIGURE 5. Population 1: PFC against SRBC at the peak of the response, in the spleens of restricted (O) or nonrestricted (●) mice at three different ages (Y = 18 to 20 weeks; M = 52 to 55 weeks, and 0 = 108 to 118 weeks). (A) Direct PFC per 10^6 spleen cells. (B) Direct PFC per spleen. (C) Indirect PFC per 10^6 spleen cells. (D) Indirect PFC per spleen. Each point represents the mean value of 5 to 8 animals. Vertical bars represent 2 SE, as in Gerbase-DeLima et al.[63]

A response was reduced at 17 weeks in the nutritionally restricted or stressed mice and only approached control values by 52 weeks. By 108 to 118 weeks of age, both dietary groups showed a considerable drop in the number of PFCs, although restricted animals manifested a slightly higher response.[63] Proliferative stimulation by PHA, Con A, and PWM was significantly higher in the old, restricted group (Figures 5 and 6). Lymphocyte transformation caused by LPS and PPD were not significantly different between controls and long-term dietary restriction. Mean life span and tenth level survivorship were the same for both groups, however, the longest living survivors were greater in the restricted group (187 vs. 163 weeks).

Gerbase-DeLima et al.[63] worked with a second population of individually caged C57 BC/6J mice which were restricted both before and after weaning. Control mice were kept five to a mother until weaning, and put on a diet of 21.6% protein, 14.5 calories, 3 to 5 g/day.[62] Restricted animals were kept nine to a mother and separated from the mother every other day. This feeding regime was continued post weaning as described briefly above.[62] Body weight, spleen weight, and spleen index were significantly lower in the restricted group as compared to controls. In response to B-cell mitogens (PWM and LPS) and T-cell mitogens (PHA, Con A, and PPD), spleen cells from restricted mice 31-weeks-old were significantly lower than controls. By 56 weeks of age the restricted group's lymphocyte transformation responses approached those of the controls, and by 75 weeks of age, the nutritionally restricted animals had significantly higher responses to each mitogen. In a study of skin allograft survival, no significant difference was present between different ages of the control mice. Within the restricted group, ability to reject skin graft significantly, improved from 24- to 28-weeks-old to 44- to 60-weeks-old and reached control levels by 68 weeks. The two groups did not differ in mean survivorship, however tenth decile survivorship was greater in the restricted groups.[2]

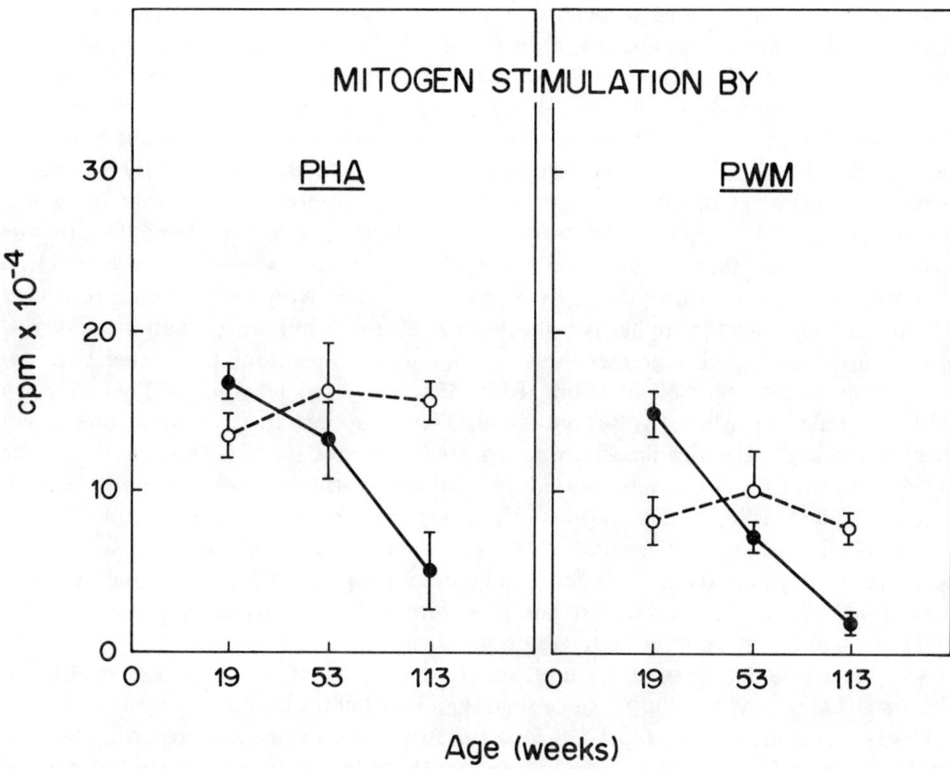

FIGURE 6. Population 1: tritiated thymidine uptake of PHA, con-A and PWM stimulated spleen cells from mice of three different ages (Y = 18 to 20 weeks; M = 52 to 55 weeks; 0 = 108 to 118 weeks) on restricted (○) or nonrestricted (●) diets since weaning. Each point represents the mean value of 10 to 12 mice. Vertical bars represent 2 SE, as in Gerbase-DeLima et al.[63]

Weindruch and co-workers[2] in an extremely comprehensive project manipulated unique dietary regimes in an effort to more thoroughly understand nutritional effect on longevity and immunity. Female (C57BL/10Sn × C_3H/HeDiSn)F1, referred to as B10C_3F, were individually caged and distinguished by the following dietary regimens; Purina® Lab Chow *ad libitum* (N/N), normal preweaning with post weaning, restricted post weaning (R/N), restricted preweaning, normal post weaning (R/R), restricted pre- and post-weaning. Each diet manifests a different life span, and longest-lived survivorship. Generally, the *ad libitum* and N/N diets showed the shortest life span with all restricted groups surviving longer. The most severely restricted group R/R maintained a survival advantage over the rest.[63] The data indicate lifelong dietary restrictions lead to more immunologically youthful animals.[63] Interestingly, the advantage seen by restricted BIOC_3Fl mice occurs much earlier in life than in C57BL/6J mice.[63] The BIOC_3Fl hybrid does not suffer the early life immunosuppression that befell the C57BL/6J. Weindruch and co-workers[2] see it as a potential strain difference, but indicate that increased survival with underfeeding, cannot always be regarded as a simple maturational effect.

The second population of female BIOC3Fl mice in this study[2] were fed diets differing only in calories: Normal (N), Diet A, (20% casein) fed just below *ad libitum* levels to produce "normally" fed mice; Restricted 28 (R28), Diet B, (28% casein) fed to allow only 70% calories of N; Restricted 35 (R35), Diet C, (35% casein) fed only 60% cal, but the same protein as N; Normal/Restricted 35 (N/R 35), fed Diet A for 1 week post weaning, and switched to Diet C until 8-months-old, then all animals were sacrificed. All deficient diets caused a reduction in body and spleen weights, and spleen indexes as compared to controls. The pattern of change of thymic indexes were opposite that of spleen indexes. At 6-weeks-old, R35 thymus glands were one seventh the weight of N mice, although by 16 weeks, N thymuses lost weight while R35 gained so that no significant differences were observed between the two groups. By 6 months, thymic weights of N and R35 mice were still the same although R35 thymic index was larger. Group R28 thymic weights were comparable at 6 months to N and R35; thymic indexes were larger than N and comparable to R35. At 6 to 7 weeks of age, R35 spleen cells were stimulated more than N by Con A and PHA. At 6 months, both restricted groups had significantly higher lymphocyte transformation indexes than the controls, with R35 responses being greater than R2. Again immunostimulation rather than immunosuppression occurred in young BIOC3F1 compared to young C57BL/6 when both are undernourished. At 8-months-old, T-cell response to PHA and Con A were measured and the diets ranked in order of greatest stimulation: N/R35, R28, N. The B-cell mitogen LPS at this age showed the reverse situation as far as lymphocyte stimulation: N/R35, R28, N. The various dietary groups showed no difference in response to the B-cell mitogens PPD, and PWM, between 4 and 6 months of age. Rectal temperatures were taken weekly between 4 and 6 months of age. All restricted diets showed lower body temperatures relative to controls, with N/R35 significantly cooler than R35 and both significantly cooler than R28 or N.

The third population in this study[2] involved male BIOC3F1 mice 1-year-old, fed Purina® Lab Chow *ad libitum* since weaning. The dietary groups were established as follows: Control animals, fed Diet A, *ad libitum*; low caloric diet receiving 94 cal/week of Diet B for 1 months, then lowered to 75 cal/week of Diet C; low calorie-low protein diet given the same number of calories as the low calorie group, but only 55% of the protein. This group was fed Diet B, except with a 15% casein content for 1 month, then switched to a modified Diet C (18.7% casein). Body temperature was similar between all groups. Spleen weight and indexes between underfed groups did not differ, although within both diets parameters were smaller than controls. Both restricted groups demonstrated greater proliferative abilities when stimulated by PHA, Con A, PWM, and MLR relative to controls; LPS and PPD equally stimulated all groups. This suggests dietary restrictions instituted after weaning can also aid in improving immune response.

Similar studies in humans are very difficult. However, there is some indication in humans that if the nutritional stress is early and severe enough, impairment of CMI responses may persist for several years. Dutz and co-workers[74,75] studied the delayed hypersensitivity response to dinitrochlorobenzene in orphans who had been severely malnourished and infected during early infancy and found significant depression of cellular immunity up to 5 years later, at a time when all were free of intercurrent disease and were well-nourished.[72-75] This may be preliminary evidence of retarded maturation of human immune system. Another recent study in Colombian children severely malnourished later in life showed a rapid restoration of cellular and secretory immunity a few weeks after initiation of a high protein diet.[76]

Clearly immunological processes basic and vital to the living organism can be manipulated and controlled by nutrition. Functions such as growth,[30,31,38,39] health,[9,65] malignancies and tumor development,[40,66,67] enzyme activity,[38,65] longevity,[55-58] and the immune response[2,61-63] have all shown a dependence on diet. The interrelationship between longevity, immunity, and diet is very complex. Changes have been indicated to be dependent on how much food is allowed, components of the diet, age, the animal is started on a diet, and duration of dietary manipulation. The first group research described above is based on two different systems; mouse strains manifesting spontaneous autoimmune diseases or cancers, and the second group, normal strains not predisposed to such malfunctions. Any explanation of the results discussed must be comprehensive enough to encompass both situations.

The results of studies involving autoimmune strains of mice can be summarized as follows: the age of onset of the disease was delayed, life span extended, and certain immune responses improved. It has been suggested that these improvements are a function of disease treatment by nutritional measures. The question remains whether processes fundamental to aging are being manipulated.[2] At least for the (NZB × NZW) F1 mouse, Gardner and co-workers[60] indicated that the disease process, i.e., production of the virus or antibodies against the virus, was unaffected. Poffenholz[67] correlating DNA repair rates of embryonic fibroblasts, to life span adds support to the idea that mice susceptible to autoimmune diseases undergo accelerated aging. Considering that in autoimmune strains of mice the disease always appears at a certain point in its life, or aging process, it follows that any agent that can slow the aging process can affect the incidence of the disease or for that matter any age-related functional change. Ross[41] also has evidence in agreement with this theory. He demonstrates a correlation between life span and activity levels of certain hepatic enzymes in the rat. When the age associated enzyme activity patterns were modified by dietary means, there were corresponding modifications in life span.

Generally, the studies involving normal mice indicate an increase in life span and immune capabilities during long periods of undernutrition. Some of this may be due to increased bacterial antigens stimulating some cellular immune systems (phagocytosis).[22,23] In addition, the increase in immune response in undernourished animals is described by Walford et al.[62] and Gerbase-DeLima[63] as being due to a delay in maturation of the immune response mediated by the dietary restrictions (Figure 7). Combining both theories, undernourishing the animal will cause a delay in the maturation of the immune system, thereby delaying the onset of the aging process as described by Walford,[68] allowing the animal to continue functionally sound. An animals life span is defined in genetic terms, and excluding death from disease, or accident, the animal will fulfill this potential. Considering the life span of an animal as finite, with immune system intrinsically involved, according to Walford,[62,68] from the point of maturation of the immune system, there is a predetermined amount of time before it begins to dysfunction, ultimately causing death. The length of life from the maturation of the immune system is limited by the immune system and depends on its own gradual loss of ability to recognize self.

The lifetime of an animal can be considered as a numberline with the immune system as a subset of this line. The end of the line (or the end of life) is determined by the midpoint of the subset (or the maturation of the immune system). Dietary restrictions cause the subset to shift down the numberline, and correspondingly extend its length, or if the dietary restrictions are severe enough, decrease it due to increased disease. No matter if delayed or not, once the immune system begins to malfunction, the aging process begins, and death due to any number of situations can occur.

ACKNOWLEDGMENTS

We recognize the support of the National Livestock and Meat Board and Wallace Genetic Foundation, for some of our research which stimulated this review. Purdue University Experiment Station Journal paper 7688.

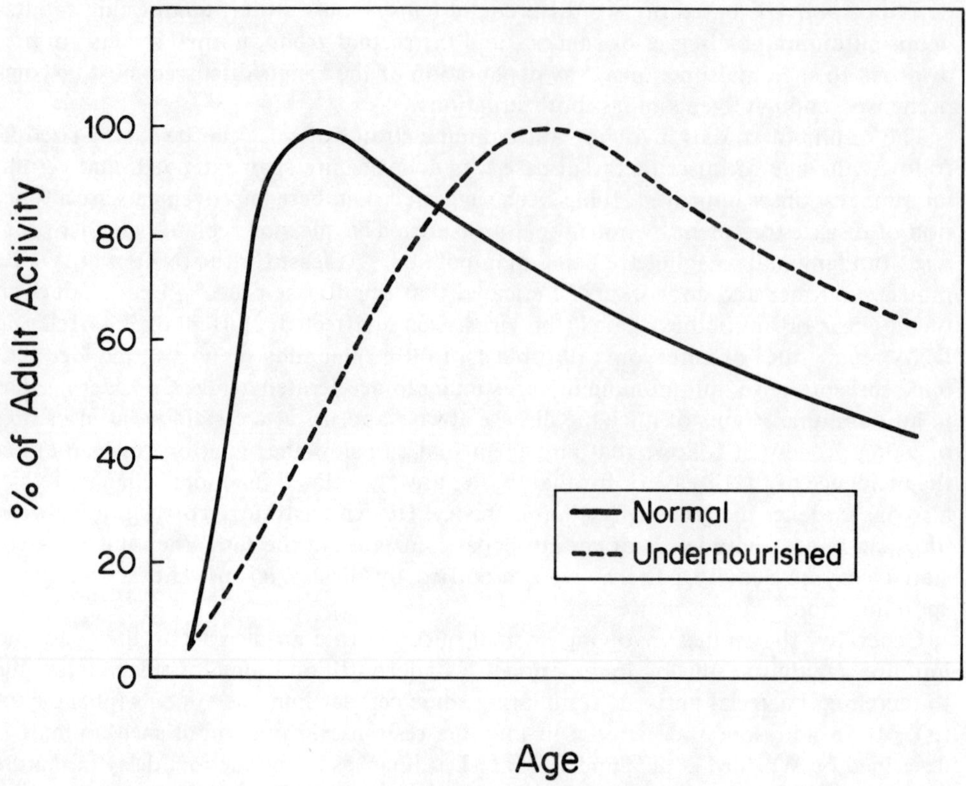

FIGURE 7. Schematic interpretation of the reversal effect. Solid curve represents immune response of mice on nonrestricted diet. If the restricted diet delays maturation of immune response capacity, then young restricted mice would show a decreased and older mice an increased reactivity compared to controls, as in Walford et al.[62]

REFERENCES

1. **Watson, R. R. and McMurray, D. N.**, Effects of malnutrition on secretory and cellular immunity, in *CRC Crit. Rev. Food Sci. Nutr.*, 12(2), 113, 1979.
2. **Weindruch, R. H., Kristie, A., Chevey, K. E., and Walford, R. L.**, Influence of controlled dietary restriction on immunologic function and aging, *Fed. Proc.*, 38, 2007, 1979.
3. **Scrimshaw, N. S., Taylor, C. E., and Gordon, J. E.**, Interactions of nutrition and infection, *WHO Monogr. Ser.*, 57, 3, 1968.
4. Nutritional Evaluation of the Population of Central America and Panama (1972): Regional Summary, INCAP and Nutrition Program, Center for Disease Control, Publ. No. HSM 72-8120, U.S. Department of Health, Education and Welfare, Washington, D.C.
5. Joint FAO/WHO Expert Committee on Nutrition, Food fortification, Protein-Calorie Malnutrition WHO Tech. Rep. Ser. No. 477, World Health Organization, Geneva, 1971.
6. **McMurray, D. N., Reyes, M. A., and Watson, R. R.**, Secretory immunoglobulins and enzymes in severely malnourished Colombian children during nutritional restoration, *Fed. Proc.*, 36, 1171, 1977, submitted.
7. **Sirisinha, S., Suskind, R., Edelman, R., Charupatana, C., and Olson, R. E.**, Complement and C3 proactivator levels in children with protein-calorie malnutrition and effect of dietary treatment, *Lancet*, 1, 1016, 1973.

8. **Peterson, B. H., Watson, R. R., and Holmes, D. H.,** Protein malnutrition and complement activity in guinea pigs, germ free and conventional rats, *J. Nutr.,* 110, 2159, 1980.
9. **Watson, R. R., Reyes, M. A., and McMurray, D. N.,** Influence of malnutrition on the concentration of IgA, lysozyme, amylase, and aminopeptidase in children's tears, *Proc. Soc. Exp. Biol. Med.,* 157, 57, 1978.
10. **Tomasi, T. B., Jr.,** Secretory immunoglobulins, *N. Engl. J. Med.,* 287, 500, 1972.
11. **McMurray, D. N., Rey, V., Casazza, L. J., and Watson, R. R.,** Effect of moderate malnutrition on concentrations of immunoglobulins and enzymes in tears of young Colombian children, *Am. J. Clin. Nutr.,* 30, 1944, 1977.
12. **Sirisinha, S., Edelman, R., Asvapaka, C., and Olson, R. E.,** Secretory and serum IgA in children with protein-calorie malnutrtion, *Pediatrics,* 55, 166, 1975.
13. **Chandra, R. K.,** Reduced secretory antibody response to live attenuated measles and poliovirus vaccines in malnourished children, *Br. Med. J.,* 2, 583, 1975.
14. **McMurray, D. N., Rey, H., Casazza, L. J., and Watson, R. R.,** Influence of malnutrition on secretory immunity in chidren, *Fed. Proc.,* 35, 588, 1976.
15. **Watson, R. R., Horton, R. G., and Clinton, J. M.,** Suppression of secretory IgA antibodies in protein malnourished guinea pigs following chlamydial eye and vaginal infection, *Fed. Proc.,* 36, 1251, 1977.
16. **Geefhuysen, J., Rosen, E. U., Katz, J., Ipp, T., and Metz, J.,** Impaired cellular immunity in kwashiorkor with improvement after therapy, *Br. Med. J.,* 4, 527, 1971.
17. **Chandra, R. K.,** Immunocompetence in undernutrition, *J. Pediatr.,* 81, 1194, 1972.
18. **Edelman, R., Suskind, R., Olson, R. E., and Sirisinha, S.,** Mechanisms of defective delayed cutaneous hypersensitivity in children with protein-calorie malnutrition, *Lancet,* 1, 506, 1973.
19. **Abbassy, A. S., Badr El-din, M. K., Hassan, A. I., Aref, G. H., Hammad, S. A., El-Araby, I. I. Badr El-din, A. A., Soliman, M. H., and Hussein, M.,** Studies of cell-mediated immunity and allergy in protein energy malnutrition. I. Cell-mediated delayed hypersensitivity, *J. Trop. Med. Hyg.,* 77, 13, 1974.
20. **Chandra, R. K.,** Rosette-forming T lymphocytes and cell-mediated immunity in malnutrition, *Br. Med. J.,* 3, 608, 1974.
21. **Watson, R. R. and Weinberg, E.,** Effect of nutritional factors on microbial pathogenicity, in *CRC Handbook Series in Nutrition and Food,* Recheigl, M., Jr., Ed., CRC Press, Boca Raton, Fla., 1979, accepted for publication.
22. **Watson, R. R., Rister, M., and Baehner, R. L.,** Superoxide dismutase activity in polymorphonuclear leukocytes and alveolar macrophages of protein malnouished rats and guinea pigs, *J. Nutr.,* 106, 1801, 1976.
23. **Cooper, W. C., Good, R. A., and Mariani, T.,** Effect of protein insufficiency on immune responsiveness, *Am. J. Clin. Nutr.,* 27, 647, 1974.
24. **Watson, R. R. and Haffer, K.,** Modification of cell-mediated immune responses by moderate dietary protein stress in immunologically immature, mature Balb/c mice, *Mech. Ageing Dev.,* 12, 269, 1980.
25. **Bistrian, B. R., Serman, M., Blackburn, G. L., Marshall, R., and Shaw, C.,** Cellular immunity in adult marasmus, *Arch. Int. Med.,* 137, 1408, 1977.
26. **Neumann, C. G., Lawlor, G. J., Stiehm, E. R., Swendseid, M. E., Newton, C., Herbert, J., Ammann, A., and Jacob, M.,** Immunologic responses in malnourished children, *Am. J. Clin. Nutr.,* 28, 89, 1975.
27. **Warren, J. V. and Hill, G. L.,** T cells and protein nutrition in hospitalized surgical patients, *Br. J. Surg.,* 64, 897, 1977.
28. **Bistrian, B. R., Blackburn, G. L., and Scrimshaw, N. S.,** Cellular immunity in semi-starved states in hospitalized adults, *Am. J. Clin. Nutr.,* 28, 1148, 1975.
29. **Berg, B. N. and Simms, H. S.,** Nutrition and longevity in the rat. II. Longevity and onset of disease with different levels of food intake, *J. Nutr.,* 71, 255, 1960.
30. **McCay, C. M., Crowell, M. F., and Maynard, L. A.,** The effect of retarded growth upon the length of life span and upon the ultimate body size, *J. Nutr.,* 10, 63, 1935.
31. **Nolen, G. A.,** Effect of various restricted dietary regimens on the growth, health and longevity of albino rats, *J. Nutr.,* 102, 1477, 1972.
32. **Stuchlikova, E., Juricova-Horakova, M., and Deyl, Z.,** New aspects of the dietary effect of life prolongation in rodents. What is the role of obesity in aging, *Exp. Gerontol.,* 10, 141, 1975.
33. **Barrows, C. H. and Kokkonen, G. C.,** Protein synthesis, development, growth and life span, *Growth,* 39, 525, 1975.
34. **Leto, S., Kokkonen, G. C., and Barrows, C. H.,** Dietary protein, life-span, and biochemical variables in female mice, *J. Gerontol.,* 31, 144, 1976a.
35. **Miller, D. S. and Payne, P. R.,** Longevity and protein intake, *Exp. Gerontol.,* 3, 231, 1968.
36. **Stoltzner, G.,** Effects of life-long dietary protein restriction on mortality, growth, organ weights, blood counts, liver aldolase and liver catalase in BALB/c mice, *Growth,* 413, 337, 1977.

37. **Segall, P. E. and Timiras, P. S.,** Pathophysiologic findings after chronic tryptophan deficiency in rats: a model for delayed growth and aging, *Mech. Ageing Dev.*, 5, 109, 1976.
38. **McCay, C. M., Maynard, L. A., Sperling, G., and Barnes, L. L.,** Retarded growth, life span, ultimate body size and age changes in the albino rat after feeding diets restricted in calories, *J. Nutr.*, 18, 1, 1939.
39. **McCay, C. M.,** Chemical aspects of ageing and the effect of diet upon ageing, in *Cowdry Problems of Ageing*, Williams & Wilkins, Baltimore, 1952.
40. **Ross, H. H. and Bras, G.,** Lasting influence of early caloric restriction on prevalence of neoplasms in the rat, *J. Natl. Cancer Inst.*, 47, 1095, 1971.
41. **Ross, M. H.,** Aging, nutrition and hepatic enzyme activity patterns in the rat, *J. Nutr.*, 97, 565, 1969.
42. **Ross, M. H.,** Protein, calories and life expectancy, *Fed. Proc.*, 18, 1190, 1959.
43. **Ross, M. H.,** Length of life on nutrition in the rat, *J. Nutr.*, 75, 197, 1961.
44. **Kay, M. M. B. and Makinodan, T.,** Immunobiology of aging: Evaluation of current status, *Clin. Immunol. Immunopathol.*, 6, 394, 1976.
45. **Makinodan, T. and Yunis, E., Eds.,** *Immunology and Aging*, Plenum Press, New York, 1977.
46. **Meredith, P. J. and Walford, R. L.,** Auto-immunity, histocompatibility, and aging, *Mech. Ageing Dev.*, 9, 61, 1979.
47. **Suskind, R. M., Ed.,** *Malnutrition and the Immune Response*, Raven Press, New York, 1977.

46. **Meredith, P. J. and Walford, R. L.,** Auto-immunity, histocompatibility, and aging, *Mech. Ageing Dev.*, 9, 61, 1979.
47. **Suskind, R. M., Ed.,** *Malnutrition and the Immune Response*, Raven Press, New York, 1977.

48. **Bell, R. G. and Hazell, L. A.,** Influence of dietary protein restriction on immune competence. I. Effect on the capacity of cells from various lymphoid organs to induce graft vs. host reactions, *J. Exp. Med.*, 141, 127, 1975.
49. **Cooper, W. C., Good, R. A., and Mariani, T.,** Effects of protein insufficiency on immune responsiveness, *Am. J. Clin. Nutr.*, 27, 647, 1974.
50. **Jose, D. G. and Good, R. A.,** Absence of enhancing antibody in cell mediated immunity to tumor heterografts in protein deficient rats, *Nature (London)*, 231, 323, 1971.
51. **Jose, D. G. and Good, R. A.,** Quantitative effects of nutritional protein and calorie deficiency upon immune response to tumors in mice, *Cancer Res.*, 33, 807, 1973.
52. **Aschkenasy, A.,** Effect of a protein free diet on lymph node and spleen cell responses in vivo to blastogenic stimulus, *Nature (London)*, 254, 63, 1975.
53. **Fernandes, G., Yunis, E. J., and Good, R. A.,** Suppression of adenocarcinoma by the immunological consequences of caloric restriction, *Nature (London)*, 263, 504, 1976.
54. **Visscher, M. B., Ball, Z. B., Barnes, R. H., and Sivertsen, I.,** The influence of caloric restriction upon the incidence of spontaneous mammary carcinoma in mice, *Surgery*, 11, 48, 1942.
55. **Fernandes, G., Yunis, E. J., and Good, R. A.,** Influence of protein restriction on immune functions in NZB mice, *J. Immunol.*, 116, 782, 1976.
56. **Fernandes, G., Yunis, E. J., Jose, D. G., and Good, R. A.,** Dietary influence on antinuclear antibodies and cell-mediated immunity in NZB mice, *Int. Arch. Allergy Appl. Immunol.*, 44, 770, 1973.
57. **Fernandes, G., Yunis, E. J., Smith, J., and Good, R. A.,** Dietary influence on breeding behavior, hemolytic anemia and longevity in NAB mice, *Proc. Soc. Exp. Biol. Med.*, 139, 1189, 1972.
58. **Fernandes, G., Yunis, E. J., and Good, R. A.,** Influence of diet on survival of mice, *Proc. Natl. Acad. Sci. U.S.A.*, 73, 1279, 1976.
59. **Dubois, E. L. and Strain, L.,** Effect of diet on survival and nephropathy of NZB/NZW hybrid mice, *Biochem. Med.*, 7, 336, 1973.
60. **Gardner, M. B., Ihle, J. N., Pillarisetty, R. J., Talal, N., Dubois, E. L., and Levy, J. A.,** Type C virus expression and host response in diet-cured NZB/W mice, *Nature (London)*, 268, 341, 1977.
61. **Jose, D. G., Stutman, O., and Good, R. A.,** Long term effect on immune responses of early nutritional deprivation, *Nature (London) New Biol.*, 241, 57, 1973.
62. **Walford, R. L., Liu, R. K., Gerbase-DeLima, M., Mathies, M., and Smith, G. S.,** Longterm dietary restriction and immune function in mice: response of sheep red blood cells and to mitogenic agents, *Mech. Ageing Dev.*, 2, 447, 1973/74.
63. **Gerbase-DeLima, M., Liu, R. K., Cheney, K. E., Mickey, R., and Walford, R. L.,** Immune function and survival in a long lived mouse strain subjected to undernutrition, *Gerontologia*, 21, 184, 1975.
64. **Nolen, G. A.,** Effects of various restricted dietary regimes on the growth, health and longevity of albino rats, *J. Nutr.*, 102, 1477, 1972.
65. **Barrows, C. H., Jr. and Roeder, L. M.,** The effect of reduced dietary intake on enzymatic activities and life span of rats, *J. Gerontol.*, 20, 69, 1965.
66. **Ross, M. H. and Bras, G.,** Influence of protein under and overnutrition on spontaneous tumor prevalence in the rat, *J. Nutr.*, 103, 944, 1973.

67. **Poffenholz, V.,** Correlation between DNA repair of embryeonic fibroblasts and different lifespan of 3 inbred mouse strains, *Mech. Ageing Dev.*, 7, 131, 1978.
68. **Walford, R. L.,** *The Immunologic Theory of Aging*, Munksgaard, Copenhagen, 1969.
69. **Walford, R. L., Liu, R. K., Mathies, M., Lipps, L., and Konen, T.,** Influence of calorie restriction on immune function, relevance for an immunologic theory of aging, *Proc. 9th Int. Congr. Nutrition*, Mexico City, Sept. 4-8, 1972.
70. **Liu, R. K., Leung, B. E., and Walford, R. L.,** Effect of temperature-transfer on growth of laboratory populations of a South American annual fish Cynolebias Bellottii, *Growth*, 39, 337, 1975.
71. **Liu, R. K. and Walford, R. L.,** Mid-life temperature-transfer effects on life-span of annual fish, *J. Gerontol.*, 30, 129, 1975.
72. **Liu, R. K. and Walford, R. L.,** The effect of lowered body temperature on life-span and immune and non-immune processes, *Gerontologia*, 18, 363, 1972.
73. **Faulk, P. W., Demgeyer, E. M., and Davies, A. J. S.,** Some effects of malnutrition on the immune response in man, *Am. J. Clin. Nutr.*, 27, 638, 1974.
74. **Dutz, W., Rossipal, E., Ghavami, H., Vessal, K., Kohout, E., and Post, C.,** Persistent cell-mediated immune-deficiency following infantaile stress during the first 6 months of life, *Europ. J. Pediatr.*, 122, 117, 1976.
75. **Dutz, W., Kohout, E., Rossipal, E., and Vessal, K.,** Infantile stress, immune modulation, and disease patterns, in *Pathology Annual*, Sommers, S. C., Ed., Appleton-Century-Croft, New York, 1976, 11, 415.
76. **McMurray, D. N., Watson, R. R., and Reyes, M. A.,** Humoral, secretory and cell-mediated immune responses during the year following renutrition of severely malnourished children, *Fed. Proc.*, 38, 613, 1979.
77. **Watson, R. R., Safranski, D., and Putt, N. J.,** unpublished data.

IMMUNITY AND MICROBIAL DISEASES

Jeffrey Galpin

INTRODUCTION

Infections may occur at any age but there is an exponential increase in incidence of infectious diseases after age 25. The aged human is more susceptible to certain infections and experiences a higher morbidity and mortality to these entities. These changes correlate with the quantitative and/or qualitative differences in specific immunologic responses that occur during the aging process. Man evolves through an early immunologic maturation and then slowly descends to physical and immunologic senescence.

In discussing infections and immunity related to aging, it is imperative to discern between those general organismal changes which enhance susceptibility and morbidity and those specific immune dysfunctions which permit unique relationships to develop between parasite and host.

Man has a continuous association with microbial organisms throughout his life span. Host defenses against infective diseases include the inherent integrity of each body system as well as the integrity of those elements of this complex organism designed particularly to ward off such invading foreign biologic units.

In discussing immunity in terms of infectious agents of the aged, the entire spectrum of its definition needs to be considered. Therefore immunity may describe the ability of a lung to clear particulate matter or the integrity of a bladder not to retain urine. Immunity may describe the function of lymphocytes or monocytes or it may define the ability of ischemic tissue to locally inhibit bacterial invasion. The complexities and interrelationships between system, organ, and tissue function in man and its defense of the body from infection is still a poorly understood concept. The relationship between aging and infection is even more embryonic in its understanding; however, the importance of its investigation increases with the desire to understand the aging process itself.

This chapter will briefly review what is known about immunity and aging as it relates to infection. It will survey infective syndromes which are more frequent or severe in the elderly and it will review some specific infectious agents which occur frequently in the aged. Wherever possible, immunologic dysfunction in its broadest definition will be related to the etiopathogenesis of the particular disease.

COMMON INFECTIOUS SYNDROMES WHICH ARE MORE FREQUENT OR SEVERE IN THE AGED

Sepsis

Gram-negative bacteremia occurs in all age groups, but attack rates and morbidity are highest in neonates and the aged. Besides age, Gram-negative bacteremia is more common in patients with chronic renal disease, cirrhosis, diabetes mellitus, both solid and hematologic malignancies, and collage vascular diseases. It is associated, therefore, with a compromised host immune system and an increased risk of infection. McCabe and Jackson[1,2] reported that the mortality from Gram-negative bacteremia is almost 84% with underlying "rapidly fatal" diseases, 48% with "ultimately fatal" diseases and about 16% with "nonfatal" diseases.

The increased morbidity, mortality, and frequency of Gram-negative sepsis within the elderly population probably represents a multifactorial etiology. The decline in immune function significantly contributes to this syndrome while the increase in respiratory and urinary tract infections and surgical wound and skin infections permits access for the pathogens to initiate a bacteremia. Clearly, it is not the bacteremic event but the status of host defense mechanisms like immune adherence,[3] serum resistance,[4,5] antiphagocytic surfaces,[6] intracellular killing,[7] susceptibility to endotoxin enzymes and toxins,[8,9] and the ability to maintain function of vital organs that are the factors deciding the outcome of any blood stream infection.

Boston City Hospital has collected data on the epidemilogy of Gram-negative sepsis for nearly 40 years from 1935 to 1972.[10] Bacteremia due to *Escherichia coli* and *Salmonella* species were the only ones seen prior to the introduction of sulfonamides, while between 1957 and 1972 the incidence of *E. coli* bacteremia per 1000 admissions rose fivefold. In 1972 *Klebsiella-Enterobacter* species were the second most common cause of bacteremic Gram-negative infection. On the other hand, by looking at underlying diseases like myelocytic leukemia or renal and bone marrow transplants, a specific organism such as *Pseudomonas aeruginosa* seems to predominate in cases of sepsis.[11-13]

The Center for Disease Control reports that between 49 and 56% of all bacteremias were caused by *Enterobacteriaceae* and *P. aeruginosa*. The mortality rate of these infections was 34%.[14]

The gastrointestinal tract is the obvious reservoir of Gram-negative bacilli; therefore, it is not surprising that *E. coli* is often isolated from aerobic blood cultures and *Bacteroides fragilis* from anaerobic cultures. There also exists a dynamic interaction between native, endogenous fecal flora and sources of Gram-negative rods acquired from environmental sources. Fecal carriage, for example, of *P. aeruginosa* increased fivefold with increasing debility or treatment of underlying diseases with neutropenia. Additionally, antimicrobial therapy with broad spectrum agents predispose to colonization by *P. aeruginosa*.[15]

Signs and symptoms of Gram-negative sepsis include fever, chills, hyperventilation, hypothermia, skin lesions, and changes in mental status; while bleeding, leukopenia, thrombocytopenia, hypotension, congestive heart failure, kidney failure, and acute respiratory distress may result. Ecthyma lesions or vesicular and bullous skin lesions may result from *P. aeruginosa, Aeromonas hydrophila, Klebsiella, Enterobacter*, and *Serratia* sepsis.[16,17] Patients may quickly progress from an initial phase of hypotension, tachycardia, and peripheral vasodilatation (warm shock), to a moribund phase of deep pallor, intense vasoconstriction, and anuria (cold shock). Cardiac rate and cardiac index are significantly lower in Gram-negative shock than in Gram-positive shock.[18]

The lipid A component of the bacterial cell wall which is a lipoidal acylated glucosamine disaccharide appears to be the toxic moiety.[19,20] After administering endotoxin with its lipopolysaccharide (LPS) component, Hageman factor is activated, Kinins are generated,[21,22] and C3 and alternative pathway factors are consumed.[23] Antibody against the "core" glycolipid antigen of LPS protect man and experimental animals against the sequelae of shock and death.[24,25] Endotoxin seems to induce three primary systems which are responsible for many of the pathophysiologic findings in Gram-negative sepsis. The complement cascade is activated leading to inflammation and activation of plasma thromboplastin antecedent (PTA) and consequent coagulation. Hageman factor activation not only stimulates PTA but activates the plasminogen system which produces fibrinolysis. Finally, Hageman factor activates Prekallikrein which cascades to bradykinin which produces, among its many effects, hypotension. Endotoxin, therefore, produces acute disseminated intravascular coagulation (DIC).

Finally, in discussing Gram-negative bacteremia, host defenses to this syndrome need to be understood. Mechanical barriers are one of the most important factors limiting the systemic invasion of the host by Gram-negative bacilli. The gastrointestinal mucosa has an important function in restricting entry of these organisms into the blood stream. Bacteremia may result from trauma, penetrating wounds, small surface ulcerations, mechanical obstruction such as caused by tumors, and ischemic necrosis of the bowel. Immunosuppressed persons may have multiple small ulcerations of the gastrointestinal mucosa. Another important host factor is the complement mediated serum bacterioloytic system. Complement-deficiency states have been reported to be associated with increased susceptibility to infection and this has been best documented with genetic deficiencies in certain complement components.[26]

The burden of clearing organisms from the blood stream falls on phagocytic cells whether they are fixed phagocytes of the reticuloendothelial system or the circulating phagocytes such as the neutrophil or monocyte.[6] There is good correlation between susceptibility to bacterial Gram-negative infections and depressed levels of circulating neutrophils. It is commonly observed that bacteremia follows neutropenia in spite of the presence of high levels of antibodies against cell wall antigens.[27]

The complement system may play an important role in deciding the pathways of C3B, the critical opsonic protein of the circulating humoral system. The alternative pathway appears to have an important function in providing nonspecific opsonic support before the availability of a specific antibody.[28] While much attention has been focused on the effect of specific antibodies as opsonins, the possibility that antibodies play a role in toxin neutralization has also been raised. As mentioned above, antibody directed against core glycolipid antigens appears to protect man and animals against the sequelae of sepsis. These antibodies appear to have a broad cross-protective activity.

It is likely that many of these host defenses are impaired in the aged. Coupled with this fact are observations concerning increased avenues of entrance for Gram-negative bacteria in the elderly as through ascending urinary tract infections or decubitus ulcers. The morbidity and mortality in the elderly increases with heart, lung, and kidney dysfunction and associated with the described immune defects in the aged, there exists a grave prognosis with this syndrome of Gram-negative sepsis.

Pneumonia

Pneumonias are perhaps the classic terminal event in the aged. Pneumonia has been described as the old man's friend. Osler[31] dubbed them "captain of the men of death". In McKeown's[29] series, bronchopneumonia was found in 11% of all autopsies. It was considered the direct cause of death in 3.6% and a terminal or contributory factor in 7.4%. It occurs more frequently as a complication in heart failure, cerebrovascular disease, and urinary tract disorders. In a study of consecutive autopsies at a chronic care facility, bronchopneumonia was felt to be the primary cause of death in 22.8% of all the deaths.[30]

When Osler described his "captain of the men of death", he was referring to the pneumococcus.[31] The prognosis in pneumococcal pneumonia is inextricably related to the patient, the extent of his disease, and the presence of bacteremia (Figure 1). Mortality increases with age. Even with penicillin therapy, the mortality of bacteremic pneumonia in patients 50 to 69 years of age may be as high as 30 to 40% and in those 70 years or older 55 to 60%[32] Mortality is higher in patients with underlying conditions such as alcoholism with delirium tremens, Laennec's cirrhosis, diabetes mellitus with acidosis, chronic renal disease, congestive heart failure, chronic obstructive pulmonary disease, and certain malignancies. Severe pneumococcal disease is also seen in patients with immunodeficiency states (B-cell defects) and splenic dysfunction or splenectomy. Secondary pneumococcal pneumonia is the most common bacterial complication of both influenza and measles.

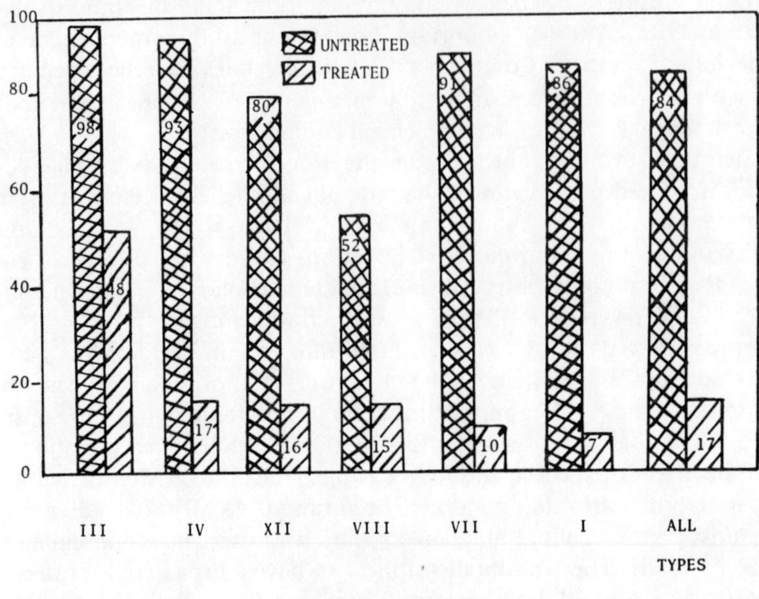

FIGURE 1. Number within bar indicates percent of fatal cases. Data for untreated cases from Tilghman and Finland (1). (From Austrian, R. and Gold, J., *Ann. Intern. Med.*, 60, 763, 1964. With permission.)

The high mortality rate in the elderly may not only reflect immune deficits or pulmonary failure but may be related to its atypical presentation. In some elderly patients, the illness may develop almost without fever and with few symptomatic complaints. By the time the diagnosis is made, antibiotic administration may be too late. The course also may be atypical. For example, pneumonia may imitate cerebrovascular accidents.[33] Mortality increases in the aged when bronchopneumonia exists rather then lobar consolidation and when leukocyte counts are below 10,000/mm 3.

The pathogenicity of pneumococci is related primarily to its capsular polysaccharide. Encapsulated organisms are virulent for man and experimental animals whereas organisms without capsular polysaccharides are not. Active or passive immunization employing ''smooth'' pneumococci protects against subsequent infection by the homologous type in animals and similar immunization of man with purified capsular polysaccharides prevents subsequent bacteremic pneumonia by the same pneumococcal type.

The development of pneumococcal pneumonia is dependent on a defect in normal host defense mechanisms, such as mucus-secreting cells, the epiglottis reflex, cilia, cough reflex, lymphatics, phagocytic leukocytes, macrophages, and opsonins. Pneumococcal pneumonia usually develops after aspiration of upper respiratory tract secretions containing pneumococci in patients with impaired host defenses.

Once the lung itself can no longer contain the organism, various suppurative complications may result. These include direct extension into the pleural or pericardial cavities, endobronchial obstruction with distal atelectasis or abscess formation, and extra pulmonary localization such as meningitis, endocarditis, or arthritis. Other complications include otitis media, mastoiditis, sinusitis, and peritonitis.

Another pathogen, *Staphylococcus aureus*, causes 1 to 10% of bacterial pneumonia.[34-36] During interepidemic periods staphylococcal pneumonia is sporadic but when influenza A or B is epidemic, *S. aureus* often is also prevelent, producing a complicating and highly lethal bronchopneumonia.[37,38] Staphlococcal pneumonia is frequent in infants and children less than 3 years of age and among older patients in the fifth and sixth decades. Males seem preferentially affected at all ages.

Antibodies to several extracellular products of the staphylococcus are found in patients with disease, or in nasal carriers, but these immunoglobulins are not protective and do not facilitate phagocytosis. Strains of *S. aureus* have two major somatic antigens, protein A and hapten, ribitol teichoic acid. Precipitins to both antigens are usual in human sera. Unlike antibodies to capsular antigen of the pneumococcus or M protein of *Streptococcus pyogenes,* antibodies are not protective. However; antiribitol teichoic acid antibodies are opsonizing.[39-41]

The epidemiology of *Staphylococcus aureus* is important. The organism is carried in the nose of up to 40% of adults and is transferred by fingers onto other areas of the skin in 20% of these carriers. Heavy carriers aerosolize staphylococci which then colonize the nasal epithelium of adjacent patients within hospitals or of others in closed environments where air exchanges with the outdoors are limited. Antecedent viral injury to respiration epithelium is paramount to the acquisition of staphylococcal pneumonia. Staphylococcal pneumonia may present as an acute hemorrhagic form during influenza epidemics or otherwise may present as a subacute chronic variety in which destruction of tissues and fibrosis is prominent. Other predisposing factors include carbuncles, pustules, abscesses, purulent conjunctivitis, mucoviscidosis, rubeola, immune deficiencies, other respiratory viruses, broad spectrum antibiotics, pregnancy, malignancy, or chronic disorders of the heart or lungs.

Not only do viruses predispose to bacterial pneumonias, but specific viruses like influenza, are themselves more severe with additional complications in the elderly. In outbreaks since 1918, primary influenza viral pneumonia has occurred predominantly among the elderly, especially when those individuals had cardiovascular disease. Other chronic disorders have also been implicated as risks for this primary pneumonia. Such patients do not respond to antibiotics and the mortality rate is high. At autopsy, findings consist of tracheitis, bronchitis, diffuse hemorrhagic pneumonia, hyaline membranes lining alveolar ducts and alveoli, and a paucity of inflammatory cells within the alveoli.[42]

Influenza attack rates are higher in children than in adults but the incidence of pulmonary complications are far higher in the elderly. New influenza mutants have produced great pandemics with characteristically high mortality in the elderly, as was observed in the 1958 to 1959 pandemic due to Hong Kong A strain.[43]

On the other hand, there was a sparing of persons 75 years of age and older in the 1968 to 1969 pandemic because of the aged individual's prior exposure to this agent in early childhood.[44] Therefore, if an elderly individual is exposed for the first time to an influenza strain antigenically shifted, mortality is high. Influenza is unique in its ability to recombine its segmented RNA to produce antigenic drift or totally change its antigenicity by recombining with an animal reservoir strain producing pandemics with true antigenic shift.

Immunity is afforded this virus, first, through secretory and serum antibody. The former is reduced in the elderly and may contribute to infectivity and morbidity wthin this group. Habershon and associates[45] showed that influenza virus used as a skin test antigen evoked a cell mediated type response in 24 to 48 hr in 12 of 42 normal subjects in whom influenza A was used as antigen and in 17 of 42 subjects when influenza B was used. There appeared to be an association of positive skin tests with prior influenzal infection. Repeated or intense stimulation is required to stimulate cell mediated immunity which may have some protective effect against infection. When influenza virus is used to stimulate thymidine uptake, an increase response of cells from patients who had been vaccinated and had contracted influenza is seen and this correlates positively with the serum hemagglutination inhibition antibody titer while it correlates negatively with interferon titers.[46]

While influenza may be inhibited by cellular immune function the organism also appears to suppress cell-mediated immunity independently during illness. Kantzler et al.[47] reported a depression in the skin test response to tuberculin and other antigens during infection of volunteers with an attenuated live influenza vaccine and during infection following challenge with a virulent strain of A2 influenza. A majority of the subjects who were infected also demonstrated suppression of thymidine uptake by their lymphocytes to simulation with phytohemagglutinin. This immune suppression could increase the hazard of reactivation of tuberculosis and other infections and possibly could increase the occurrence of neoplasia.

Finally, there is evidence in animals that cell mediated immunity can actually be deleterious during illness. Antithymocyte serum reduced mortality with experimental influenza in mice and it reduced lung consolidation although viral titers were not lowered.[48]

Influenza is only one of several viruses whose presentation is more severe in the elderly. Outbreaks of respiratory syncytial virus (RSV) infection have been associated, for example, with a particularly high proportion developing bronchopneumonia in the aged population.[49,50] In one study of hospitalized older patients (most of 70 years of age), two thirds developed pneumonia. In a recent outbreak of RSV in a nursing home, 25% of the women and 5% of the men were infected. Forty seven percent developed pneumonia and 87% had fever.[50]

Other types of pneumonia-like necrotizing Gram-negative pneumonia occur more frequently in the elderly because of the underlying disease which allows access to the lower respiratory tract and because of poor clearance and immunity in the pulmonary organ itself. Pneumonia in the aged is thus a multiparametric syndrome dependent on organ integrity, immune competence, and other predisposing factors being present. The factors may or may not be related primarily to the aging process. Accepting the same multifactorial predisposition in the aged, true opportunistic pathogens like the fungi would also be expected to occur more frequently; yet, evidence is at present only suggestive. Tuberculosis, however, clearly is more frequent in the elderly although one factor unrelated to susceptibility is the predominant exposure rate of our elderly population when they were young. However, accepting this, the elderly still have increased reactivation of tuberculosis.[51,52] Extrapulmonary cases are also of greater frequency in the elderly. About 50% of extrapulmonary disease occurs over age 45. More than 62% of pulmonary cases are in this age category. In older age groups the pleural site is predominant with the lymphatics remaining prominent and genitourinary tract becoming prominent especially in the very old.[53-55] The age of patients with skeletal tuberculosis tends to be increasing, as it is for patients with other forms of extrapulmonary disease.[56] Finally the age of patients with miliary tuberculosis appears to be increasing.[57]

The mean age of 69 Americans with miliary tuberculosis from 1954 to 1970 reviewed by Munt was 50 years.[58] It is in the older group of patients that the diagnosis is less obvious,[59] and may remain an enigma until autopsy unless adequate diagnostic tests are performed.

Pneumonia in the aged may evolve through several etiologies in the same individual. Therefore, viral infection may predispose to bacterial pneumonia and the latter may permit reactivation of a tuberculosis site. Coupling this phenomena with the subtle difficulties of diagnosis in the elderly creates a major challenge for the care of this type of patient.

Urinary Tract Infections

Urinary tract infections have long been associated as a cause of high morbidity and mortality in the elderly. Its prevalence varies according to environmental effects like private household living vs. residential homes vs. a hospital.

Urinary infection is present in about 20% of all women over 65. Brocklehurst and co-workers[60] studied women aged 45 to 64 in the same population by the same criteria and found infection in 3%. There seems therefore, to be a marked increase in urinary infection in women in the seventh decade and in men 5 to 10 years later.[61,62] Previous prostatic surgery was a related factor in men, but previous pelvic surgery in women was not related. The presence of residual urine in old patients is probably one of the most important etiologic factors.[63]

Experimental studies have shown that the more organisms delivered to the kidneys, the greater the chance of infection.[64] Very few organisms are needed to infect the medulla while 10,000 times that are needed to infect the cortex.[65] The etiology of this differential relates to inceased medullary ammonia which is due to high osmolality, low blood flow, and and acidic environment.[66,67]

In addition to inoculum size and local environs, other factors participate in producing urinary tract infections. Certain organisms such as specific serogroups of *E. coli* seem to cause most infections.[68,69] Some of these *E. coli* possess specifie K antigens, which again are somehow associated with a predilection to infect.[70,71] The presence of pili on infecting organisms may be significant in permitting attachment of pathogens to the urinary tract epithelium.[72,73] Other qualities related to the ability to produce pyelonephritis include an organism's motility or capability to split urease exemplified by *proteus* species.[74,75]

The host is equally important as the organism in permitting infection to take place. The urine itself possesses some antibacterial activity. The pH and osmolality of urine inhibits some bacteria. The presence of glucose, on the other hand, makes urine a better culture medium.[76] Prostatic fluid added to urine is inhibitory. Overall, urine has been shown to inhibit migrating, adhering, and killing functions of polymorphonuclear leukocytes.[77,78]

On a more functional level, the flushing mechanism of the kidney is somewhat protective.[79] The mucosal surface of bladders also has some inherent resistance to invasion unless it is damaged.[80]

The role of humoral immunity is poorly understood but bacteria do produce specific IgM and then IgG against the O antigen of Gram-negative bacilli.[81,82] The antibodies have not been shown to be protective in man but animal studies have demonstrated some protection afforded by antibodies to the K antigen.[83] Specific IgA and IgG antibodies are found more frequently in the urine of patients with upper urinary tract infection than in those with lower urinary tract infections. Hanson[81] found that serum sensitive strains are less virulent and at most cause asymptomatic bacteriuria.

Delayed hypersensitivity has yet to be indicted as a major immune component in urinary tract infections[82] but several investigators have found bacterial antigen persistence in kidneys and have speculated on the role of autoimmunity in this disease state.[84] Patients with pyelonephritis have, for example, increased quantities of antibody against Tamm-Horsfall protein.[85] Aoki et al.[86] looked at kidneys from patients with pyelonephritis and found antigen in kidneys from all of those studied.

Resistance to infection is also decreased by abnormalities of the urinary tract. Any cause of obstruction to urinary flow whether localized within the kidney or distal in ureter, bladder, or urethra increases the frequency of infection. Therefore, congenital anomalies of the ureter or urethra-like valves, stenosis or bands, calculi, ureteral compression, benign prostatic hypertrophy, polycystic kidney disease, hypokalemic nephropathy, and renal lesions from sickle cell tract or disease all increase the frequency of infection.[87] Calculi may increase the frequency of infection through obstruction and irritation or they may actually form secondary to primary infections with organisms like *proteus* or *klebsiella* species.[88] Organisms may also persist deep in calculi despite antibiotics. Finally, vesicoureteral reflux, and neurogenic dysfunction of the bladder also increase susceptibility to infection.[89,90]

Urinary tract infections are, indeed, more frequent in the elderly. The reasons are again multifactorial and include both kidney and bladder dysfunction, overall immune depression, and decreased resistance of local barriers. In addition to these factors, one must include the effects of other underlying diseases and other organ failure.

Infective Endocarditis

The mean age of patients with infective endocarditis (IE) has increased in the modern era partially due to the use of antibiotics. In 1926 the median age was less than 30 years;[91] by 1943 this had increased to 39 years, and today over 50% of patients are older than 50 years.[92,93] Currently 21% of cases occurs in persons older than 60 years.[94] Another reason for this shift stems from the decline in rheumatic heart disease with the rise in degenerative heart disease of the eldery. Second, the age of the population is increasing with increased survival of individuals with rheumatic or congenital heart disease. Another type of endocarditis in the aged secondary to therapeutic modalities like intravenous catheters, hyperalimentation lines, pacemakers, and dialysis shunts has also emerged in the modern era. Twenty eight percent of endocarditis cases recently reviewed in Seattle were nosocomial in origin.[95] The degenerative cardiac lesions like calcific nodular lesions secondary to arteriosclerotic cardiovascular disease or post-myocardial infarction thrombus are important precursors of infections in those individuals without valvular disease and they occur with an increased incidence in the elderly. Prosthetic valve endocarditis (PVE) is rising rapidly in incidence. Early PVE complicates 0.5 to 1% of valve implantations while late PVE occurs in 0.2 to 0.5% per year.[96-98] Staphylococci, aerobic Gram-negative bacilli, Candida, and Aspergillus are important pathogens of early PVE. Other diseases in adults and especially the elderly which predispose to IE include idiopathic hypertrophic subaortic stenosis (IHSS)[99,100] and mitral prolapse.[101]

The pathogenesis of endocarditis requires several events to occur in an almost cascade fashion. Nonbacterial thrombotic endocarditis (NBTE) is an important event which permits an early lesion to develop where organisms can adhere and grow, sitting on fibrin-platelet deposits, overlying interstitial edema and cellular distortion. This area is produced by many types of mechanical, toxic, or infectious injuries to the endothelium.[102-104] Systemic stress producing injury may also take the form of blood turbulence.[105,106] Once NBTE is established, transient bacteremia is required to produce IE.[107] This invasion usually occurs when a mucosal barrier is breached as dental extraction or gastrointestinal, urologic, and gynecologic procedures.[108,109] Part of this colonization is dependent on the ability or avidity of certain organisms to adhere to this platelet mesh. Gould et al.[110] showed that organisms frequently associated with IE like enterococci, viridans Streptococci, *S. aureus, S. epidermidis,* and *P. aeruginosa* adhere more avidly in animal models. Oral streptococci produce a complex extracellular polysaccharide dextran which allows it to adhere to enamel and possibly plays a role in adherence in IE.[111] Some strains of bacteria like IE producing staphylococci and streptococci also stimulate platelet aggregation which probably plays a role in the pathogenesis of IE.[112]

Immunologically, IE stimulates both humoral and cellular immunity. Antibody may either stimulate the production of bacterial agglutination and increase valve colonization or it may inhibit IE by improving clearance of bacteria.[113] Infective endocarditis confers constant intravascular antigenic challenge with development of rheumatoid factor, opsonic IgG, agglutinating IgG, IgM and complement fixing (IgG, IgM) antibodies, cryoglobulins, and even macroglobulins.[114-116] Using a Raji cell or Clq technique, circulating immune complexes have been found associated with IE with marked elevation in chronic infection, when extravascular manifestations occur, or when there is hypocomplementemia. Levels fall with good therapy.[117] Patients may also present with immune complex glomerulonephritis as a primary extracardiac complication.[118]

Clinically, the elderly patient frequently presents in similar manner to younger individuals. There are differences, however, for as noted earlier many elderly IE patients have no prior history of valvular disease.[119] Roberts and Buchbinder, for example,[120] noted anatomically normal valves in 53% of their patients. A minority of infecting agents in the elderly are of low virulence while the remainder are pathogenic organisms like coagulose-positive *Staphylococci enterococci, Streptococcus pneumonia,* and *Escherica coli.*[121-123] Antecedent staphylococcal infections are very important in the aged.[124-127] In one study 45% of patients had no fever during their hospitalization.[128] The elderly patient also not infrequently presents with no leukocytosis. Occasionally the elderly present with abacteremia although blood cultures are useful in the majority of cases.[122,128,130] Finally, despite antibiotics the mortality rate is far greater in the older patient.[121,126,131]

In summary, endocarditis affects all ages but the aged are becoming more frequent targets. The etiopathogenesis of this disease is complicated and its elements relate to valvular endothelial competence, immunologic competence, and host mucosal integrity. It is not unreasonable to expect dysfuncion in these elements with age but the exact interactions of bacteria and valvular infection in the aged requires further study.

Skin and Soft Tissue Infections

Three major syndromes which affect the elderly will be briefly reviewed. Candidiasis is probably the most common fungal infection of the elderly. This is an adventitial pathogen which needs either a local or a systemic abnormality before it manifests itself. By far the most important cutaneous viral infection in the elderly is herpes zoster caused by the varicella-zoster virus. In children it presents as varicella while in adults it is a reactivated disease whose origin stems from dorsal root ganglia latency. Finally, decubitus ulcers probably account for the greatest morbidity and mortality in the elderly in terms of skin infections. This infection is of multiple etiology and is related mostly to immobility and decreased immunity of the host.

Candidiasis

Candida organisms are grouped with the fungi imperfect (Deuteromycetes) since a sexual stage has not been identified. They are small (4 — 6 μm) thin walled ovoid cells that reproduce by budding. Seven species are regularly recovered from man. They are *Candida albicans, C. guillermondii, C. krusei, C. parapsilosis, C. stellatoidea, C. tropicalis,* and *C. pseudotropicalis.*

Intact integument is an important immunologic barrier to Candida invasion and any process causing skin maceration or vascular insufficiency leaves the site susceptible to this organism. Normal resistance to cutaneous candidiasis probably requires intact T-cell functions, as suggested by the syndrome of chronic mucocutaneous candidiasis

(CMC).[132] CMC is a cellular T-cell immunodeficiency characterized by persistent *Candida* infection of the mucous membranes, skin, hair, and nails. There is an associated endocrinopathy in half the cases and it is familiar in one fifth. The cellular defect is narrow and includes *C. albicans* and a few antigenically similar fungi. Since other host defenses are normal in this syndrome, systemic candidiasis does not occur. Pearsall et al.[133] reported that mitogen-stimulation lymphocytes produced a lymphokine that killed *C. albicans.* Diamond[134] suggested that certain blood mononuclear leukocytes could kill another yeast *Cryptococcus neoformans* extracellularly. Lymphocyte or lymphocyte-mononuclear phagocyte dysfunction is probably most important in mucocutaneous or cutaneous candidiasis syndromes like thrush, candida esophagitis, gastrointestinal candidiasis, candidia vaginitis, candida folliculitis, and balanitis, paronychia, onychomycosis, intertrigo, and macronodular or genralized candidiasis.

Once the organism breaches the blood stream, polymorphonuclear cells play a major role in host defense. Neutrophils and monocytes lacking myeloperoxidase or the capacity to generate hydrogen peroxide or superoxide anion fail to kill *Candida albicans* effectively.[135,136] Chymotrypsin, like cationic proteins, act by increasing the membrane permeability of the yeast and is part of neutrophil granules.[137,138]

The role of macrophages is not clear because although Cohen and Cline[139] reported human alveolar macrophage inability to kill *C. albicans,* Lehrer[140] found human macrophages did indeed kill. Taschdjian et al.[141] showed by immunofluorescence that organisms were sequestrated in tissue macrophages throughout the human body in cases of disseminated candidiasis.

Both heat stable and heat labile serum components enhance the ingestion of *C. albicans* by neutrophils.[142] Complement may exert an influence on the rate of *C. albicans* uptake by neutrophils[143] but it does not effect the subsequent killing of these organisms.[142,144] Serum iron binding proteins have also been shown to inhibit the growth of this organism.[145,146] Other humoral factors induce *C. albicans* to form pseudohyphae and to clump the organisms in vitro.[147]

There are certain underlying conditions which also predispose to candida infection. Diabetes mellitus predisposes to cutaneous but not disseminated disease while antibiotics, especially those like tetracycline which not only select out candida but actually inhibit phagocytosis, predispose to disseminated candidiasis. Patients with leukemia lose mucosal integrity and frequently develop esophageal and gastrointestinal candidiasis.[148,149] Other factors allowing this infection to disseminate include hyperalimentation, polyethylene catheters, and implantation of prosthetic materials like cardiac valves.[150] A summary of immunologic factors is found in Table 1.

Herpes Zoster

The varicella-zoster virus is a herpes virus that measures 45 to 50 μm and contains DNA. There is a surrounding capsid and an outer envelope. The virus is pathogenic only for man and apes. Zoster is a disease rare in childhood and most frequently seen in individuals over the age of 50 years. More than 50% of individuals reaching 85 years of age have had at least one attack of herpes zoster. Rates are even higher in individuals with malignancies, diabetes mellitus, or those who are immunosuppressed.[151] In some cases reactivation is triggered by these underlying factors. Other important predisposing factors include local X-irradiation, trauma, treatment with arsenicals, neurosyphilis, or tumor entrapment of the dorsal root ganglia or nerve root. It is thought that the primary decline of immunity with age and the lack of exposure to children with chicken pox promotes reactivation.[152] Most disease remains in one dermatome but 2% disseminate and these occur more frequently in individuals with underlying malignancies.

Table 1
IMMUNOLOGIC FINDINGS IN CHRONIC MUCOCUTANEOUS CANDIDIASIS

Common abnormalities
- Cutaneous anergy to *Candida* antigens
- Decreased migration inhibition factor production
- Decreased or absent lymphocyte transformation to *Candida*

Uncommon abnormalities
- Cutaneous anergy to other antigens
- Serum inhibitor to *Candida* transformation
- Secretory IgA[a] deficiency
- Monocyte chemotactic defect
- Suppressor T-cell abnormality

Other abnormalities
- Thymic abnormalities: thymoma, hypertrophy, dystrophy
- Complement deposition in skin

Normal findings
- Normal B- and T-cell numbers
- Normal PHA[b] and mixed leukocyte culture responses
- Normal complement levels
- Normal or elevated immunoglobulins
- Normal or elevated *Candida* antibody titers
- Normal phagocytic function

[a] IgA = immunoglobulin A.
[b] PHA = phytohemagglutinin.

Edwards, J. E. Jr., Lehrer, R I., Stiehm, E. R., Fischer, T. J., and Young, L. S., *Ann. Intern. Med.*, 89, 98, 1978. With permission.

As is true of most herpes virus, varicella-zoster (V-Z) virus produces a latent infection. Initially the infection produces chicken pox but in later life reactivation in the form of zoster occurs. Examination of ganglia in patients dying right after onset of acute zoster reveals degeneration of ganglion cells, satellite cells, Schwann cell, and nerve fibers, with infiltration of lymphocytes and polymorphonuclear cells and blood vessel congestion.[153-155] Antigen has been demonstrated by immunofluorescence in satellite and Schwann cells but not in ganglion cells.[156,157]

A variety of humoral and cell mediated immune mechanisms are recruited during primary and reactivated V-Z disease. Antibodies like complement fixing IgG are produced in response, but these are probably not effective because of the cell to cell type of nonproductive infection that exists[158] Determination of antibody against membrane antigen by fluorescence microscopy (FAMA) or immune adherence hemagglutination (IAHA) is best for determining susceptibility to this virus.[159-161] Primary immune protection is probably produced by K-lymphocytes or natural killer cells although further studies are required.

Decubitus Ulcers

This syndrome represents the "too common" pressure sores seen in the elderly or debilitated patient. The elderly who acquire this wound are predisposed to sepsis and osteomyelitis. Those individuls over the age of 65 years who develop septicemia secondary to decubitus ulcers have an inordinately high mortality. There is even a higher morbidity and mortality in these individuals when they are anemic and have low albumin levels. There is a polymicrobial flora in these wounds yet sepsis primarily is attributed to the Bacteroides species, Staphylococci, and β hemolytic Streptococci. These organisms are probably selected out because of their ability to invade tissue and reach the blood.[162-163] *B. fragilis* is an almost universal inhabitant of decubitus ulcers and is found in many cases of diabetic foot ulcers. Anaerobic bacteria are now held to be the major pathogens in these latter conditions although *Staphylococcus aureus* remains the other important pathogen.[164]

Decubitus ulcers are preventable with good care. Immunity in this syndrome is considered on a broader perspective. The barrier trespassed upon is the skin. If the patient is poorly nourished or has small vessel disease, soft tissue is easier to invade. If a patient remains immobilized on a bony prominence, the likelihood of a decubitus forming is enormous. If the skin is neurologically anaesthetic the frequency of pressure sores also increases.

It is easier to prevent a decubitus ulcer than to treat it. Once developed the ulcer develops ischemic low redox potential areas suitable for bacterial colonization and invasion. Immune deficits at this point permit easy access for pathogens and sepsis is also inevitable. The two complications beside sepsis to be aware of with this syndrome include polymicrobial meningitis and osteomyelitis.

Summary

The examples of infectious syndromes described in this chapter are those which have been studied the most comprehensively as to their pathogenesis and as to host immune defenses. There are many other infectious syndromes found more frequently or presenting more severely in the age. Meningitis, for example, is more severe in the elderly and may present in an insidious manner in this age group. Because biliary tract disease is more frequent in the aged, cholecystitis and peritonitis are more frequent.

Similarly, diverticulitis is more common because of the increased frequency of diverticulosis. Viral hepatitis, although less common in the aged, carries with it a high mortality in this group when it does occur. The aged have a high incidence of achlorhydria and because of this lack of gastric acidity many organisms like tuberculosis, salmonella, and even listeriosis may be more frequent. Finally, even newly recognized diseases like Legionnaires' disease has a higher morbidity and mortality in the aged.

In discussing infection and immunity in the aged, it is still too early to fully understand the interrelationships that exist between pathogen and host. Man in aging not only is immunologically descending but develops unique immune parameters which cannot be equated with the immature stage. Therefore, the intracacies of infection upon the organism, man, must be appreciated not only as occurring within senescent function but occuring in a unique milieu. Some infections, as described, may actually contribute to this dysfunction and perhaps be responsible for some of the aging processes, while other infections may merely take advantage of the dysfunctions.

In understanding these associations, a further awareness of aging itself occurs and other diseases like those of the central nervous system, heart, lung, kidney, and other organ systems can be further clarified. A great deal of work is required in this area before substantive information can really be conveyed. This chapter represents more of an outline which we hope can be used to initiate the research required to expand our early awareness of the role of infections in adulthood and the aged.

REFERENCES

1. **McCabe, W. R. and Jackson, G. G.**, Gram-negative bacteremia. I, *Arch. Intern. Med.*, 110, 847, 1962.
2. **McCabe, W. R. and Jackson, G. G.**, Gram-negative bacteremia. II. Clinical, laboratory, and therapeutic observations, *Arch. Intern. Med.*, 110, 856, 1962.
3. **Salit, I. E. and Gotschlich, E. C.**, Type 1, Escherichia Coli pili: characterization of binding to monkey kidney cells, *J. Exp. Med.*, 146, 1182, 1977.
4. **Roantree, R. J. and Ranta, L. A.**, A study of the relationship of the normal bactericidal activity of human serum to bacterial infection, *J. Clin. Invest.*, 39, 72, 1960.
5. **Fierer, J., Finley, H., and Braude, E.**, A plaque assay on agar for detection of gram negative bacilli sensitive to complement, *J. Immunol.*, 109, 1156, 1972.
6. **Young, L. S. and Armstrong, D.**, Human immunity to Pseudomonas aeruginosa. I. In vitro interaction of bacteria, polymorphonuclear leukocytes, and serum, factors, *J. Infect. Dis.*, 126, 257, 1972.
7. **Miller, R. M., Garbus, J., and Hornick, R. B.**, Lack of enhanced oxygen consumption by polymorphonuclear leukocytes on phagocytosis of virulent *Salmonella typhi, Science,* 175, 1010, 1972.
8. **Liu, P. V.**, Extracellular toxins of Pseudomonas aeruginosa, *J. Infect. Dis.*, 130 (Suppl.), S-94, 1974.
9. **Wretlind, B. and Wodstron, T.**, Purification and properties of a protease with elastase activity from Pseudomonas aeruginosa, *J. Gen. Microbiol.*, 103, 319, 1977.
10. **McGowan, J. E., Barnes, M. W., and Finland, M. W.**, Bacteremia at Boston City Hospital: occurrence and mortality during 12 selected years (1935—1972) with special reference to hospital acquired cases, *J. Infect. Dis.*, 132, 316, 1975.
11. **Armstrong, D., Young, L. S., Meyer, R. D., Blevins, A. H.**, Infectious complications of neoplastic disease, *Med. Clin. North Am.*, 55, 729, 1971.
12. **Leigh, D. A.**, Bacteraemia in patients receiving human cadaveric renal transplants, *J. Clin. Pathol.*, 24, 295, 1971.
13. **Winston, D. J., Gale, R. P., Meyer, D. V., Young, L. S.**, Infectious complications of human bone marrow transplantation, *Medicine,* 58, 1, 1979.
14. National Nosocomial Infections Study Report, Annual Summary 1976, Center for Disease Control, Atlanta, 1978.
15. **Buck, A. C. and Cooke, E. M.**, The fate of ingested Pseudomonas aeruginosa in normal persons, *J. Med. Microbiol.*, 2, 521, 1969.
16. **Ketover, B. P., Young, L. S., and Armstrong, D.**, Septicemia due to *Aeromonas hydrophila:* clinical and immunologic aspects, *J. Infect. Dis.*, 127, 284, 1973.
17. **Fisher, K. W., Gerger, B., and Keusch, T. T.**, Subepidermal bullae due to *E. coli, Arch. Dermatol.*, 11, 105, 1974.
18. **Gunnar, R. M., Leob, H. S., Winslow, E. J., Blain, C., Robinson, J.**, Hemodynamic measurements in bacteremic and septic shock in man, *J. Infect. Dis.*, 128, 295, 1973.
19. **Galanos, C., Lüderitz, O., Rietschel, E. T.**, Newer aspects of the chemistry and biology of bacterial lipopolysaccharides with special r eference to their lipid A component. International review of biochemistry, *Biochem. Lipids II,* 14, 239, 1977.
20. **Lüderitz, O.**, Endotoxins and other cell wall components of gram negative bacteria and their biological activities, in *Microbiology,* American Society for Microbiology, Washington, D.C., 1977, 239.
21. **Kimball, H. R., Melmon, K. L., and Wolff, S. M.**, Endotoxin induced kinin production in man, *Proc. Soc. Exp. Biol. Med.*, 139, 1078, 1972.
22. **Nies, A. S., Forsyth, R. P., Williams, H. E., Melmon, K. L.**, Contribution of kinins to endotoxin shock in unanesthetized Rhesus monkeys, *Circ. Res.*, 22, 155, 1968.
23. **Ulevitch, R. J., Cochrane, C. G., Henson, P. M., Morrison, D. C., Doe, W. F.**, Mediation systems in bacterial lipopolysaccharide-induced hypotension and disseminated intravascular coagulation. I. The role of complement, *J. Exp. Med.*, 142, 1570, 1975.
24. **Ziegler, E. J., Douglas, H., Sherman, J. E., Davis, C. E., Bravde, A. I.**, Treatment of E. Coli and Klebsiella bacteremia in granulocytic animals with antiserum to a UDP-GAL epimerase-deficient mutant, *J. Immunol.*, 11, 433, 1973.
25. **Young, L. S., Ingram, J., and Stevens, P.**, Functional role of antibody against core glycolipid of *Enterbacteriaceae, J. Clin. Invest.*, 56, 850, 1975.
26. **Agnello, V.**, Complement deficiency states, *Medicine,* 57, 1, 1978.
27. **Young, L. S., Meyer, R. D., and Armstrong, D.**, *Pseudomonas aeruginosa* vaccine in cancer patients, *Ann. Intern. Med.*, 79, 518, 1973.
28. **Johnston, R. B., Newman, M. S., and Struth, A. G.**, An abnormality of the alternate pathway of complement activation in sickle-cell disease, *N. Engl. J. Med.*, 288, 803, 1973.
29. **McKeown, F.**, *Pathology of the Aged,* Butterworths, London, 1965, 361.
30. **Rossman, I., Rodstein, M., and Bornstein, A.**, Undiagnosed diseases in an aging population, *Arch. Intern. Med.*, 33, 366, 1974.

31. **Osler, W.,** Lobar Pneumonia, in *Osler's Textbook Revisited,* Harvey, A. M. and McKusick, V. A., Eds., Appleton-Century-Crofts, New York, 1976, 75.
32. **Austrian, R. and Gold, J.,** Pneumococcal bacteremia with a special reference to bacteremic pneumococcal pneumonia, *Ann. Intern. Med.,* 60, 759, 1964.
33. **Zeman, F. D. and Wallach, K.,** Pneumonia in the aged, *Arch. Intern. Med.,* 77, 678, 1946.
34. **Chickering, H. T. and Park, J. H.,** *Staphylococcus aureus* pneumonia, *JAMA,* 72, 618, 1919.
35. **Ede, S., Davis, G. M., and Holmes, F. H.,** Staphylococcic pneumonia, *JAMA,* 170, 638, 1959.
36. **Sullivan, R. J., Jr., Dowdle, W. R., Marine, W. M., and Hierholzer, J. C.,** Adult pneumonia in a general hospital. Etiology and host risk factors, *Arch. Intern. Med.,* 129, 935, 1972.
37. **Finland, M., Peterson, O. L., and Strauss, E.,** Staphlococcic pneumonia occuring during an epidemic of influenza, *Arch. Intern. Med.,* 70, 183, 1942.
38. **Jensen, K. and Lassen, H. C.,** Fulminating staphylococcal infections treated with fucidin and penicillin or semisynthetic penicillin, *Ann. Intern. Med.,* 60, 790, 1964.
39. **Mudd, S.,** Resistance against *Staphylococcus aureus, JAMA,* 218, 1671, 1971
40. **Singleton, L, Ross, G. W., and Kohn, J.,** Staphylococcal teichoic acid antibody in the sera of patients with burns, *Nature (London),* 263, 1173, 1964.
41. **Martin, R. R. and White, A.,** The in vitro release of leukocyte histamine by staphylococcal antigens, *J. Immunol.,* 102, 437, 1969.
42. **Louria, D. B., Blumenfeld, H. L., Ellis, J. T., Kilbourne, E. D., Rogers, D. E.,** Studies on influenza in the pandemic of 1957—1958. II. Pulmonary complications of influenza, *J. Clin. Invest.,* 38, 213, 1959.
43. **Housworth, J. and Langmuir, A. D.,** Excess mortality from epidemic influenza 1957—1966, *Am. J. Epidemiol.,* 100, 40, 1974.
44. **Housworth, J. and Spoon, M.,** The age distribution of excess mortality during A2 Hong Kong influenza epidemics compared with earlier A2 outbreaks, *Am. J. Epidemiol.,* 94, 348, 1971.
45. **Habershon, R. B., Molyneaux, M. E., Slavin, G., Loewi, G., and Tyrell, D. A. J.,** Skin tests with influenza virus, *J. Hyg. Camb.,* 71, 755, 1973.
46. **Cate, T. R. and Kelly, J. R.,** Hong Kong influenza antigen sensitivity and decreased interferon response of peripheral lymphocytes, in *Antimicrobiol Agents and Chemotherapy, 1970,* Hobby, G. L., Ed., American Society for Microbiology, Bethesda, Md. 1971, 156.
47. **Kantzter, G. B., Lanteria, S. F., Cusumano, C. L., Lee, J. D., Ganguly, R., and Waldman, R.,** Immunosuppression during influenza virus infection, *Infect. Immun.,* 1, 996, 1974.
48. **Suzuki F., Ohya, J., and Ishida, N.,** Effect of antilymphocyte serum on influenza virus infection in mice, *Proc. Soc. Exp. Biol. Med.,* 146, 78, 1974.
49. **Fransen, H., Sterner, G., Forsgren, M.,** Acute lower respiratory illness in elderly patients with respiratory syncytial virus infection. *Acta Medica Scand.,* 182, 323, 1967.
50. Center for Disease Control, Respiratory syncytial virus-Missouri, *Morbid. Mortal. Weekly Rep.,* 26, 351, 1977.
51. **Sweany, H. C.,** The pathology of primary tuberculosis infection in the adult, *Am. Rev. Tuberc.,* 39, 236, 1939.
52. **Stead, W. S., Kerby, G. R., and Schlueter, D. P.,** The clinical spectrum of primary tuberculosis in adults. Confusion with reinfection in the pathogenesis of chronic tuberculosis, *Ann. Intern. Med.,* 68, 731, 1968.
53. **Sibley, J. C.,** A study of 200 cases of tuberculosis pleurisy with effusion, *Am. Rev. Tuberc.,* 62, 314, 1950.
54. **Dhancl, S., Fisher, M., and Fewell, J. W.,** Intrathoracic tuberculosis lymphadenopathy in adults, *JAMA,* 241, 505, 1979.
55. **Christensen, W. I.,** Genitourinary tuberculosis: review of 102 cases, *Medicine,* 53, 377, 1974.
56. **Davidson, P. T. and Horowitz, I.** Skeletal tuberculosis. A review with patient presentation and discussion, *Am. J. Med.,* 48, 77, 1970.
57. **Gelf, A. F., Liffler, C., and Brewin, A.,** Miliary tuberculosis, *Am. Rev. Respir. Dis.,* 108, 1329, 1973.
58. **Munt, P. W.,** Miliary tuberculosis in the chemotherapy era: with a clinical review of 69 American adults, *Medicine,* 51, 139, 1971.
59. Miliary tuberculosis in the elderly, editorial, *Br. Med. J.,* 2, 265, 1965.
60. **Brocklehurst, J. C., Fry, J., Griffiths, L., and Kalton, G.,** Urinary infection and symptoms of dysuria in women aged 45-64 years: their relevance to similar findings in the elderly, *Age Ageing,* 1, 41, 1972.
61. **Akhtar, H. R., Andrews, G. R., Caird, F. I., and Fallon, R. J.,** Urinary tract infection in the elderly — a population study, *Age Ageing,* 1, 48, 1972.
62. **Brocklehurst, J. C., Dillane, J. J., Griffiths, L., and Fry, J.,** The prevalence and symptomatology of urinary infection in an aged population, *Gerontol. Clin.,* 10, 242, 1968.

63. **Brocklehurst, J. C., Bee, P., Jones, D. M., and Palmer, M. K.,** Bacteriuria in geriatric hospital patients — its correlates and management, *Age and Ageing,* 6, 240, 1977.
64. **Guze, L. B., Goldner, B. H., and Kalmanson, G. M.,** Pyelonephritis, 1. Observations on the course of chronic non-obstructed enterococcal infection in the kidney of the rat, *Yale J. Biol. Med.,* 33, 372, 1961.
65. **Freedman, L. R. and Beeson, P. B.** Experimental pyelonephritis IV. Observations on infections resulting from direct inoculation of bacteria in different zones of the kidney, *Yale J. Biol. Med.,* 30, 406, 1958.
66. **Beeson, P. B. and Rowley, D.,** The anticomplementary effect of kidney tissue. Its association with ammonia production, *J. Exp. Med.,* 110, 685, 1959.
67. **Rochu, H. and Fekety, F. R.,** Acute inflammation in the renal cortex and medulla following thermal injury, *J. Exp. Med.,* 119, 131, 1964.
68. **Gruneberg, R. N., Leigh, D. A., and Brumfitt, W.,** *Escherichia coli* serotypes in urinary tract infection: studies in domicilliary, antenatal and hospital practice, in *Urinary Tract Infection,* O'Grady, F. and Brumfitt, W., Eds., Oxford University Press, London, 1968, 68.
69. **Olling, S., Hanson, L. A., and Holmgren, J.,** The bactericidal effect of normal human serum on E. Coli strains from normals and from patients with urinary tract infections, *Infection,* 1, 24, 1973.
70. **Glynn, A. A., Brumfitt, W., and Howard, C. J.,** K antigen and its relation to urinary tract infections, *Lancet,* 1, 514, 1971.
71. **Kaijser, B.,** Immunology of *Escherichia coli* K antigen and its relation to urinary tract infection, *J. Infect. Dis.,* 127, 670, 1973.
72. **Silverblatt, F. S.,** Host-parasite interaction in the rat renal pelvis: a possible role of pili in the pathogenesis of pyelonephritis, *J. Exp. Med.,* 140, 1696, 1974.
73. **Salit, I. E. and Gothschlich, E. C.,** Characterization of *E. coli* pili binding sites on mammalian cell membranes. Sixteenth Interscience Conf. Antimicrobial Agents Chemotherapy, Abstr. 10, Chicago, 1976.
74. **Braude, A. I.,** Current concepts of pyelonephritis, *Medicine,* 25, 257, 1973.
75. **Musker, D. M., Griffith, D. P., and Yaun, D.,** Role of *Urease* in pyelonephritis resulting from urinary tract infection with *Proteus, J. Infect. Dis.,* 131, 177, 1975.
76. **Kaye, D.,** Antibacterial activity of human urine, *J. Clin. Invest.,* 47, 2374, 1968.
77. **Stamey, T. A., Fair, W. R., and Timothy, M. M.,** Antibacterial nature of prostatic fluid, *Nature (London),* 218, 444, 1968.
78. **Bryant, R. E., Sutcliffe, M. C., and McGee, F. A.,** Human polymorphonuclear leukocyte function in urine, *Yale, J. Biol. Med.,* 46, 113, 1973.
79. **Cox, C. E., and Hinman, F., Jr.,** Experiments with induced bacteriuria, vesical emptying and bacteria growth on the mechanism of bladder defense to infection, *J. Urol.,* 86, 739, 1961.
80. **Cobbs, C. G. and Kaye, D.,** Antibacterial mechanism in the urinary bladder, *Yale J. Biol. Med.,* 40, 93, 1967.
81. **Hanson, L. A.,** Host parasite relationships in urinary tract infections, *J. Infect. Dis.,* 127, 726, 1973.
82. **Miller, T. E. and North, J. D.,** Host response in urinary tract infections, *Kidney Int.,* 5, 179, 1974.
83. **Hanson, L. S., Ahlstedt, S., and Fasth, A.,** Antigens of *Escherichia coli,* human immune response, and the pathogenesis of urinary tract infections, *J. Infect. Dis.,* 126, S-944, 1977.
84. **Susin, M. and Becker, E. L.,** The pathology of pyelonephritis, in *Urinary Tract Infection and Its Management,* Kaye, D., Ed., C. V. Mosby, St. Louis, 1972, 65.
85. **Hanson, L. A., Fasth, A., and Jodal, U.,** Autoantibodies to Tamm-Horsfall protein, a tool for diagnosing the level of urinary tract infection, *Lancet,* 1, 226, 1976.
86. **Aoki, S., Imamura, S., and Aoki, M.,** Abacterial and bacterial pyelonephritis. Immunofluorescent localization of bacterial antigen, *N. Engl. J. Med.,* 281, 1375, 1969.
87. **Rocha, H.,** Pathogenesis and clinical manifestations of urinary tract infection in *Urinary Tract Infection and Its Management,* Kaye, D., Ed., C. V. Mosby, St. Louis, 1972, 6.
88. **Cotran, T. S., Vivaldi, E., and Zangwill, D. P.,** Retrograde pyelonephritis in rats, *J. Pathol.,* 43, 1, 1963.
89. **Smellie, J. M. and Normand, I. C. S.,** Experience of followup of children with urinary tract infection, in *Urinary Tract Infection,* O'Grady, F. and Brumfitt, W., Eds., Oxford University Press, London, 1968, 123.
90. **Smellie, J. M. and Normand, I. C. S.,** Bacteriuria reflux and renal scarring *Arch. Dis. Child,* 50, 581, 1975.
91. **Thayer, W. S.,** Studies on bacterial (infective) endocarditis, *Johns Hopkins Hosp. Rep.,* 22, 1, 1926.
92. **Durack, D. T. and Petersdorf, R. G.,** Changes in the epidemiology of endocarditis, in *Infective Endocarditis, An American Heart Association Symposium,* Kaplan, E. L., Taranta, A. V., Eds., The American Heart Association, Dallas, 1977, 3.
93. **Garvey, G. J. and Neu, H. C.,** Infective endocarditis: an evolving disease, *Medicine,* 57, 105, 1978.

94. **Watanakunakorn, C.**, Changing epidemiology and newer aspects of infective endocarditis, *Adv. Intern. Med.*, 22, 21, 1977.
95. **Pelletier, L. L. and Petersdorf, R. G.**, Infective Endocarditis: a review of 125 cases from the University of Washington Hospitals, 1963—1972, *Medicine*, 56, 287, 1977.
96. **Dismukes, W. E., Karchmer, A. W., and Buckley, M. J.**, Prosthetic valve endocarditis: analysis of 38 cases, *Circulation*, 48, 365, 1973.
97. **Amoury, R. A., Bowman, F. O., Jr., and Malra, J. R.**, Endocarditis associated with intracardiac prostheses: diagnosis, management and prophylaxis, *J. Thorac. Cardiovasc Surg.*, 51, 36, 1966.
98. **Petheram, I. S. and Boyce, J. M. H.**, Prosthetic valve endocarditis: a review of 24 cases, *Thorax*, 32, 478, 1977.
99. **Cardelia, J. V., Befeler, B., and Hildner, F. J.**, Hypertrophic subaortic stenosis complicated by aortic insufficiency and subacute bacterial endocarditis, *Am. Heart J.*, 81, 543, 1971.
100. **Wang, K., Gobel, F. L., and Gleason, D. F.**, Bacterial endocarditis in idiopathic hypertrophic subaortic stenosis, *Am. Heart J.*, 89, 359, 1975.
101. **Corrigan, D., Bolen, J., and Hancock, E. W.**, Mitral valve prolapse and infective endocarditis, *Am. J. Med.*, 63, 215, 1977.
102. **Angrist, A. A. and Oka, M.**, Pathogenesis of bacterial endocarditis, *JAMA*, 183, 249, 1963.
103. **Durack, D. T.**, Experimental bacterial endocarditis. IV. Structure and function of very early lesions, *J. Pathol.*, 115, 81, 1975.
104. **Weinstein, L. and Schlesinger, J. J.**, Pathoanatomic, pathophysiologic, and clinical correlations in endocarditis. I., *N. Engl. J. Med.*, 291, 832, 1974.
105. **Rodbard, S.**, Blood velocity and endocarditis, *Circulation*, 27, 18, 1963.
106. **Lepeschkin, E.**, On the relation between the site of valvular involvement in endocarditis and the blood pressure resting on the valve, *Am. J. Med. Sci.*, 224, 318, 1952.
107. **Okell, C. C. and Elliott, S. D.**, Bacteremia and oral sepsis. With special reference to the aetiology of subacute endocarditis, *Lancet*, 2, 869, 1935.
108. **Everett, E. D. and Hirschmann, J. V.**, Transient bacteremia and endocarditis prophylasis, a review, *Medicine*, 56, 61, 1977.
109. **Loesche, W. J.**, Indigenous human flora and bacteremia, in *Infective Endocarditis, An American Heart Association Symposium*, Kaplan, E. L. and Taranta, A. V., Eds., The American Heart Association, Dallas, 1977, 40.
110. **Gould, K., Ramirez-Ronda, C. H., and Holmes, R. K.**, Adherence of bacteria to heart valves in vitro, *J. Clin. Invest.*, 56, 1364, 1975.
111. **Gibbons, R. J. and Nygaard, M.**, Synthesis of insoluble dextran and its significance in the formation of gelatinous deposits by plaque-forming streptococci, *Arch. Oral Biol.*, 13, 1249, 1968.
112. **Clawson, C. C. and White, J. G.**, Platelet interaction with bacteria, I. Reaction phases and effects of inhibitors, *Am. J. Pathol.*, 63, 367, 1971.
113. **Mair, W.**, Pneumococcal endocarditis in rabbits, *J. Pathol. Bacteriol.*, 26, 426, 1923.
114. **Messner, R. P., Laxdal, T., and Quie, P. G.**, Rheumatoid factors in subacute bacterial endocarditis-bacterium, duration of disease, or genetic predisposition?, *Ann. Intern. Med.*, 68, 746, 1968.
115. **Laxdal, T., Messner, R. P., and Williams, R. C.**, Opsonic agglutinating and complement-fixing antibodies in patients with subacute bacterial endocarditis, *J. Lab. Clin. Med.*, 71, 638, 1968.
116. **Horwitz, D., Quismorio, F. P., and Friou, G. J.**, Cryoglobulinemia in patients with infectious endocarditis, *Clin. Exp. Immunol.*, 19, 131, 1975.
117. **Bayer, A. S., Theofilopaulos, A. N., Eisenberg, R., et al.**, Circulating immune complexes in infective endocarditis, *N. Engl. J. Med.*, 295, 1500, 1976.
118. **Gutman, R. A., Striker, G. E., and Gilliland, B. C.**, The immune complex glomerulonephritis of bacterial endocarditis, *Medicine*, 51, 1, 1972.
119. **Robinson, M. J.**, Infective endocarditis at autopsy 1965—1969, *Am. J. Med.*, 52, 492, 1972.
120. **Roberts, W. C. and Buchbinder, N. A.**, Left sided valvular active infective endocarditis, *Am. J. Med.*, 53, 20, 1972.
121. **Cummings, V., Furman, S., and Dunst, M.**, Subacute bacterial endocarditis in the older age group, *JAMA*, 172, 137, 1960.
122. **Cherubin, C. S. and Neu, H. C.**, Infective endocarditis at the Presbyterian Hospital in New York City from 1938—1967, *Am. J. Med.*, 51, 83, 1971.
123. **Hughes, P.**, Bacterial endocarditis a changing disease, *Q. J. Med.*, 140, 511, 1966.
124. **Lerner, P. I. and Weinstein, L.**, Infective endocarditis in the antibiotic era, *N. Engl. J. Med.*, 274, 199, 1966.
125. **Wallach, J. B., Glass, M., Lukash, L., and Angust, A. A.**, Bacterial endocarditis in the aged, *Ann. Intern. Med.*, 42, 1206, 1955.
126. **Jackson, J. F. and Allison, F.**, Bacterial endocarditis, *South. Med. J.*, 54, 1331, 1961.
127. **Osler, W.**, Malignant endocarditis, *Lancet*, 1, 415, 459, 505, 1885.

128. **Applefeld, M. M. and Hornick, R. B.,** Infective endocarditis in patients over age 60, *Am. Heart J.,* 88, 90, 1974.
129. **Gleckler, W. J.,** Diagnostic aspects of subacute bacterial endocarditis in the elderly, *Arch. Intern. Med.,* 102, 761, 1959.
130. **Blout, J. C.,** Bacterial endocarditis, *Am. J. Cardiol.,* 38, 909, 1965.
131. **Anderson, H. T. and Staffurth, J. J.,** Subacute bacterial endocarditis in the elderly, *Lancet,* 1, 1055, 1955.
132. **Stiehm, E. R.,** Chronic cutaneous candidiasis, clinical aspects, in UCLA Conference, Severe Candida Infections: Clinical Perspective, Immune Defense Mechanisms and Current Concepts of Therapy (Edwards, J. E., Jr., Moderator), *Ann. Intern. Med.,* 89, 91, 1978.
133. **Pearsall, N. N., Sundsmo, J. S., and Weiser, R. S.,** Lymphokine toxicity for yeast cells, *J. Immunol.,* 110, 1444, 1973.
134. **Diamond, R. D.,** Antibody-dependent killing *Cryptococcus neoformans* by human peripheral blood mononuclear cells, *Nature (London),* 247, 148, 1974.
136. **Lehrer, R. I.,** The fungicidal mechanisms of human nonocytes. 1. Evidence for myeloperoxidase-linked and myeloperoxidase independent candidacidal mechanisma, *J. Clin. Invest.,* 55, 338, 1975.
136. **Lehrer, R. I.,** Measurement of candidacidal activity of specific leukocyte types in mixed cell populations. II. Normal and chronic granulomatous disease eosinophils, *Infect. Immun.,* 3, 800, 1971.
137. **Lehrer, R. I.,** Functional aspects of a second mechanism of candidacidal activity by human neutrophils, *J. Clin. Invest.,* 51, 2566, 1972.
138. **Lehrer, R. I., Ladra, K. M., and Hake, R. B.,** Non-oxidative fungicidal mechanisms of mammalian granulocytes: demonstration of components with candidacidal activity in human, rabbit, and guinea pig leukocytes, *Infect. Immun.,* 11, 1226, 1975.
139. **Cohen, A. B. and Cline, M. J.,** The human alveolar macrophages: isolation, cultivation in vitro and studies of morphologic and functional characteristics, *J. Clin. Invest.,* 50, 1390, 1971.
140. **Lehrer, R. I.,** Host defense mechanisms against disseminated candidiasis in UCLA Conference, Severe Candida Infections: Clinical Perspective, Immune Defense Mechanisms and Current Concepts of Therapy (Edwards, J. E., Jr., Moderator), *Ann. Intern. Med.,* 89, 91, 1978.
141. **Taschdjian, C. L., Toni, E. F., and Hsu, K. C.,** Immunofluorescence studies of Candida in human reticuloendothelial phagocytes: implications for immunogenesis and pathogenesis of systemic candidiasis, *Am. J. Clin. Pathol.,* 56, 50, 1971.
142. **Lehrer, R. I. and Cline, M. J.,** Interaction of *Candida albicans* with human leukocytes and serum, *J. Bacteriol.,* 98, 996, 1969.
143. **Morelli, R. and Rosenberg, L. T.,** The role of complement in the phagocytosis of *Candida albicans* by mouse peripheral blood leukocytes, *J. Immunol.,* 107, 476, 1971.
144. **Kernbaum, S.,** Pouvoirs phagocytaire et fongicide envers *Candida albicans* des polynucleaires neutrophiles humains en presence de serum depourvu de C3 et C4, *Ann. Microbiol. (Paris),* 126A, 75, 1975.
145. **Schade, A. L. and Caroline, L.,** An iron-binding component in human blood plasma, *Science,* 104, 340, 1966.
146. **Esterly, N. B., Brammer, S. R., and Crounse, R. G.,** In vitro inhibition of candidal growth by human serum, *J. Invest. Dermatol.,* 49, 246, 1967.
147. **Louria, D. B., Smith, J. K., and Brayton, R. G.,** Anti-Candida factors in serum and their inhibitors. I. Clinical and laboratory observation, *J. Infect. Dis.,* 125, 102, 1972.
148. **Lehrer, R. I.,** Inhibition by sulfonamides of the candidacidal activity of human neutrophils, *J. Clin. Invest.,* 50, 2498, 1971.
149. **Forsgren, A., Schmeling, D., and Quie, P. G.,** Effect of tetracycline on the phagocytic function of human leukocytes, *J. Infect. Dis.,* 130, 412, 1974.
150. **Curry, C. R. and Quie, P. G.,** Fungal septicemia in patients receiving parenteral hyperalimentation, *N. Engl. J. Med.,* 285, 1221, 1971.
151. **Hope-Simpson, R. E.,** The nature of Herpes-zoster. I. A long-term study and a new hypothesis, *Proc. R. Soc. Med.,* 58, 9, 1965.
152. **Lucy, J. P.,** Varicella-zoster virus, *J. Invest. Dermatol.,* 61, 212, 1973.
153. **Esire, M. M. and Tomlinson, A. H.,** Herpes zoster: demonstration of virus in trigeminal nerve and ganglion by immunofluorescence and electron microscopy, *J. Neurol. Sci.,* 15, 35, 1972.
154. **Ghatak, N. R., and Zimmerman, H. M.,** Spinal ganglion in herpes zoster, *Arch. Pathol.,* 95, 411, 1973.
155. **Bastian, F. O., Rabson, A. S., and Yee, C. L.,** Herpesvirus varicellae: isolated from human dorsal root ganglia, *Arch. Pathol.,* 97, 331, 1974.
156. **Shibuta, H., Ishikawa, T., and Hondo, R.,** Varicella virus isolation from spinal ganglion, *Arch. Gesamte Virusforsch.,* 45, 382, 1974.
157. **Brunell, P. A., Gershon, A. A., Uduman, S. A.,** Varicella-zoster immunoglobulins during varicella, latency and zoster, *J. Infect. Dis.,* 132, 49, 1975.

158. **Brunell, P. A. and Casey, H. L.**, A crude tissue culture antigen for the determination of varicella-zoster complement fixing antibody, *Public Health Rep.*, 79, 839, 1964.
159. **Williams, V., Gershon, A., and Brunell, P. A.**, Serologic response to varicella-zoster membrane antigens measured by indirect immunofluorescence, *J. Infect. Dis.*, 130, 669, 1974.
160. **Kaltzer, A. G., Steinberg, S., and Gershon, A. A.**, Immune adherence hemagglutination: further observations on demonstration of antibody to varicella-zoster virus, *J. Infect. Dis.*, 135, 1010, 1977.
161. **Galpin, J. E., Chow, A. W., and Guze, L. B.**, Sepsis associated with decubitus ulcer, *Am. J. Med.*, 61, 346, 1976.
162. **Chow, A. W., Galpin, J. E., and Guze, L. B.**, Clindamycin treatment of sepsis caused by decubitus ulcer, *J. Infect. Dis.*, 135, 565, 1977.
163. **Louie, T. J., Bartlee, J. G., and Talley, F. P.**, Aerobic and anaerobic bacteria in diabetic foot ulcer, *Ann. Intern. Med,*. 85, 461, 1976.

IMMUNOSUPPRESSION, AUTOIMMUNITY, AND PRECOCIOUS AGING: OBSERVATIONS AND SPECULATIONS*

H. Hugh Fudenberg

OBSERVATIONS

We have previously described two patients with various symptoms of "precocious aging". The patients and their first-degree relatives were studied for several immunologic parameters. The first patient, a white female first seen at age 15 years, had very short stature, onset of menses at age 4, breast development and pubic hair at age 9, and progeric nuclear bilateral sclerotic ("senile") cataracts at age 9. Immunologic studies showed that her peripheral blood lymphocyte populations were abnormal: 14% active T-cells (normal level; 28 ± 6%) and 45% total T-cells (normal; 65 ± 5%), as determined by rosette formation with nonenzyme-treated sheep red blood cells. Her mother had normal active and total T-cells (29% and 63.5%). Her father had moderately depressed levels of active and total T-cells (19% and 53.5%), and one of her three half-siblings had low active T-cells (13%) as did the mother of the half-siblings, the patient's stepmother (18% active T-cells). The patient developed osteosarcoma 1 year later, and further family studies (Figure 1) revealed a very high prevalence of malignancy and of moderately decreased active T-cells on both the paternal and maternal sides of the family.[1] Lack of cooperation by the family made HLA, autoantibody, and suppressor T-cell studies impossible.

In a second family, the proband, a black male 15-years-old with short stature (height 132 cm), had many stigmata of precocious aging: prematurely gray hair, sparse hair, generalized periodontitis, osteoporosis (by X-ray), carcinomatous changes of the oral mucosa, and changes in skin strength and elasticity of the type seen in aged individuals, but much more severe. The patient fulfilled some of the diagnostic criteria of the dyskeratosis congenita syndrome, a premalignant cutaneous disease. One sibling with similar physical features of precocious aging had died with the same clinical syndrome before the time of study; the propositus and sibling (his elder sister) were products of a second-cousin marriage. Active and total T-cells were decreased in the proband, as was a subpopulation of T-cells binding to a B lymphoblastoid cell line (T-BLCL). These parameters were also studied in seven siblings and in several other relatives in three generations (Figure 2). The mother had dermatomyositis, and the maternal grandmother and her sister reportedly had rheumatoid arthritis. Family studies revealed a high prevalence of deficiency in active T-cells and in T-BLCL, in some cases severe enough to result in a decrease in total T-cells. [In an earlier study,[2] we had shown a significant inverse correlation between levels of T-BLCL and circulating immune complexes in patients with multiple sclerosis.] We concluded from these data that an apparently genetically determined defect in cell-mediated immunity was associated with, and perhaps the cause of, the symptoms of precocious aging in the patient, and we hypothesized that an abiotrophy of one or another subpopulation of T-cells may result in physiologic aging.[3] We did not preclude the possibility that the immunologic defect might be a consequence of other (e.g., endocrine) factors.

* Publication No. 400 from the Department of Basic and Clinical Immunology and Microbiology, Medical University of South Carolina. Research supported in part by USPHS Grants HD-09938 and CA-25746. Editorial assistance provided by Charles L. Smith.

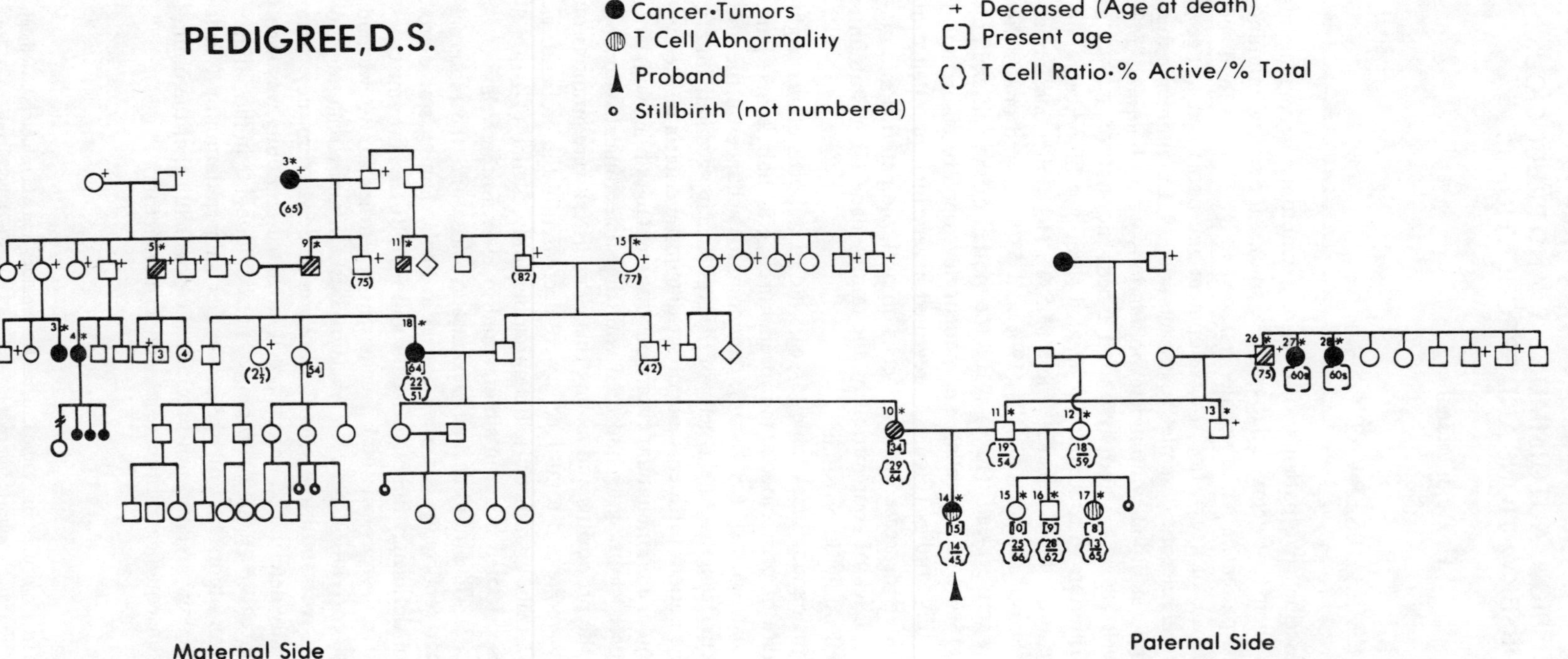

FIGURE 1. Pedigree of a proband with multiple symptoms of precocious aging, showing high incidence of malignancy and of T-cell abnormalities in family members. (From Fudenberg, H. H., Schuman, S. H., Goust, J. M., and Jorgenson, R., *Gerontology*, 24, 266, 1978, S. Karger AG, Basel. With permission.)

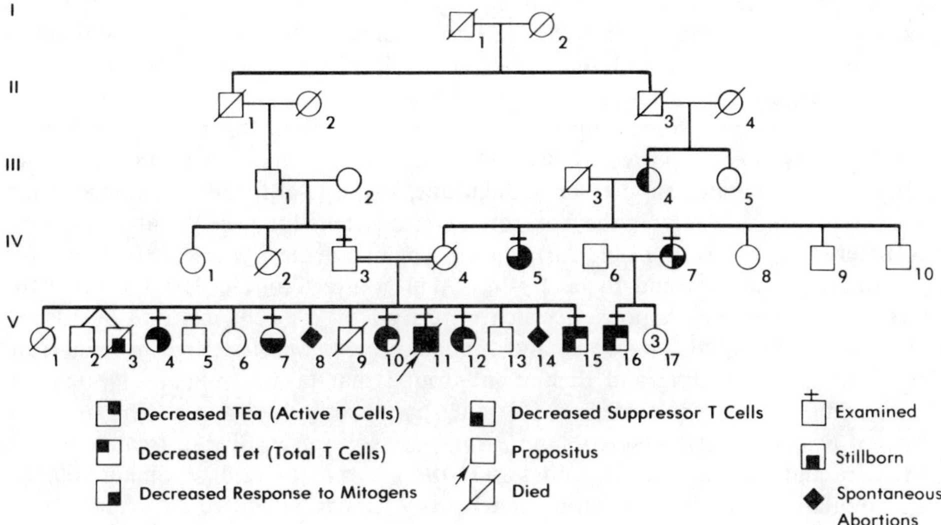

FIGURE 2. Pedigree of a second proband with symptoms of precocious aging. The proband (V-11) and his older sister (V-1) had dyskeratosis congenita. Their mother (IV-4) had dermatomyositis. (From Fudenberg, H. H., Schuman, S. H., Goust, J. M., Vesole, D. H., and Salinas, C. F., *Gerontology*, 24, 268, 1979, S. Karger AG, Basel. With permission.)

IMMUNOLOGIC AND GENETIC FACTORS IN AGING

Studies over the past 10 years have given rise to a multitude of theories on aging (e.g., References 4 to 8). Investigations of a variety of biological systems have been initiated and expanded in attempts to find methods that eventually might be used to delay the onset of human aging or lessen the severity of its physiologic effects, as well as for preventing some of the diseases associated with aging. Among the theories of aging are those proposing an immunologic cause of aging, since most organ-specific autoantibodies are increased in frequency in aged populations as compared with young populations.[4]

In order to test the hypothesis that autoimmunity has an important role in age-associated diseases, we performed experiments in the past (1966 to 1969) using RF/Un mice, which only late in life (30 months) develop abnormal urinary findings and small deposits of IgG and C3 of the "lumpy-bumpy" type in the kidney, morphologically very similar to those found in patients with systemic lupus erythematosus and in NZB/NZW hybrid mice.[9] Neonatal thymectomy resulted in the appearance of marked renal antigen-antibody complex deposition at 3 to 6 months of age and early death from renal failure. These observations suggested to us that a thymic suppressor factor might function to delay the appearance of autoantibodies and/or development of autoimmune disease in these mice; we postulated that autoimmune disease results when the function and/or numbers of nonspecific suppressor T-cells are diminished, with consequent marked rise in immunoglobulin levels and autoimmune clones (both humoral and cellular).[10] Our own studies of human populations indicated that all normal individuals have *low* levels of various autoantibodies, presumably monitored by normal T suppressor functions.[11,12] The relevance of this finding to the aging process is suggested by the findings of Mackay,[13] who has shown in several population studies that individuals with significantly elevated levels of autoantibodies (but without clinical autoimmune disease) had shorter life spans than did individuals of similar age, sex, and ethnic origin with "no" autoantibodies (as defined by his level of sensitivity).

Until recently, the concept of "suppressor T-cells" was viewed as heretical; however, an explosion of the literature in this area has produced a host of reports supporting their existence in mice and in humans (a recent critical review and discussion can be found in Reference 14). Gershon et al.[15] have suggested that suppressor T-cells inhibit not only B-cells but also some subpopulation(s) of T-cells (i.e., "helper" T-cells). Similar findings have been reported by Benacerraf and co-workers (reviewed in Reference 16). In studies of isolated suppressor populations, Vadas et al.[17] found that the Ly and Ia phenotypes of mouse lymphocytes from several strains involved in different functions differed. T-cells responsible for delayed-type cutaneous hypersensitivity and for *helper* functions were found to be Ly-1$^+$, 2$^-$, in contrast to T-cells responsible for *suppression* of antibody responses, which were Ly-1$^-$, 2$^+$. T-cells involved in delayed cutaneous hypersensitivity were Ia$^-$, and suppressor cells were Ia$^+$.[17] Using cells from CBA/J mice, Hämmerling and Eichmann[18] found that Ia determinants, present on both unprimed and primed antibody-forming precursor cells, were absent from the surface of helper T-cells, whereas suppressor T-cells were sensitive to treatment with anti-Ia sera and complement, demonstrating the presence of Ia determinants on this T-cell population. Similiarly, Cantor and Boyse[19,20] have identified two functionally distinct murine T-cell subclasses on the basis of their expression of discrete thymus-dependent Ly alloantigens. The Ly-1 phenotype was found to be expressed by T-cells responsible for helper activity, delayed hypersensitivity, and mixed lymphocyte reactivity to Ia determinants, and the Ly-23 phenotype on T-cells that exert suppressor effects and also cytotoxic effects.[19-21] Thus, the fact that suppressor T-cells are a separate and distinct subpopulation of T-cells in both mice and rats is well established. Indeed, in studies of 1-month-old NZB/W mice, Gerber and Steinberg[22] were able to physically separate thymocytes that showed suppressor but not helper effects from those that showed help but no suppression, using unit gravity sedimentation and a graft-vs.-host assay for thymocyte function.

Earlier, Gerber et al.[23] had shown that suppressor cells are lost as NZB/W mice age, and that suppressor function is lost before helper function. Morton et al.,[24] using mice of the same strain, showed a spontaneous loss of thymic suppressor cells and subsequent development of autoimmunity and lymphoreticular hyperplasia with increasing age. Restoration of suppressor cells by treatment with 2-week-old syngeneic thymocytes every 2 weeks, starting at 4 weeks of age, retarded all the major disease manifestations usually observed (i.e., positive direct Coombs' tests, renal disease, and lymphoreticular proliferation).

Genetic differences in longevity have been shown to be correlated with diminished suppressor function in several strains of inbred mice. For example, Ranney and Steinberg[25] studied the age-dependent release of a low-molecular-weight suppressor of DNA synthesis by cultured thymocytes and spleen cells from C57BL/6 and BALB/c ("normal") mice and by cells from the lymphoid organs of NZB/W ("autoimmune") mice. They found that spleen cells from the "normal" strains released high levels of the soluble suppressor early in life and gradually decreasing quantities with increasing age, whereas the NZB/W cells released only low levels even early in life.

In studies using spleen cells from DA rats, Folch and Waksman[26] showed that suppressor activity was present in normal animals but absent in doubly thymus-deprived animals, and that the spleens of older rats differed from those of younger ones by a variable loss of suppressor cells. In rabbits, Kamin, Henry, and Fudenberg[27] have shown that high concentrations of suppressor T-cells are present in the appendix, moderate concentrations in the spleen, and none in the thymus itself at 3 months. In contrast, in newborn rabbits high concentrations of suppressor cells were present in the thymus; and in 2-year-old rabbits, levels in the appendix and spleen were markedly reduced in comparison with those at 3 months (Kamin and Fudenberg, unpublished observations).[27a] [In humans, using thymuses obtained at cardiac surgery, we have found the concentration of suppressor T-cells in the thymus to be much lower in individuals 15- to 30-years-old than in infants and children 2- to 8-years-old.[27b] Similar results were obtained using peripheral blood.]

Kurnick et al.[28] have demonstrated PHA-induced activation of suppressor T-cells in normal human peripheral blood lymphocytes, and the existence of suppressor T-cells in humans has been further supported by the studies of Witemeyer et al.[29] on the suppression of normal B-cell maturation by peripheral blood cells from patients with "acquired" hypogammaglobulinemia and from normal neonates. Further, the role of suppressor cells in the pathogenesis of common variable hypogammaglobulinemia and the immunodeficiency associated with monoclonal gammopathy has been documented by Waldman et al.,[30] who suggested a block in B-cell maturation by suppressor cells as a possible mechanism for the humoral immune deficiency in both disorders. Recent reports suggest that (a) human patients with systemic lupus erythematosus (SLE), a disease closely similar to the autoimmune disease in NZB/W mice, *lack* suppressor T-cells in their peripheral blood, but that suppressor activity is regained as the clinical symptoms diminish with corticosteroid therapy[31] and (b) that suppressor cell activity in symptomatic SLE patients receiving corticosteroid therapy was significantly reduced as compared to both normal controls and non-SLE patients receiving similar doses of corticosteroids.[32] In the latter study it was suggested that the presence of B-cell hyperfunction in SLE might be secondary to depressed suppressor cell activity. On the basis of these and similar findings, we proposed (e.g., Reference 1) that a decline in suppressor T-cells was intimately associated with physiologic aging, and indeed might be the cause thereof. Subsequently, Hallgren and Yunis[33] reported that Concanavalin A (Con A)-activated lymphocytes derived from an aging human population differed from those of young individuals in showing a variable loss of suppressor activity.

Aging and Cellular Immunity: Studies in Animals

Studies of thymectomized and untreated mice have produced several lines of evidence to suggest that thymic involution invariably accompanies the aging process and results in a loss of function of thymus-derived lymphocytes. The thymus apparently is the only gland in which extreme involution occurs as a concomitant of normal aging.[34] [We have shown in humans that parathyroid hormone levels decline in elderly normal individuals in a fashion closely paralleling the decline in thymus size[35].] Aging varies considerably in different inbred strains of mice, as measured by several parameters, and genetic differences in longevity have been described in a number of studies. Three of the strains that live *the longest* are the LP, 129, and C57BL strains; these strains are all homozygous H^{2b} at the major histocompatibility complex (MHC) of the mouse,[36] and few animals of these long-lived strains develop "autoimmune" phenomena. Some investigators have therefore suggested that it is important to distinguish between long-lived and short-lived inbred mouse strains and between autoimmune-susceptible and nonsusceptible strains in interpreting data on aging, since true senescence of a particular function may be detectable only in the long-lived strains. However, low-level "autoimmunity" may also be an integral part of the normal aging process, responsible for removal of aged and/or damaged tissues, as suggested by us some years ago.[10-12]

Studies of cellular immunity performed in aging mice have revealed that within the same batch of mice, increasing age may be associated with increased capabilities in some parameters of cellular immunity and decreased capabilities in others.[37] The exact role of the immune system in aging is not clear, but a genetically programmed process seems to be involved. Some changes in cell-mediated immunity in long-lived $BC3F_1$ mice associated with thymic involution and aging are the loss by thymic tissues of the capacity to influence the following functions: (a) lymphocyte repopulation of the T-cell-dependent areas of lymph nodes, (b) mitogenic reactivity of splenic cells to T-cell-specific mitogens phytohemagglutinin (PHA) and concanavalin A (Con A), (c) number of θ-antigen-positive splenic lymphocytes and splenic T-cell helper function, and (d) mitogenic reactivity of splenic T-cells to allogeneic lymphocytes.[38] It has also been found that in inbred rats, changes in the antibody response with age can be seen in highly responding strains but not in poorly responding strains, suggesting that factors influencing antibody formation at different ages modulate the genetically set capability of the immune system.[39]

A high incidence of certain "autoantibodies" has been reported in various mouse strains.[40] For example, Friou and Teague[41] found antibodies to nucleoprotein in 34% of multiparous mice of the A/J strain and in 13% of the males of the same strain in mice at age 6 to 12 months. No antinuclear factors were found in the sera of 16 other mouse strains of comparable age, although subsequent studies showed these to be present in the serum of aged mice of other strains.[42] Other "autoantibodies" (i.e., positive Coombs' tests) have been observed in increasing frequency with increasing age in NZB/W hybrid mice by many observers (e.g., see Reference 43). Immunologic renal disease and antinuclear antibodies have also been found in a high percentage of NZB/W hybrids by many observers (e.g., see References 44 and 45) and in varying prevalence in different strains of neonatally thymectomized mice,[46,47] as has an increase in renal lysozyme excretion,[48] an invariant concomitant of aging and a very sensitive indicator of "wasting disease".[49] Recently, Sacher and Duffy[50] estimated the average life spans for the male progeny from 21 of the 25 possible matings of 5 inbred mouse strains, and correlated this with a new metabolic parameter; their data suggest the existence of a genetically determined "longevity factor" dependent on the partition of energy between the phasic metabolism of activity and the continuous maintenance metabolism.[50] Although the 21 genotypes varied greatly in susceptibility to neoplastic disease, the authors indicated that the excess mortality due to these diseases was of secondary importance in determining survival time.

We showed in 1969[51] that neonatal thymectomy results in deposition of IgG and complement in the kidneys of young RF/Un mice; these deposits are histologically identical to those seen in normal aged mice of the strain studied and in young NZB/W mice.[9] It is of considerable interest that the inbred mice in which wasting disease was experimentally induced (by injection of the parental strain with lymphoid cells of F_1 hybrid offspring) developed not only the serologic features mentioned above but also thymic atrophy, atrophy of thymus-dependent lymphoid tissue, and amyloidosis.[52]

Other experimental evidence indicates that a decline in cellular immunity occurs with aging in C57BL mice.[53] Callard and Basten[54] have also shown that in CBA/H mice there is a T-cell defect in old mice. They concluded that the defect was more likely to be qualitative than quantitative, but since they used only mitogenic response to PHA to assess T-cell function, a quantitative defect in one or another T-cell subpopulation cannot be excluded. Indeed, the authors stated that their data "although arguing against a quantitative defect in total T-cell numbers, do not exclude the possibility of selective depletion of a reactive subpopulation of T-cells." Goidl et al.[55] have reported that there is an apparent *loss* of thymic *helper* cells and an *increase* in *suppressor* activity in C57BL/6 mice,[55] but others have questioned those results on the basis that the methods used were inadequate to justify the conclusions reached.[56] In $B6CF_1$ mice, Brennan and Jaroslow[57] have reported an age-associated decline in theta antigen on splenic T-cells, and Rose and Girardi[58] have shown that the age of the host is important in detecting tumor-associated transplantation antigens on cultured cells from BALB/c mice immunized with transformed cell lines.[58]

Fabris, Pierpaoli and Sorkin[59] reported some time ago that hypopituitary dwarf mice (Snell-Bagg strain), with a usual life span of 3 to 5.5 months, lived for >12 months when treated with lymph node lymphocytes (but not bone marrow cells) from normal mice or when treated simultaneously with both somatropic hormone (growth hormone) and thyrotropic hormone (thyroxine). The authors concluded that optimal thymic function is directly related to survival, with the possible explanation that immunosurveillance by T-cells against foreign matter or against modified self components increases survival. Sorkin[59a] now believes that the pituitary defect is due to a defect in one or another hypothalamic function, but in any event T-cells are necessary to prolong life in these mice. Furthermore, a recent study by Dilman[60] suggests that the hypothalamic defect which he assumes is responsible for the immunologic and metabolic defects resulting in aging is secondary to a decrease in pineal function. In preliminary experiments, injection of crude pineal extracts increased the life span of rodents,[60] using both healthy, aged animals and animals with chemically induced carcinomas. In both cases, the injection of semipurified pineal extract extended life as compared with untreated control groups. In this context, it is noteworthy that Greenberg and Weiss[61] have shown a reduced number of β-adrenergic receptors in the pineal gland of aged rats as compared with 3-month-old rats.

Aging and Cellular Immunity: Studies in Humans

HLA heterozygosity has been suggested as a genetic marker of long-term survival in humans in studies by Gerkins et al.,[62] who found that old, healthy persons had a larger number of HLA specificities than did cancer patients or young, healthy persons. However, their results remain controversial.

Serologic data for aged, presumably normal subjects show a high incidence of serologic abnormalities of the "autoimmune" variety similar to those observed in mice with thymic atrophy (induced either by injection of F_1 lymphoid cells into inbred parents or neonatal treatment with cortisone acetate), and to those seen in neonatally thymectomized mice.[63,64] Total T-cells have been reported by Smith et al.[65] to be at the lower limits of normal in aged populations (70-87 years), but "active" T-cells were not measured in this study. In one study,[66] a comparison of aged (>65 years) and young (<25 years) people showed significant depression of T-cell immune responses in the aged as measured by cutaneous delayed hypersensitivity (skin tests) to five antigens, in vitro lymphocyte PHA response, and late IgG response to 5 μg flagellin. Further, the mortality of very old people (>80 years) hyporesponsive in skin tests was significantly greater over a 2-year period than that of normally responsive very old people.

Lymphocyte response to PHA in vitro has repeatedly been reported to decrease with age in humans (e.g., References 67 and 68). However, Foad et al.[69] have shown that although the response is low in aged as compared with young subjects at 3 days, it is significantly higher at 5 days of culture when high concentrations of the mitogen (0.1 to 0.2 mg per culture) are used. The latter findings suggest a different interpretation of earlier studies of PHA responsiveness in relation to age and/or immune deficiency states (and also indicate the need for age-matched controls in lymphocyte cultures when evaluating immune deficiency). Ben-Zwi et al.[70] have found that the proportion of E-rosette-forming lymphocytes (total T-cells) was significantly lower among elderly individuals than among young adults or children 3- to 15-years-old. Cells forming "stable" E rosettes (resistant to prolonged incubation at 37°C) were found among elderly lymphocytes but could not be found among those from children over 1 year of age or from young adults.[70] Previous studies by Galili and Schlesinger[71] indicated that the proportion of *thymus* cells forming stable E rosettes decreased with increasing age in a strictly linear correlation for thymus donors from 4 to 55 years of age (however, the function of stable rosette-forming T-cells is unknown). Another report has shown that a subpopulation of human peripheral blood lymphocytes capable of binding with human (autologous or allogeneic) erythrocytes to form ''autorosettes'' are part of the T-cell population, and that the determinants on the erythrocyte surface which are involved in autorosette formation are expressed to a lesser extent on aging than on young red cells.[72]

In one recent study, Girard et al.[73] found evidence for both absolute decrease and functional impairment of total T-cells (negative skin tests to 100 IU tuberculin and to three other thymus-dependent antigens, poor in vitro lymphocyte [^{3}H]thymidine incorporation in response to PHA, and in some, failure of lymphocytes to produce leukocyte migration inhibition factor (LIF) in vitro) in 59 of 880 patients *hospitalized in a geriatric hospital* but with no obvious signs of active disease. Indeed, all of the results described above, although highly provocative, are difficult to interpret. In spite of the number of studies of various immune parameters which have been performed previously in attempts to define age-associated changes in man, no definite conclusions can be drawn because (a) the results of studies by different investigators often disagree, (b) in most studies the number of individuals examined has been too small to permit effective statistical comparisons, and (c), most importantly, the ''normal'' aged individuals studied have for the most part been selected from elderly people living in nursing homes, as opposed to active, healthy individuals living in the same community setting as individuals in the younger age groups studied. As a further example, in one very recent study of suppressor activity in elderly as compared with young individuals, the group of young people consisted almost exclusively[16-18] of healthy volunteers, whereas the study population of 25 elderly people were almost all drawn from individuals in hospital neurology clinics, with such disorders as seizures, cerebral vascular disease, dementia, amyotropic lateral sclerosis, and Parkinsonism.[74] This problem has been well stated by Epstein[75] in a recent report of the effects of aging on the kidney, who pointed out two important sources of error in cross-sectional studies comparing groups of different age: (a) first, that elderly subjects without overt disease may often have subclinical impairments (detectable by laboratory tests) which, though unnoticed, may adversely affect test results and (b) second, that subjects over the age of 75 represent a sample of biologically ''superior'' survivors from a cohort that has experienced at least 75% mortality (the ''selective mortality'' concept developed by Andres[76]), so that a cross-sectional study will seem to show age-related differences that do not exist. Cleary, as pointed out by Shock,[77] the best way to avoid these problems is to perform longitudinal studies of a single population over a long period, where repeated observations are made on the same subjects as they age, improving the possibility of identifying changes that are associated with aging rather than disease.

The need for longitudinal studies cannot be overemphasized. Again, an excellent summary is provided in a recent report on age and immune cell parameters by Zighelboim and co-workers:[78] ''The detection of age differences in a particular biological parameter is not necessarily indicative of actual age-dependent functional changes. Age differences could result from the action of confounding variables which were introduced into the study design by mismatching young and old study groups on a critical determinant such as health status or any other variable which could potentially affect immune status. In prior studies, the epidemiological characteristics of the study groups were not defined, and in many cases comparisons were made between healthy laboratory workers and geriatric individuals obtained from rest homes, asylums, and outpatient clinics. The latter groups cannot be considered representative of community-dwelling individuals, either young or old, because of the obvious differences in natural history. Thus, it may be that the age effects on immune status observed in these studies were artifacts caused by confounding environmental or personal variables. When interpreting the available data on immune status and age, it must be kept in mind that all of these studies have been cross-sectional in design, and thus the groups compared have been confounded on the date of birth. Under these conditions, any data obtained must be considered provisional until sufficient evidence is provided to support the validity of the comparisons attempted. Direct proof that age differences in a parameter equal age changes must come ultimately from a longitudinal investigation.''

Aging and Immunoglobulins: Studies in Humans

In a study of 73 apparently normal Swiss volunteers over 95-years-old, Radl et al.[79] found idiopathic monoclonal proteins in 19%. Sera of individuals without paraproteinemia had an increase in IgA and IgG levels; an increase in the IgG_1 and IgG_3 subclasses was shown to be responsible for the elevated IgG levels. They concluded that aging in humans is accompanied by selective changes in the extent of the antibody-immunoglobulin ''repertoire.'' (Alternatively, we believe this might reflect a decline in Ig class-specific suppressor T-cells, as suggested by Waldmann's results.) Buckley et al.,[80] in longitudinal observations of IgG, IgA, and IgM levels for healthy individuals 40 years and older, found increasing levels of IgG and IgA in approximately two thirds of the subjects studied (but subnormal levels in others). They hypothesized an association of increased serum IgA and IgG levels with longevity (survival to older age) and a selective mortality of aged persons with relatively lower immunoglobulin levels (see also Reference 68). Studies of cellular immune function and autoantibodies were not performed.

Rowley et al.[81] found antinuclear antibodies (against DNA, RNA, histone, or other factors) in 45% of normal individuals between the ages of 70 and 79, but in only 5% of women and 2% of men between the ages of 20 and 29. Antiparietal cell antibodies were found in 26% of elderly patients (average age 76) without overt clinical disease but in only 7% of patients of an average age of 25.[82] Whether this is a consequence of the atrophic gastritis that occurs with aging is unknown. The incidence of antithyroid antibodies is also increased in aged individuals.[83] We have obtained similar data on organ-specific antibodies but not on antinuclear antibodies in an aged population shown to be normal by history, physical examination, chest film, electrocardiograms, and SMA-12.[84] Hallgren et al.[68] have also reported increased levels of autoantibodies in people >80 years of age, and especially in those with low lymphocyte responsiveness to PHA.

Need for Further Immunogenetic Studies

We are attempting in our ongoing studies of patients with symptoms of precocious aging to correlate the laboratory findings in such patients with HLA genotypes, allotypes of IgA,[85] IgM,[86] and IgG,[87] and the ''B-cell alloantigens''[88,89] serologically defined by HLA-DR typing.[90] These markers, alone or in combination, may be linked not only to immunologic responsiveness to various antigens in man (as the H-2 genotypes seem to be in mice) but also to aging. Indeed, HLA-B8 is associated with a wide variety of autoimmune disorders in humans (e.g., see Reference 91 for review), and Mackay's group[13] has obtained data indicating that autoantibodies to nuclear and tissue-specific antigens increase in prevalence with aging; furthermore, in their study, subjects with autoantibodies, as mentioned earlier above, had a shorter life span than those without in the population studied. The HLA antigens presumably are linked to

Ir genes determining the height not only of B-cell but also of T-cell responses to various antigens, as are the H-2 antigens in mice;[92] furthermore, as indicated above, the H-2 locus in mice, which has considerable polymorphism, is analogous to the HLA complex in man; mice homozygous for H^{2b} are essentially devoid of detectable autoantibodies and are long-lived.[36]

The MHC in the mouse is on the same chromosome as are genes for various complement components and the immune response genes in the *Ir* gene subregion; separate loci exist for Ir-A, Ir-B, Ir-C, and Ir-E. Genes at these loci produce helper effects to various antigens. This is true for both humoral and cellular immunity, as shown by Fachet and co-workers,[93,94] who also showed that there was an inverse correlation between cellular and humoral immune responses to a given antigen, controlled by the same Ir-linked genes; this is compatible with the concept of an increase in suppressor T-cell activity causing a decrease in humoral immunity. Genes at another closely linked locus, Ir-J, produce *suppressor* effects in cell-mediated immunity, and Fachet (personal communication)[94a] considers this likely in explaining his data. In man, the four HLA loci investigated to date are the loci for complement components C2 and C4 of the classical pathway, for Bf of the alternate complement pathway, and C6 and C8 of the final common pathway. These are present on chromosome six, as are the three known loci for B-cell alloantigens (including HLA-DR). Although immune response genes have not been proven to exist in man, there is inferential evidence for their existence; as discussed above, it is now almost certain that these will be closely linked to HLA. Presumably, human Ir genes governing antigen-specific *suppression,* at a sublocus analogous to mouse I-J, will also be found to be linked to HLA. If control of suppressor activity is multifactorial, the Gm, Km, or other allotype loci might also be involved. In any event, a search for *linkage* of lymphocyte subpopulation abnormalities in precocious aging seems warranted.

In our previous studies we have shown that Gm phenotypes are related to the height of the immune response to flagellin and to longevity. Furthermore, recent studies suggest that certain rare Gm phenotypes are associated with neuroblastoma (although typing was limited to 4 of the 24 known Gm markers).[95] Double-blind studies of Gm type in relation to frequency of tumors and resistance or response to therapy are currently in progress in our laboratories; the results so far have shown (a) a dramatic increase in the frequency of Gm(2) in Whites with malignant melanoma[96] and (b) a significant association between heterozygosity for Km(1) and Km(3) allotypes and humoral immune response to breast cancer.[97] Furthermore, we recently reported a highly significant difference in response to *H. influenzae* and meningococcus polysaccharide vaccines in patients with a given Km allotype as compared with those lacking this allotype.[98] In regard to B-cell alloantigens, it has been shown by others that for certain diseases associated with a greatly increased incidence of a given HLA antigen, the association with a given B-cell alloantigen may be even more striking — e.g., multiple sclerosis,[99,100] celiac disease and dermatitis herpetiformes,[101] and diabetes.[102]

Finally, thymosin levels have been reported to be decreased with age.[103] However, few attempts have been made to correlate this finding with specific T-cell subpopulations, and none with immunogenetic markers. It is conceivable that certain of the above genotypes could be present in high frequency in patients with both low thymosin levels and precocious aging. The possibility of such an *association* warrants a search for *linkage* of low thymosin levels in these individuals with various immunogenetic markers, although it is unclear at present whether the decrease in thymosin is a primary event associated with a decrease in active and suppressor T-cells or is merely a concomitant of the thymic involution which occurs with aging. This point merits detailed studies.

To our knowledge, studies in man correlating autoantibodies, quantitative and qualitative aberrations in immunoglobulins, quantitative measurements of cellular immunity, thymosin levels, and various immunogenetic markers with physiologic aging have not hitherto been performed, nor have studies correlating these with number and/or function of various T-cell subpopulations and thymosin levels. Such studies should provide meaningful information as to the immunologic mechanisms involved in precocious aging, and hopefully their genetic basis. This would be especially valuable if a clear correlation were found between one or another immunogenetic marker (a "genetic predisposition marker") and endocrine findings characteristic of physiologic aging. For example, if a genetic predisposition *linked* to a deficiency in suppressor T-cells is found, this may suggest a genetically determined immunologic defect as directly involved in the pathogenesis of aging (whether primary or secondary to a pituitary, hypothalamic, or pineal defect) rather than a concomitant thereof.

Endocrine Factors in Aging

Functional changes of the pituitary are known to occur with aging. The classic change is the menopausal syndrome, in which gonadal hypofunction is followed by a period of marked increase in gonadotropin [i.e., luteinizing hormone and follicle stimulating hormone (LH and FSH)] levels.[104] Pituitary function, other than gonadotropin release and synthesis, is likewise altered in clinically normal older individuals as compared with younger individuals. Pituitary adenomas are present in approximately 6% of autopsied pituitaries from patients who die after 80 years of age, and many of these glands contain prolactin granules,[105] suggesting that unrecognized prolactins may be present in many elderly people. [Cohen et al.[106] have also reported that in their postmortem studies of 113 outbred male rats of strain Crl:CD(SD)BR, 12- to 39-months-old, neoplasms of endocrine organs were encountered at least three times more frequently than were neoplasms in any other organ system.] Serum prolactin levels in elderly normal subjects, both men and women, are frequently elevated, as has also been found in rats.[107]

Pituitary responsiveness to a variety of releasing substances has been studied in elderly patients. Growth hormone (GH) responds to insulin-induced hypoglycemia in approximately 80% of older individuals, but the response is diminished in comparison with that seen in younger subjects.[108] Similarly, the GH response to arginine is decreased.[109] It has also been shown that sleep-related increases in GH do not occur in the elderly.[110] The thyrotropin (TSH) response to thyrotropin-releasing factor is also decreased to about 40% of that seen in younger individuals.[111] Corticotropin (ACTH) release following metyrapone is probably normal in older people, although when urinary excretion of steroids rather than plasma steroid levels is used as the index of ACTH secretion, the response appears to be decreased.[112]

In males, it appears that some degree of Leydig cell hypofunction begins at around 45 to 50 years of age, becoming more pronounced after age 70. The concomitant elevation in plasma FSH and LH levels at this time indicates that this is due to a primary decline in testicular function and is not secondary to pituitary hypofunction.[113] However, in spite of the reduced Leydig cell function, plasma testosterone levels do not show a broad decline until around the age of 70, at least in part due to an increase in the blood concentration of sex hormone binding globulin (SHBG), resulting in an increase in testosterone binding, reduced metabolic clearing rate, and hence accumulation of testosterone in the blood.[114] There is a highly significant correlation between free testosterone concentration and LH and FSH levels, suggesting that gonadotropin secretion is regulated via *free* rather than *total* testosterone levels.[115] The reasons for Leydig cell hypofunction are not properly understood. If testicular function, as defined by testosterone production capacity, is a consequence of changes in the activity of one or several enzymes, this should result in a change in the ratio of 17-OH-progesterone to testosterone. Indeed, in one study of normal young adults, the ratio of 17-OH-progesterone to testosterone in the plasma was found to be 0.33 ± 0.02.[116]

Although many studies of individual hormone responses to different stimuli have been reported in a variety of syndromes, little or no data is available on the results of dynamic pituitary testing of children with precocious aging syndromes. In one progeric child studied by Rosenbloom et al.,[117] growth hormone responsiveness was reported to be normal. Interpretation of provocative testing of pituitary function in many of these syndromes is extremely difficult because of the frequent occurrence of obesity, dementia (or mental retardation), and/or hypogonadism. Obesity leads to hyperinsulinism,[118,119] often accompanied by decreased growth hormone responses.[120-122] Similarly, altered mentation suggests possible defects in the synthesis, release, or function of one or more neurotransmitters throughout the brain. Such defects could involve the hypothalamus and pituitary, altering the effects of exogenous stimuli. Hypogonadism, on the other hand, could reflect either failure of development or precocious aging; in either case, LH and FSH would be altered. These limitations must be kept in mind in undertaking a systematic examination of anterior pituitary reserve in individuals who share one or another feature of precocious aging.

Finch[123] has recently reviewed neuroendocrine mechanisms and aging, including evidence gathered in both humans and rodents. His survey indicated that the available data are consistent with hypotheses that hypothalamic aging changes contribute to, and possibly control, aging changes in diverse target tissues. He suggested that possibly pacemakers of aging reside in neural loci such as the hypothalamus, which by their commanding role in physiologic regulation serve to regulate cellular aging changes in distant target tissues.

SPECULATIONS

Decrease in one parameter of T-cell function, namely, active T-cells, has been found by us in two cases of markedly precocious aging, along with significant decreases thereof in approximately half of the first-degree relatives in both families.[1,3] Autoimmune disease was present in one patient, and malignancy developed in the other. There was a remarkable incidence of malignancy on the maternal and paternal sides of the families of both probands, and of autoimmune disease in the family of one.

As indicated above, aging is accompanied by changes in immune function. These have been documented in mice, but in man it has been difficult to obtain unequivocal results for *normal* aging populations, because of the small sample sizes and differences in environmental and personal histories, and the lack of longitudinal studies (see above). We intuitively believe that a diminution in suppressor T-cells is present in precocious aging and is also present in, and probably involved in the pathogenesis of, normal physiologic aging. We also believe that this results from a genetically determined abiotrophy in T-cell effector function and in the number and/or function of nonspecific suppressor T-cells. Evidence for the involvement of T-cells is provided by the experiments of Sorkin and co-workers,[59] discussed above, using hypopituitary dwarf mice of the Snell-Bagg strain. Their studies showed that endocrinological deficiencies in such mice are associated with a lack of normal development of the lymphoid system, as evidence by marked hypotrophy of the thymus with progressive loss of small lymphocytes in the cortex, hypotrophy of the spleen and peripheral lymph nodes (par ticularly in their thymus-dependent areas), decreased numbers of peripheral blood lymphocytes, and marked deficiency of cell-mediated immune reactions. Physiologically, these animals, according to the authors, "can be considered to be much older than their chronological age. The process of ageing in these animals is precocious and accelerated." The average life span of these mice is only 4.5 months, as opposed to 20 months for normal mice. By 4 months, they show many characteristic signs of aging, including hair loss and discoloration, atrophy of the skin and loss of normal elasticity, and often bilateral cataracts. This process of accelerated aging could be prevented in two ways: (1) When the dwarf mice were treated at 1 month with a single intraperitoneal injection of 150×10^6 peripheral lymph node lymphocytes from normal 40-day-old Snell-Bagg mice, they survived for more than 12 months. In contrast, injection of thymocytes (as stated earlier, suppressor T-cells are no longer present in the thymus in middle-aged mice) or bone marrow cells had no effect. (2) When the dwarf mice were treated during the postweaning period with 250 μg of bovine somatotropic hormone and L-thyroxine for 30 days, their life span was similarly extended, and their physical appearance was normal (although they remained small). However, this treatment was ineffective when preceded by thymectomy. Thus, it would appear that the symptoms of precocious aging in Snell-Bagg hypopituitary dwarf mice result directly from thymic deficiency, which in turn results from endocrine deficiency (cells producing somatotropic growth hormone are scanty or sometimes absent, and the total content of somatotropic hormone in the pituitary glands is 1/1000 of that in normal animals). It is likely that the somatotropic hormone used may have been "contaminated" by a pituitary thymotropic hormone, since it was not made by peptide synthesis.

In terms of possible mechanisms for accelerated aging both in experimental animals and in humans, we have postulated previously that a decrease in suppressor cells and in other parameters of the efferent limb of cell-mediated immunity would result in increased autoantibody levels and in malignancy. Immune complexes consisting of autoantibody plus antigen (e.g., thyroglobulin)[124,125] and antibody plus tumor antigen[126,127] have been reported to be present in normal kidney; deposition of such complexes in the kidney is one possible explanation for the decrease in renal function which occurs with aging. Similarly, reductions in pulmonary elasticity and thus pulmonary function occur with age, and this could be due to the deposition of antigen-antibody complexes in the lung, or to diminution of alpha-1-antitrypsin concentration or function, so that minor infections would liberate neutrophil and macrophage proteases which would not be bound by this anti-protease, leading to digestion of lung elastin and/or collagen. Furthermore, α-1-antitrypsin has been shown in several studies to have a role in immunoregulation, and an age-related decline in its biological activity might contribute to the well-documented decline in immune function with age. For example, Lipsky et al.[128] have reported that lymphocytes which have undergone mitogen-induced (Con A) blastogenic transformation in tissue culture have α-1-antitrypsin on their surfaces, whereas unstimulated cells do not. This is of particular interest in view of the fact that human lymphocytes activated by Con A have been shown to suppress the response of normal lymphocytes to mitogens, antigens, and allogeneic cells,[129] and the report by Hallgren and Yunis[33] that Con A-activated lymphocytes derived from an aging human population differed from those of young individuals in showing a variable loss of suppressor activity. In addition, Arora et al. [130] have shown that α-1-antitrypsin has a suppressive effect on the formation of hemolytic plaques by anti-SRBC producing cells when injected into mice in vivo or when added to cultured spleen cells in vitro. It is also of interest that the loci for Pi and Gm are linked.[131]

Many of the symptoms attributable to physiologic aging (e.g., diminution in renal function, decrease in mental function, etc.) may be due to impaired blood flow to the regions involved. Whether or not atherosclerosis should be considered a part of physiologic aging or merely a concomitant "disease" has been the subject of considerable debate. Nonetheless, atherosclerosis is the one pathologic hallmark most consistently increased with advancing age. Little attention has been paid to the possible immunologic etiology of atherosclerosis, but deposition of antigen-antibody complexes in the small blood vessels of the kidney and of the brain as well as in the coronary arteries and large arteries would provide a basis for an immunologic theory of atherosclerosis. The evidence for the involvement of immunological factors in the development of atheromatous arterial lesions has been reviewed recently by Beaumont and Beaumont.[132] First, Mathews[133] has reported that the national death rate from ischemic heart disease in Australia is significantly correlated with the population frequency of the HLA haplotype 1-8; HLA-B8 has been found to be linked to genes that predispose to several "autoimmune" diseases, such as myasthenia gravis, chronic active hepatitis, Addison's disease, juvenile-onset diabetes, and Graves' disease.[91,92] Second, it is well known that injury to arterial tissue results from repeated injections of antigens in models of experimental chronic serum sickness, and it has been shown that the histological lesions are due to trapping of soluble circulating antigen-antibody complexes in the arterial wall,[134-136] including deposition of immune complexes in the aorta and coronary arteries at sites where hydrodynamic conditions are favorable.[137] Further, typical atherosclerotic plaques can be induced in rabbits by the combination of an immunization course and a long-term cholesterol diet, even when the enriched diet is given after the end of the immunizing process.[138,139]

In humans, typical coronary and aortic atherosclerosis with subsequent ischemia has been described in patients with systemic lupus erythematosus, and autopsies following death from myocardial infarction have shown widespread coronary arteritis and typical occlusive atheroslerotic plaques.[140-143] There is little doubt that this atherosclerosis was due to the SLE, because it happened before 30 years of age, often in women and in the absence of other risk factors. Another example of possible immune atherosclerosis in man is the arterial disease that sometimes develops in heart or kidney homotransplants.[144-146] Thus, atherosclerosis may be the result of a variety of autoimmune complex diseases, including antibodies to elastin or other components of the arterial wall.[138]

Finally, it may also be possible that a defect in suppressor cells, if proven in normal and/or accelerated aging, could result from a lack of thymosin. As discussed above, thymosin levels have been shown to decrease with age[103] and in patients with autoimmune disease accompanied by diminished suppressor T-cell function. Thymosin administration restores (perhaps indirectly) suppressor T-cell activity to normal.[147] Further, in NZB/W hybrid mice, thymosin not ony restores suppressor T-cell numbers to normal but also prolongs life.[148] Whether additional thymic epithelial hormones act on other subpopulations of T-cells is unknown, but this possibility merits investigation.

As stated above, Sorkin and co-workers[59] have attributed the accelerated aging and diminished T-cell function in hypopituitary dwarf mice to the genetically determined pituitary defect. If this is true, it may imply a defect in a pituitary hormone (as yet unidentified) which acts specifically on the thymus. This in turn may conceivably be due to a defect in a hypothalamic releasing factor which acts on thymic epithelium. If so, it might be anticipated that other pituitary hormones and the hormones secreted by their target tissues (adrenal, thyroid, etc.), as well as the pituitary hormones responsible for their release (FSH, LH, prolactin, etc.), would be present in normal amounts; that is, it might be expected that in accelerated (and/or normal) aging, there is a selective deficiency of a pituitary thymotropic hormone or a hypothalamic releasing factor for such a postulated hormone. Indeed, two investigators have provided data suggesting that there may be a defect at a still higher level, namely, in a pineal gland hormone which acts on the hypothalamus. As discussed previously, Dilman[60] has postulated that the sensitivity of the hypothalamus to homeostatic stimuli is increased in normal aging, and that this is responsible for age-related "immunodepression". Furthermore, it is his personal belief (Reference 60, and personal communication) that this is secondary to an abiotrophy of the pineal gland. In this context, Greenberg and Weiss[61] have shown that in aged rat brain, β-adrenergic receptors are reduced in number, and that the capacity of the pineal gland to develop supersensitivity on exposure to light is reduced. They feel that the reduced responsiveness to catecholamines in aged rats is due to the decreased number of β-adrenergic receptors, which in turn may be caused by an impairment of the capacity of the receptors in aged animals to adapt to changes in adrenergic neuronal input. [In the case of steroid hormones, decreased responsiveness to these hormones in aged individuals is accompanied by a decline in the number but not in the affinity of steroid receptors in target tissues;[149] diminished β-adrenergic responsiveness to catecholamine hormones has also been found in tissues from senescent rodents and humans.[150]] Finch has also suggested that hypothalamic changes are the fundamental factor in the aging process.[123]

The studies described here, in patients with marked symptoms of precocious aging, should begin to provide data relevant to the above possibilities. On the basis of these findings, it may be possible to design a large-scale longitudinal study of *normal* individuals, concentrating on genetic, immunologic, and endocrine factors which can be shown to be correlated with physiologic aging.

REFERENCES

1. **Fudenberg, H. H., Schuman, S. H., Goust, J. M., and Jorgenson, R.**, T cells, precocious aging, and familial neoplasia, *Gerontology*, 24, 266, 1978.
2. **Goust, J. M., Chenais, F., Carnes, J. E., Hames, C. G., Fudenberg, H. H., and Hogan, E. L.**, Abnormal T cell subpopulations and circulating immune complexes in the Guillain-Barre syndrome and multiple sclerosis, *Neurology*, 28, 421, 1978.
3. **Fudenberg, H. H., Goust, J. M., Vesole, D. H., and Salinas, C. F.**, Active and suppressor T cells: diminution in a patient with dyskeratosis congenita and in first-degree relatives, *Gerontology*, 25, 231, 1979.
4. **Walford, R. L.**, *The Immunologic Theory of Aging*, Munksgaard, Copenhagen, 1969.
5. **Comfort, A.**, *Ageing, the Biology of Senescence*, Routledge and Kegan Paul, London, 1964.
6. **Krohn, P. L., Ed.**, *Topics in the Biology of Aging*, Interscience, New York, 1966.
7. **Burch, P. R. J.**, *Growth, Disease and Aging*, University of Toronto Press, Canada, 1969.
8. **Burnet, F. M.**, Autoimmunity and ageing, in *Progress in Immunology II*, Vol. 5, Brent, L. and Holborow, J., Eds., North-Holland, Amsterdam, 1974, 27.
9. **Guttman, P. H., Wuepper, K. D., and Fudenberg, H. H.**, On the presence of gamma-G and beta-1C globulins in renal glomeruli of aging and neonatally x-irradiated mice, *Vox Sang.*, 12, 329, 1967.
10. **Fudenberg, H. H. and Wells, J. V.**, Pathogenesis of autoimmune diseases, in *Recent Advances in Rheumatology*, Buchanan W. W., and Dick, W. C., Eds., Churchill Livingstone, London, 1976, 171.
11. **Fudenberg, H. H.**, Genetically determined immune deficiency as the predisposing cause of "autoimmunity" and lymphoid neoplasia, *Am. J. Med.*, 51, 295, 1971.
12. **Fudenberg, H. H.**, Are autoimmune diseases and malignancy due to selective T cell deficiencies? in *Critical Factors in Cancer Immunology*, Vol. 10, Schultz, J. and Leif, R. C., Eds., Academic Press, New York, 1975, 179.
13. **Mackay, I. R.**, Ageing and immunological function in man, *Gerontologia*, 18, 285, 1972.
14. **Gershon, R. K.**, Immunoregulation by T cells, in *Molecular Approaches to Immunology*, Smith, E. E. and Ribbons, D. W., Eds., Academic Press, New York, 1975, 267.
15. **Gershon, R. K., Maurer, P. H., and Merryman, C. F.**, A cellular basis for genetically controlled immunologic unresponsiveness in mice: tolerance induction in T-cells, *Proc. Natl. Acad. Sci. U.S.A.*, 70, 250, 1973.

16. **Kapp, J. A., Pierce, C. W., Theze, J., and Benacerraf, B.,** Modulation of immune responses by suppressor T cells, *Fed. Proc.,* 37, 2361, 1978.
17. **Vadas, M. A., Miller, J. F. A. P., McKenzie, I. F. C., Chism, S. E., Shen, F. W., Boyse, E. A., Gamble, J. R., and Whitelaw, A. M.,** Ly and Ia antigen phenotypes of T cells in delayed-type hypersensitivity and in suppression, *J. Exp. Med.,* 144, 10, 1976.
18. **Hämmerling, G. J. and Eichmann, K.,** Expression of Ia determinants on immunocompetent cells, *Eur. J. Immunol.,* 6, 565, 1976.
19. **Cantor, H. and Boyse, E. A.,** Functional subclasses of T lymphocytes bearing different Ly antigens. I. The generation of functionally distinct T-cell subclasses is a differentiative process independent of antigen, *J. Exp. Med.,* 141, 1376, 1975.
20. **Cantor, H. and Boyse, E. A.**Functional subclasses of T lymphocytes bearing different antigens. II. Cooperation between subclasses of Ly+ cells in the generation of killer activity, *J. Exp. Med.,* 141, 1390, 1975.
21. **Jandinski, J., Cantor, H., Tadakuma, T., Peavy, D. L., and Pierce, C. W.,** Separation of helper T cells from suppressor T cells expressing different Ly components. I. Polyclonal activation: suppressor and helper activities are inherent properties of distinct T-cell subclasses, *J. Exp. Med.,* 143, 1382, 1976.
22. **Gerber, N. L. and Steinberg, A. D.,** Physical separation of "suppressor" from "helper" thymocytes, *J. Immunol.,* 115, 1744, 1975.
23. **Gerber, N. L., Hardin, J. A., Chused, T. M., and Steinberg, A. D.,** Loss with age in NZB/W mice of thymic suppressor cells in the graft-vs-host reaction. *J. Immunol.,* 113, 1618, 1974.
24. **Morton, R. O., Goodman, D. G., Gershwin, M. E., Derkay, C., Squire, R. A., and Steinberg, A. D.,** Suppression of autoimmunity in NZB mice with steroid-sensitive x-radiation-sensitive syngeneic young thymocytes, *Arth. Rheum.,* 19, 1347, 1976.
25. **Ranney, D. F. and Steinberg, A. D.,** Differences in the age-dependent release of a low molecular weight suppressor (LMWS) and stimulators by normal and NZB/W lymphoid organs, *J. Immunol.,* 117, 1219, 1976.
26. **Folch, H. and Waksman, B. H.,** The splenic suppressor cell. I. Activity of thymus-dependent adherent cells: changes with age and stress, *J. Immunol.,* 113, 127, 1974.
27. **Kamin, R. M., Henry, C., and Fudenberg, H. H.,** Suppressor cells in the rabbit appendix, *J. Immunol.,* 113, 1151, 1974.
27a. **Kamin, R. M. and Fudenberg, H. H.,** unpublished observations.
27b. **Goust, J. M. and Fudenberg, H. H.,** unpublished data.
28. **Kurnick, J. T., Bell, C., and Grey, H. M.,** PHA-induced activation of suppressor cells in normal human peripheral blood lymphcoytes, *Scand. J. Immunol.,* 5, 771, 1976.
29. **Witemeyer, S. B., Bankhurst, A. D., and Williams, R. C. Jr.,** Studies on the suppression of normal B-cell maturation by peripheral blood cells from patients with acquired hypogammaglobulinemia and from neonates, *Clin. Immunol. Immunopathol.,* 6, 312 1976.
30. **Waldmann, T. A., Broder, S., Krakauer, R., MacDermott, R. P., Durm, M., Goldman, C., and Meade, B.,** The role of suppressor cells in the pathogenesis of common variable hypogammaglobulinemia and the immunodeficiency associated with myeloma, *Fed. Proc.,* 35, 2067, 1976.
31. **Bresnihan, B. and Jasin, H. E.,** Suppressor dunciton of peripheral blood mononuclear cells in normal individuals and in patients with systemic lupus erythematosus, *J. Clin. Invest.,* 59:106, 1977.
32. **Newman, B., Blank, S., Lomnitzer, R., Disler, P., and Rabson, A. R.,** Lack of suppressor cell activity in systemic lupus erythematosus, *Clin. Immunol. Immunopathol.,* 13, 187, 1979.
33. **Hallgren, H. M. and Yunis, E. J.,** Suppressor lymphocytes in young and aged humans, *J. Immunol.,* 118, 2004, 1977.
34. **Greenberg, L. J. and Yunis, E. J.,** Immunologic control of aging: a possible primary event, *Gerontologia,* 18, 247, 1972.
35. **Roof, B. S., Piel, C. F., Hansen, J., and Fudenberg, H. H.,** Serum parathyroid hormone levels and serum calcium levels from birth through senescence, *Mech. Ageing Develop.,* 5, 289, 1976.
36. **Storer, J. B.,** Longevity and gross pathology at death in 22 inbred mouse strains, *J. Gerontol.,* 21, 404, 1966.
37. **Walters, C. S. and Claman, H. N.,** Age-related changes in cell-mediated immunity in BALB/c mice, *J. Immunol.,* 115, 1438, 1975.
38. **Hirokawa, K. and Makinodan, T.,** Thymic involution. Effect on T cell differentiation, *J. Immunol.,* 114, 1659, 1975.
39. **Kunz, H. W., Gill, T. J., and Corson, J. M.,** Effects of age and genetic background on the antibody response in inbred rats, *Gerontologia,* 20, 88, 1974.
40. **Norins, L. C. and Holmes, M. C.,** Antinuclear factor in mice, *J. Immunol.,* 93, 148, 1964.
41. **Friou, G. J. and Teague, P. O.,** Spontaneous autoimmunity in mice: antibodies to nuclcoprotein in strain A/J, *Science,* 143, 1333, 1964.

42. **Teague, P. O., Friou, G. J., and Myers, L. L.,** Anti-nuclear antibodies in mice. I. Influence of age and possible genetic factors on spontaneous and induced responses, *J. Immunol.*, 101, 791, 1968.
43. **Burnet, F. M. and Holmes, M. C.,** Thymic changes in the mouse strain NZB in relation to the autoimmune state, *J. Pathol. Bacteriol.*, 88, 229, 1964.
44. **Mellors, R. C.,** Autoimmune and immunoproliferative diseases of NZB/B1 mice and hybrids, *Int. Rev. Exp. Pathol.*, 5, 217, 1966.
45. **Lambert, P. H. and Dixon, F. J.,** Pathogenesis of the glomerulonephritis of NZB/W mice, *J. Exp. Med.*, 127, 507, 1968.
46. **de Vries, M. J., Van Putten, L. M., Balner, H., and Van Bekkum, D. W.,** Lésions suggérant une réactivité auto-immune chez des souris atteintes de la "runt disease" aprés thymectomie néonatale, *Rev. Fr. Etud. Clin. Biol.*, 9, 381, 1964.
47. **Teague, P. O., Yunis, E. J., Rodey, G., Fish, A. J., Stutman, O., and Good, R. A.,** Autoimmune phenomena and renal disease in mice, *Lab. Invest.*, 22, 121, 1970.
48. **Troup, G. M. and Walford, R. L.,** Transplantation disease, renal lysozyme, and aging, *Transplantation*, 5, 43, 1967.
49. **Troup, G. M., Wagner, I., and Walford, R. L.,** Liver pigment, liver histidase, and renal lysozyme changes in relation to age in normal and irradiated Syrian hamsters, *Radiat. Res.*, 29, 489, 1966.
50. **Sacher, G. A. and Duffy, P. H.,** Genetic relation of life span to metabolic rate for inbred mouse strains and their hybrids, *Fed. Proc.*, 38, 184, 1979.
51. **Guttman, P. H., Davis, W. C., Fudenberg, H. H., and Merigan, T. C.,** Effect of interferon on the course of spontaneous and radiation-induced renal lesions in the RF/Un mouse, *Vox Sang.*, 17, 278, 1969.
52. **Bradbury, S. and Micklem, H. S.,** Amyloidosis and lymphoid aplasia in mouse radiation chimeras, *Am. J. Pathol.*, 46, 263, 1965.
53. **Metcalf, D.,** The nature and regulation of lymphopoiesis in the normal and neoplastic thymus, in *The Thymus: Experimental and Clinical Studies*, Wolstenholme, G. E. W. and Porter, R., Eds., Little, Brown, Boston, 1966, 242.
54. **Callard, R. E. and Basten, A.,** Immune function in aged mice. I. T-cell responsiveness using phytohemmaglutinin as a functional probe, *Cell. Immunol.*, 31, 13, 1977.
55. **Goidl, E. A., Innes, J. B., and Weksler, M. E.,** Immunological studies of aging. II. Loss of IgG and high avidity plaque-forming cells and increased suppressor cell activity in aging mice, *J. Exp. Med.*, 144, 1037, 1976.
56. **Makinodan, T. and Yunis, E., Eds.,** *Immunology and Ageing*, Vol. 1, Plenum Press, New York, 1978.
57. **Brennan, P. C. and Jaroslow, B. N.,** Age-associated decline in theta antigen on spleen thymus-derived lymphocytes of $B6CF_1$ mice, *Cell. Immunol.*, 15, 51, 1975.
58. **Rose, W. and Girardi, A. J.,** Importance of age and host in detecting tumor-associated transplantation antigens, *J. Immunol.*, 113, 1058, 1974.
59. **Fabris, N., Pierpaoli, W., and Sorkin, E.,** Lymphocytes, hormones and ageing, *Nature (London)*, 240, 557, 1977.

59a. **Sorkin, E.,** personal communication.

60. **Dilman, V. M.,** Metabolic immunodepression which increases the risk of cancer, *Lancet*, 2, 1207, 1977.
61. **Greenberg, L. H. and Weiss, B.,** Beta-adrenergic receptors in aged rat brain: reduced number and capacity of pineal gland to develop supersensitivity, *Science*, 201, 61, 1978.
62. **Gerkins, V. R., Ting, A., Menck, H. T., Casagrande, J. T., Terasaki, P. I., Pike, M. C., and Henderson, B. E.,** HL-A heterozygosity as a genetic marker of long-term survival, *J. Natl. Cancer Inst.*, 52, 1909, 1974.
63. **Morton, J. I. and Siegel, B. V.,** Response of NZB mice to foreign antigen and development of autoimmne disease, *J. Reticuloendothel. Soc.*, 6, 78, 1969.
64. **Whittingham, S. F.,** Fluorescence Microsopic and Serological Data in Human Autoimmune Disease. Ph.D. thesis, University of Melbourne, Australia, 1970.
65. **Smith, M. A., Evans, J., and Steel, C. M.,** Age-related variation in proportion of circulating T cells, *Lancet*, 2, 922, 1974.
66. **Roberts-Thomson, I. C., Whittingham, S., Youngchaiyud, U., and Mackay, I. R.,** Ageing, Immune response, and mortality, *Lancet*, 2, 368, 1974.
67. **Weksler, M. E. and Hütteroth, T. H.,** Impaired lymphocyte function in aged humans, *J. Clin. Invest.*, 53, 99, 1974.
68. **Hallgren, H. M., Buckley, C. E., Gilbertsen, V. A., and Yunis, E. J.,** Lymphocyte phytohemmaglutinin responsiveness, immunoglobulins and autoantibodies in aging humans, *J. Immunol.*, 111, 1101, 1973.
69. **Foad, B. S. I., Adams, L. E., Yamauchi, Y., and Litwin, A.,** Phytomitogen responses of peripheral blood lymphocytes in young and older subjects, *Clin. Exp. Immunol.*, 17, 657, 1974.

70. **Ben-Zwi, A., Galili, U., Russell, A., and Schlesinger, M.,** Age-associated changes in subpopulations of human lymphocytes, *Clin. Immunol. Immunopathol.,* 7, 139, 1977.
71. **Galili, U. and Schlesinger, M.,** Subpopulations of human thymus cells differing in their capacity to form stable E-rosettes and in their immunologic reactivity, *J. Immunol.,* 115, 827, 1975.
72. **Gluckman, J. P. and Montambault, P.,** Spontaneous auto-rosette-forming cells in man. A marker for a subset population of T lymphocytes?, *Clin. Exp. Immunol.,* 22, 302, 1975.
73. **Girard, J. P., Paychère, M., Cuevas, M., and Fernandes, B.,** Cell-mediated immunity in an ageing population, *Clin. Exp. Immunol.,* 27, 85, 1977.
74. **Antel, J. P. and Arnason, B. G. W.,** Suppressor cell function in man: evidence for altered sensitivity of responder cells with age, *Clin. Immunol. Immunopathol.,* 13, 119, 1979.
75. **Epstein, M.,** Effects of aging on the kidney, *Fed. Proc.,* 38, 168, 1979.
76. **Andres, R.,** Physiological factors of aging significant to the clinician, *J. Amer. Geriat. Soc.,* 17, 274, 1969.
77. **Shock, N. W.,** Systems physiology and aging: introduction, *Fed. Proc.,* 38, 161, 1979.
78. **Portaro, J. K., Glick, G. I., and Zighelboim, J.,** Population immunology. Age and immune cell parameters, *Clin. Immunol. Immunopathol.,* 11, 339, 1978.
79. **Radl, J., Sepers, J. M., Skvaril, F., Morell, A., and Hijmans, W.,** Immunoglobulin patterns in humans over 95 years of age, *Clin. Exp. Immunol.,* 22, 84, 1975.
80. **Buckley, C. E., Buckley, E. G., and Dorsey, F. C.,** Longitudinal changes in serum immunoglobulin levels in older humans, *Fed. Proc.,* 33, 2036, 1974.
81. **Rowley, M. J., Buchanan, H., and Mackay, I. R.,** Reciprocal change with age in antibody to extrinsic and intrinsic antigens, *Lancet,* 2, 24, 1968.
82. **Herbeuval, R., Duheille, J., Cuny, G., and Haagen, A.,** Anticorps anti-estomac et vieillissement, *Presse Med.,* 75, 731, 1967.
83. **Goudie, R. B., Anderson, J. R., and Gray, K. G.,** Complement-fixing antithyroid antibodies in hospital patients with asymptomatic thyroid lesions, *J. Pathol. Bacteriol.,* 77, 389, 1959.
84. **Pandey, J. P., Fudenberg, H. H., Ainsworth, S. K., and Loadholt, C. B.,** Autoantibodies in healthy subjects of different age groups, *Mech. Ageing Develop.,* 10, 399, 1979.
85. **Vyas, G. N. and Fudenberg, H. H.,** Am(1), the first genetic marker of human immunoglobulin A, *Proc. Natl. Acad. Sci. U.S.A.,* 64, 1211, 1969.
86. **Wells, J. V., Bleumers, J. F., and Fudenberg, H. H.,** Human anti-IgM iso-antibodies: detection of IgM allotypic markers, *Proc. Natl. Acad. Sci. U.S.A.,* 70, 827, 1973.
87. **Fudenberg, H. H. and Warner, N. L.,** Genetics of immunoglobulins, *Adv. Hum. Genet.,* 1, 131, 1970.
88. **Mann, D. L., Abelson, L., Harris, S., and Amos, D. B.,** Detection of antigens specific for B-lymphoid cultured cell lines with human alloantisera, *J. Exp. Med.,* 142, 84, 1975.
89. **Terasaki, P. I., Opelz, G., Park, M. S., and Mickey, M. R.,** Four new B lympocyte specificities, in *Histocompatibility Testing 1975,* Kissmeyer-Nielsen, F., Ed., Munksgaard, Copenhagen, 1975, 657.
90. **Scott, D. W. and Amos, D. B.,** Tissue transplantation, in *Immunological Disease,* Vol. 1, Samter, M., Ed., Little, Brown, New York, 1978, 341.
91. **Galbraith, R. M. and Fudenberg, H. H.,** Autoimmunity in chronic active hepatitis and diabetes mellitus: a review, *Clin. Immunol. Immunopathol.,* 8, 116, 1977.
92. **Fudenberg, H. H., Pink, R. L., Wang, A. C., and Douglas, S. D.,** *Basic Immunogenetics,* 2nd ed., Oxford University Press, New York, 1978.
93. **Fachet, J. and Andó, I.,** Genetic control of contact sensitivity to oxazolne in inbred, H-2 congenic and intra-H-2 recombinant strains of mice, *Eur. J. Immunol.,* 7, 223, 1977.
94. **Andó, I. and Fachet, J.,** Genetic control of two different types of antibody responses to oxazolone, *Eur. J. Immunol.,* 7, 516, 1977.
94a. **Fachet, J.,** personal communication.
95. **Morell, A., Scherz, R., Käser, H., and Skvaril, F.,** Evidence for an association between uncommon Gm phenotypes and neuroblastoma, *Lancet,* 1, 23, 1977.
96. **Pandey, J. P., Fudenberg, H. H., Hersh, E., and Gutterman, J.,** Allotype studies in malignant melanoma, 1979, in preparation.
97. **Pandey, J. P., Holton, O. D., and Fudenberg, H. H.,** Preponderance of IG3 subclass and Gm and Km allotype preference in breast cancer patients with anti-tumor antibodies, 1979, in preparation.
98. **Pandey, J. P., Fudenberg, H. H., Virella, G., Gotschlich, E. C., Parke, J. C., Loadholt, C. B., Kyong, C. U., and Galbraith, R. M.,** Association between immunoglobulin allotypes and immune responses to *Haemophilus influenzae* and meningococcus polysaccharides, *Lancet,* 1, 190, 1979.
99. **Winchester, R. J., Ebers, G., Fu, S. M., Espinosa, L., Zabriskie, J., and Kunkel, H. G.,** B-cell alloantigen Ag 7a in multiple sclerosis, *Lancet,* 2, 814, 1975.
100. **Compston, D. A., Batchelor, J. R., and McDonald, W. I.,** B-lymphocyte alloantigens associated with multiple sclerosis, *Lancet,* 2, 1261, 1976.

101. **Terasaki, P. I., Park, M. S., Opelz, G., and Ting, A.,** Multiple sclerosis and high incidence of a B lymphocyte antigen, *Science,* 193, 1245, 1976.
102. **Bodmer, J. G., Mann, J., Hill, A., Hill, H., Young, D., and Winearls, B.,** The association of Ia antigens with juvenile onset diabetes and rheumatoid arthritis, *Tissue Antigens,* 10, 197, 1977.
103. **Goldstein, A. L., Hooper, J. A., Schulof, R. S., Cohen, G. H., Thurman, G. B., McDaniel, M. C., White, A., and Dardenne, M.,** Thymosin and the immunopathology of aging, *Fed. Proc.,* 33, 2053, 1977.
104. **Wide, L., Nillius, S. J., Gemzell, C., and Roos, P.,** Serum levels and urinary excretion of FSH and LH in healthy men and women 17 to 76 years of age, *Acta Endocrinol. (Copenhagen) Suppl.,* 174, 41, 1973.
105. **Kovacs, K., Ryan, N., Horvath, E., Singer, W., and Ezrin, C.:** pituitary adenomas in old age, *J. Gerontol.,* 35, 16, 1980.
106. **Cohen, B. J., Anver, M. R., Ringler, D. H., and Adelman, R. C.,** Age-associated pathological changes in male rats, *Fed. Proc.,* 37, 2848, 1978.
107. **Llewellyn, A., Singer, W., Chan, A., Dolson, J., and Grife, C.,** Pituitary dysfunction in old age, *Ann. R. Coll. Phys. Surg. Can.,* 12, 41, 1979.
108. **Laron, Z., Doron, M., and Amikan, B.,** Plasma growth hormone in men and women over 70 years of age, in *Medicine and Sport,* Vol. 4, Brunner, D. and Jokl, E., Eds., Karger, New York, 1970, 126.
109. **Dudl, R. J. and Ensinck, J. W.,** The role of insulin, glucagon and growth hormone in carbohydrate homeostasis during aging, *Diabetes,* 21, 357, 1972.
110. **Carlson, H. E., Gillin, J. C., Gordon, P., and Snyder, F.,** Absence of sheep-related growth hormone peaks in aged normal subjects in acromegaly, *J. Clin. Endocrinol. Metab.,* 34, 1102, 1972.
111. **Snyder, P. J. and Utiger, R. D.,** Response to thyrotropin releasing hormone (TRH) in normal man, *J. Clin. Endocrinol. Metab.,* 34, 380, 1972.
112. **Jensen, H. K. and Blichert-Toft, M.,** Pituitary-adrenal function in old age evaluated by the intravenous metyrapone test, *Acta Endocrinol. (Copenhagen),* 64, 431, 1970.
113. **Stearns, E. L., MacDonnell, J. A., Kaufman, B. J., Padua, R., Lueman, T. S., Winter, J. S. D., and Faiman, C.,** Declining testicular function with age: hormonal and clinical correlates, *Am. J. Med.,* 57, 761, 1974.
114. **Vermeulen, A., Rubens, R., and Verdonck, L.,** Testosterone secretion and metabolism in male senescence, *J. Clin. Endocrinol. Metab.,* 34, 730, 1972.
115. **Rubens, R., Dhont, M., and Vermeulen, A.,** Further studies on Leydig cell function in old age, *J. Clin. Endocrinol. Metab.,* 39, 40, 1974.
116. **Mathur, R. S., Sagel, J. S.,Williamson, H. O., Colwell, J. A., and Nair, R. M. G.,** Evaluation of the pituitary-gonadal axis using gonadotropin releasing hormone and its superactive analogues, in *Hypothalamic Hormones: Chemistry, Physiology and Clinical Applications,* Gupta, D. and Voelter, W., Eds., Verlag Chemie, Weinheim, 1978, 509.
117. **Rosenbloom, A. L., Karacan, I. J., and DeBusk, F. L.,** Sleep characteristics and endocrine response in progeria, *J. Pediat.,* 77, 692, 1970.
118. **Vajda, B., Heald, F. P., and Mayer, J.,** Intravenous glucose tolerance in obese adolescents, *Lancet,* 1, 902, 1964.
119. **Berkowitz, D.,** Metabolic changes associated with obesity before and after weight reduction, *JAMA,* 187, 399, 1964.
120. **Roth, J., Glick, S. M., Yalow, R. S., and Berson, S. A.,** Secretion of human growth hormone: physiologic and experimental modification, *Metabolism,* 12, 577, 1963.
121. **Rabinowitz, D,.** Hormonal profile and forearm metabolism in human obesity, *Am. J. Clin. Nutr.,* 21, 1438, 1968.
122. **Beck, P., Koumans, J. H. T., Winterling, C. A., Stein, M. F., Danghaday, W. H., and Kipnis, D. M.,** Studies of insulin and growth hormone secretion in human obesity, *J. Lab. Clin. Med.,* 64, 654, 1968.
123. **Finch, C. E.,** Neuroendocrine mechanisms and aging, *Fed. Proc.,* 38, 178, 1979.
124. **Jordan, S. C., Johnston, W. H., and Bergstein, J. M.,** Immune complex glomerulonephritis mediated by thyroid antigens, *Arch. Pathol. Lab. Med.,* 102, 530, 1978.
125. **Ploth, D. W., Fitz, A., Schnetzler, D., Seidenfeld, J., and Wilson, C. B.,** Thyroglobulin — antithyroglobulin immune complex glomerulonephritis complicating radioiodine therapy, *Clin. Immunol. Immunopathol.,* 9, 327, 1978.
126. **Jones, J. W., Levin, A., and Fudenberg, H. H.,** Glomerular antigen complexes associated with transitional cell carcinoma, *Surg. Gynecol. Obstet.,* 140, 896, 1975.
127. **Lewis, M. G., Loughridge, L. W., and Phillips, T. M.,** Immunologial sudies in nephrotic syndrome associated with extrarenal malignant disease, *Lancet,* 2, 134, 1971.

128. **Lipsky, J. J., Berninger, R. W., Hyman, L. R., and Talamo, R. C.,** Presence of alpha-1-antitrypsin on mitogen-stimulated human lymphocytes, *J. Immunol.*, 122, 24, 1979.
129. **Shou, L., Schwartz, S. A., and Good, R. A.,** Suppressor cell activity after concanavalin A treatment of lymphocytes from normal donors, *J. Exp. Med.*, 143, 1100, 1976.
130. **Arora, P. K., Miller, H. C., and Aronson, L. D.,** Alpha$_1$-antitrypsin is an effector of immunological stasis, *Nature (London)*, 274, 589, 1978.
131. **Gedde-Dahl, T., Cook, P. J. L., Fagerhol, M. K., and Pierce, J. A.,** Improved estimate of the Gm-Pi linkage, *Ann. Hum. Genet.*, 39, 43, 1975.
132. **Beaumont, J. L. and Beaumont, V.,** Immunological aspects of atherosclerosis, *Atherosclerosis Rev.*, 3, 133, 1978.
133. **Mathews, J. D.,** Ischaemic heart disease: possible genetic markers, *Lancet*, 2, 681, 1975.
134. **Saphir, O., Stryzak, D., and Ohringer, L.,** Hypersensitivity changes in coronary arteries of rabbits and their relationship to arteriosclerosis, *Lab. Invest.*, 7, 434, 1958.
135. **Germuth, F. G., Senterfit, L. B., and Pollack, A. D.,** Immune complex disease. I. Experimental acute and chronic glomerulonephritis, *Johns Hopkins Med. J.*, 120, 225 251, 1967.
136. **Cochrane, C. G.,** The role of immune complexes and complement in tissue injury, *J. Allerg.*, 42, 113, 1968.
137. **Kniker, W. I. and Cochrane, C. G.,** Pathogenic factors in vascular lesions of experimental serum sickness, *J. Exp. Med.*, 122, 83, 1965.
138. **Minick, C. R. and Murphy, G. E.,** Experimental induction of athero-arteriosclerosis by the synergy of allergic injury to arteries and lipid-rich diet. II. Effect of repeatedly injected foreign protein in rabbits fed a lipid-rich cholesterol-poor diet, *Am. J. Pathol.*, 73, 265, 1973.
139. **Scebat, L., Renais, J., Groult, N., Iris, L., and Lenegre, J.,** Lésions artérielles produites chez le lapin par des injections de broyats d'aorte de rat, *Rev. Fr. Etud. Clin. Biol.*, 11, 806, 1966.
140. **Meller, J., Conde, C. A., Deppisch, L. M., Donoso, E., and Dack, S.,** Myocardial infarction due to coronary atherosclerosis in three young adults with systemic lupus erythematosus, *Am. J. Cardiol.*, 35, 309, 1975.
141. **Kong, T. Q., Kellum, R. E., and Hazerick, J. R.,** Clinical diagnosis of cardiac involvement in systemic lupus erythematosus: a correlation of clinical and autopsy findings in thirty patients, *Circulation*, 26, 7, 1962.
142. **Tsakraklides, V. G., Blieden, L. C., and Edwards, J. E.,** Coronary atherosclerosis and myocardial infarction associated with systemic lupus erythematosus, *Am. Heart J.*, 87, 637, 1974.
143. **Brigden, W., Bywaters, E. G. L., Lessof, M. H., and Ross, I. P.,** The heart in systemic lupus erythematosus, *Br. Heart J.*, 22, 1, 1960.
144. **Hadjiisky, P., Scebat, L., Renais, J., Cachera, J. P., Dubost, C., and Lenegre, J.,** Altérations morphologiques des vaisseaux coronaires de deux homotransplants cardiaques de longue durée chez l'homme, *Rev. Fr. Etud. Clin. Biol.*, 16, 596, 1971.
145. **Dempster, W. J.,** Atheroma in a transplanted heart, *Lancet*, 2, 1247, 1969.
146. **Kosek, J. C. and Biebler, C. H.,** Atheroma in a transplanted heart, *Lancet*, 1, 563, 1970.
147. **Horowitz, S., Borcherding, W., Moorthy, A. V., Chesney, R., Schulte-Wisserman, H., Hong, R., and Goldstein, A. L.,** Induction of suppressor T cells in systemic lupus erythematosus by thymosin and cultured thymic epithelium, *Science*, 197, 999, 1977.
148. **Dauphinee, M. J., Talal, N., Goldstein, A. L., and White, A.,** Thymosin corrects the abnormal DNA synthetic response of NZB mouse thymocytes, *Proc. Natl. Acad. Sci. U.S.A.*, 71, 2637, 1974.
149. **Kanungo, M. S., Patnaik, S. K., and Koul, O.,** Decrease in 17-beta-oestradiol receptor in brain of ageing rat, *Nature (London)*, 253, 366, 1975.
150. **Ericsson, E. and Lundholm, L.,** Adrenergic beta-receptor activity and cyclic AMP metabolism in vascular smooth muscle: variations with age, *Mech. Ageing Develop.*, 4, 1, 1975.

EXPERIMENTAL NEOPLASIA OF THE MURINE IMMUNE SYSTEM*

Neal K. Clapp

INTRODUCTION

The organs which are presently recognized as contributing to the function of the immune system develop neoplasms which are grouped under the term of reticular tissue tumors (or more commonly called leukemias). Considerable variation exists in tumor incidences and types between species and even between the large number of inbred and noninbred mouse strains, in which most of the experimental work has been performed. Our research experience has primarily involved studies of murine leukemias (primarily radiation-induced); therefore, we will restrict our discussions to this area with the hope it will especially benefit the experimental gerontologist.

The mouse thymus is extremely sensitive to certain physical (especially ionizing radiation) and chemical agents and develops a very characteristic thymic lymphoma with which much experimental work has been performed to elucidate disease characteristics as well as mechanisms of induction. While some similarities exist between spontaneous and induced leukemias in experimental animals and those observed "spontaneously" in humans, many differences are also obvious. With the possible exception of myeloid leukemia, animal experimenters still lack an exact duplicate for even one of the several human types of leukemia. However, experimental efforts continue to inform us of inducing agents, modifying factors (i.e., environmental conditions, viruses, etc.), and possible mechanistic inferences. Various agents have been incriminated and most, if not all, have enjoyed popularity with researchers seeking mechanisms to explain the process of leukemogenesis.

The discovery of the radiation inducibility of neoplasms of the reticular tissues, has provided an excellent tool for explaining the biological dangers of radiation exposure and for studying the pathogenesis of reticular neoplasia. The mouse is an extensively used experimental model for aging studies which have shown that the induction of leukemias is the primary contributing factor in explaining radiation-associated life-shortening.[1-3] Since most of the data in experimental leukemogenesis have been obtained from murine studies, we will emphasize these findings and attempt to correlate the interpretations.

It is not within the scope of this chapter to deal extensively with human leukemias. Human data have primarily been available (1) after accidental exposures; especially of radiation workers, (2) intentional exposures which include radiation therapy for a variety of human diseases, and (3) the follow-up observations on Hiroshima and Nagasaki survivors from the atomic detonations in Japan. Some difficulties which arise in interpreting human data are (1) the accuracy of dosimetry is often difficult, if not impossible, to determine and consequently the actual exposure dose is uncertain, and (2) the difficulty of obtaining adequate control populations with which comparisons must be made.

NEOPLASIA OF RETICULAR TISSUE (EXPERIMENTAL)

The reticular tissues which comprise the immune system include tissues in which

* Research sponsored by the Office of Health and Environmental Research, U.S. Department of Energy, under contract W-7405-eng-26 with the Union Carbide Corporation.

developing progenitor cells are recognized as well as those that are well enough differentiated to be associated with immune response. These tissues may or may not be the ones in which the cells will later perform their immune activity. Included in this scope will be the bone marrow, thymus, lymph nodes, liver, spleen, and Peyer's patches, with some reference to any or all of these cells or their related "sister" cells which may have localized or become fixed within other tissues.

In the literature, neoplasms of the cells which comprise the immune system in mammals have generally been listed under the broad heading of "leukemias" or neoplasms of the reticular tissue. We will discuss the various leukemias as to cell type and pathogenesis and also their response or development as a result of physical (ionizing radiation) insults to the animal. A great variation exists in any single disease from one animal to another and, consequently, any or all of the symptoms may be present in an animal with the particular disease. The rapidity of onset, the general health of the animal, the environment in which it is maintained, and many other factors may influence not only the incidence but also the actual course of the disease. Here we will simply try to recognize and categorize the disease, realizing that there are many differences of opinions among experimental and human pathologists; we will try only to simplistically discuss an admittedly complicated area of disease recognition, development, and progression. Descriptions of morphology and pathogenesis and typical cases are reported elsewhere.[4,5]

Types of Murine Leukemias

Thymic Lymphoma

The thymus is an organ which is located in the anterior mediastinum of the mammalian thoracic cavity. It is quite extensive in neonatal animals but rapidly involutes with age to a relatively small organ throughout most of adult life. The organ is composed of a cortex and a medulla, the denser cortex containing the larger numbers of lymphocytes. Dunn[5] reports that Hassal's bodies are less well-defined in the mouse than in man and cannot be recognized in some strains.

Most mouse strains develop spontaneous thymic lymphomas which range from very low incidences[6-10] in certain strains (BALB/c, RF, etc.) to very high incidences approaching 100% in AKR mice.[11] In thymic lymphoma, the thymus can enlarge to five to ten times that found in the normal animal. Depending upon the time course of the disease, it may be confined only to the thorax, or it may extend to include almost any tissue in the body. Most often, in a fulminating course of the disease, the thymus will be markedly enlarged and may occupy up to one half of the total space in the thoracic cavity. The animal often dies of suffocation due to excessive intrathoracic pressure. Likewise, hydrothorax often contributes to the demise of the affected animal.

The leukemic cells, which are immature but readily recognizable as lymphocytes, usually infiltrate the pericardium and pleura and follow the vascular and bronchial tree into the lung parenchyma, where they form a cuffing of leukemic cells which typically is located around the bronchioles and smaller pulmonary arteries and arterioles. When the disease is slower in developing, leukemic cells may infiltrate almost any tissue in the body; preferentially, the reticular tissues of the spleen, liver, lymph nodes, and Peyer's patches which are most often involved in a thymic lymphoma that has become generalized. In addition, the uterus, ovary, and kidney are also frequent sites of metastatic leukemic infiltration. As in the lung, the infiltration in the liver and kidney is most often perivascular, although leukemic cells may also be found within the sinusoids of the liver. In the spleen, the lymphoma cells will usually infiltrate the red pulp and cause a typical homogeneous microscopic appearance with almost total obliteration of the normal splenic architecture; the gross appearance of both liver and spleen is very smooth. In the irradiated female, radiogenic thymic lymphomas often infiltrate the ovary and a differential diagnosis must be made between actual ovarian tumors and marked enlargement due to infiltration by leukemic cells into the ovarian tissue; however, ovarian tumors and thymic lymphoma infiltration may occur concurrently.

In mouse strains which have a relatively low incidence of spontaneous lymphomas (i.e., RF and BALB/c), thymic lymphomas are slightly more prevalent in females than in males[8,10,11] but incidences for both sexes approximate ≤ 5% (Table 1). With whole body irradiation of 50 rads or more (Figure 1), incidences of thymic lymphomas increased approximately linearly through 300 rads with no further increase in incidences at 400 rads. Other investigators have observed similar results.[7,8,10,11] In a study using 60-MeV protons (Figure 1), there were slightly higher incidences in the 300 to 400 rad range with X-rays as compared with protons even though these sources as used in the study have a similar linear energy transfer.[1] Females are more responsive to radiation induction of thymic lymphomas than males.[8,10,11]

Radiation causes the temporal advancement of thymic lymphomas with mean survival times generally decreasing with increasing dose through 300 to 400 rads; maximum lymphoma incidences in the 35 to 40% range are observed in females. This neoplasm lends itself well to a study of causation and effects due to ionizing radiation since it occurs very early (9 to 12 months of age) with few intercurrent diseases to complicate the mortality picture. In a typical study, the mean survival time for thymic lymphomas in controls was 455 days with a maximum temporal advancement to 268 days following 300 rads of X-rays (Table 1).

Myeloid Leukemia

Myeloid leukemia is an uncontrolled proliferative disease of the granulocytic elements from the bone marrow and may involve any of the three cell types: neutrophils (the most common cell type by far), basophils, or eosinophils. The disease resembles chronic myelogenous leukemia in man, and Furth and co-workers[11] developed the RF strain of mouse as a model for the study of this disease. The site of origin of the leukemia is still open to question, but the bone marrow where the myelogenous cells are maturing and differentiating is in all probability the place of origin. The most common locations for the development of the leukemia are the spleen and liver, and all of the lymph nodes may become involved when the leukemia becomes generalized.[4] As in thymic lymphoma, the liver and spleen with myeloid leukemia are grossly very smooth; the cells proliferate primarily within the red pulp of the spleen and, in the liver, tend to be perivascular but also extensively involve the sinusoids of the liver. Within the liver, myeloid leukemia is spread more diffusely through the sinusoids and parenchyma than are thymic lymphoma cells. In contrast with observations in thymic lymphoma, extremely high white blood cells counts are seen in the peripheral blood, reaching several hundred thousand cells per mm^3 and forming emboli which readily metastasize to the lung parenchyma and occlude vessels therein. These emboli cause petechial hemorrhages in the lung and result in bone marrow necrosis in the sternum.[4]

Myeloid leukemia spontaneous incidences are slightly lower in female RF mice[12] than in males (∼1% vs. ∼5%). When compared with thymic lymphoma, myloid leukemia occurs later in the life of the RF mouse, the mean survival time averaging approximately 622 days for spontaneous cases (Table 1). After whole-body ionizing radiation, incidences are increased and also temporally advanced; incidences in females are increased to 20 to 25% at 250 to 300 rads and then decline with sublethal doses above 300 rad (Figure 2). The decline beyond 200 to 300 rads may be due to cell killing (this effect overrides the cell transformation effect which is expressed as leukemia) after the radiation insult.[12] With increasing doses through 400 rads the mean survival time is

Table 1

INCIDENCES AND MEAN SURVIVAL TIMES (MST) FOR RETICULAR TISSUE NEOPLASMS IN RF FEMALE MICE. X-RADIATION (300 RADS) GIVEN AT 8 WEEKS OF AGE

Treatment	No. of mice	MST days	Thymic lymphoma		Myeloid leukemia		Reticulum cell sarcoma		Nonthymic lymphoma		Total leukemia incidences (%)
			%	MST days	%	MST days	%	MST days	%	MST days	
0	427	636	4.0	455	0.9	622	56.2	659	7.0	697	68.1
300 R	216	435	35.6	268	15.7	393	21.7	599	4.2	467	67.2

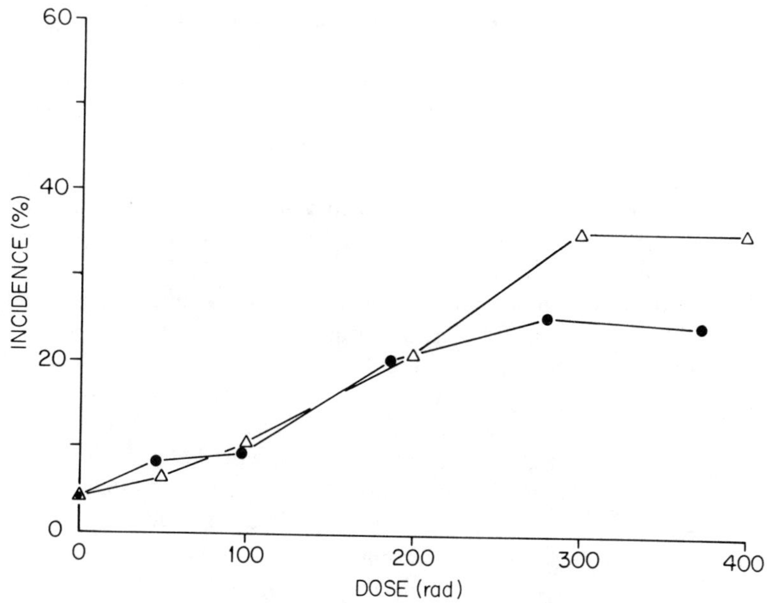

FIGURE 1. Incidences of thymic lymphoma in female RF mice as a function of radiation dose after 60-Mev protons (●) or 300 kVp X-rays (△). (From Clapp, N. K., Darden, E. G., Jr., and Jernigan, M. C., *Radiat. Res.*, 57, 158, 1974. With permission.)

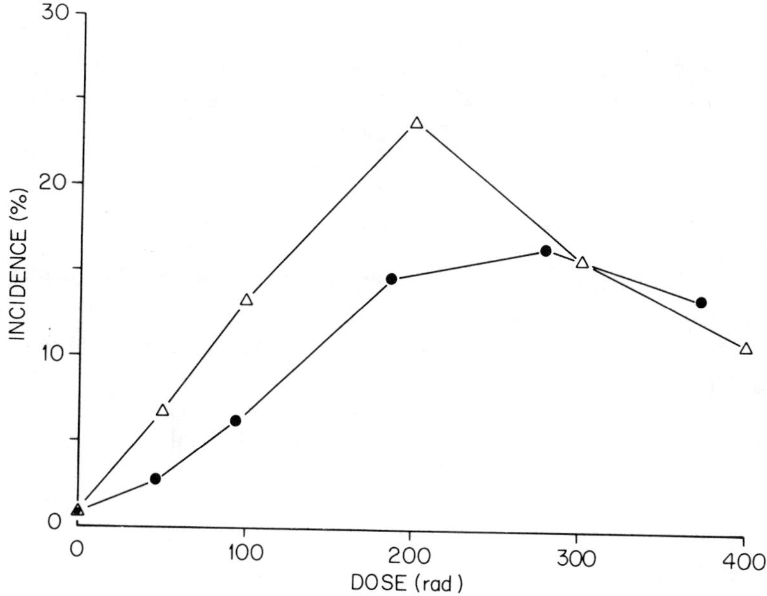

FIGURE 2. Incidences of myeloid leukemia in female RF mice as a function of radiation dose after 60-Mev protons (●) or 300 kVp X-rays (△). (From Clapp, N. K., Darden, E. B., Jr., and Jernigan, M. C., *Radiat. Res.*, 57, 158, 1974. With permission.)

shortened about 200 days.[1] A similar dose-response curve was seen following X-rays or γ-rays by Upton et al.[12] except their maximum incidences were observed at 300 rads.

One interesting observation regarding the inducibility of myeloid leukemia has been that mice raised in a conventional environment are more susceptible to myeloid leukemia induction by radiation than those raised in barriers or isolators.[7,9,13,14] When a large low-level irradiation study was performed in the Biology Division of the Oak Ridge National Laboratory, a barrier was established for breeding and maintaining the animals.[15] Prior to this time, most studies had been carried out in conventional facilities, and incidences of myeloid leukemia were similar to those reported in this paper. However, when animals with well-defined and controlled microbial flora were irradiated in the barrier, a dramatic reduction in incidences of myeloid leukemia (failure of induction) was observed[15] as compared with incidences in animals maintained in conventional facilities. In a similar but smaller study, Walburg et al.[14] observed a similar decline with a reduction in microbial flora (e.g., myeloid leukemia incidences for isolator < barrier < "clean" conventional < "dirty" conventional). In addition to the reduced ability of radiation to induce myeloid leukemia, we also observed that there was a comparable increase in the number of barrier animals developing thymic lymphoma following whole-body ionizing radiation. It would appear that there is some maximum percentage of animals that are able to develop leukemias (65 to 70% in some studies) in a given population of RF mice after irradiation (Table 1). When animals are in a controlled bacterial environment, those animals which would develop myeloid leukemia if maintained in a conventional environment apparently developed thymic lymphomas instead. We observed approximately the *same total number* of leukemias regardless of whether the animals were housed in a barrier or in conventional facilities.[1] The mechanism behind the shift in incidences is not understood but may relate to the increased cell turnover because of contaminating infectious organisms, viruses, etc., within animals maintained in conventional facilities.

Reticulum Cell Sarcoma

Reticulum cell sarcoma is a late occurring disease in most mouse strains and is characterized by a nonfulminating development and a chronic course. Because of the chronicity of this disease, animals dying late in life from other causes have a relatively high incidence of reticulum cell sarcoma as an incidental finding. Animals dying spontaneously with the disease will have a mean survival time of 600 to 650 days and incidences in untreated controls will reach or exceed 50% (Table 1).

Reticulum cell sarcomas have been characterized by Dunn.[5] She described a type A (or monocytic) type of reticulum cell sarcoma leukemia which could either be localized or generalized and was derived from either monocytes or histiocytes. A reticulum cell sarcoma type B was described as being similar to Hodgkin's disease in humans. However, in our experience, the extremely wide variation is not only in cell types but also in the general pathogenesis of the disease which has made it very difficult to categorize all reticulum cell sarcomas observed in our RF and BALB/c mice into these two categories.

There is considerable variation in the degree and frequency of involvement of different organs by this neoplasm. The disease may be totally confined within the abdomen and involve exclusively the mesenteric lymph node, a common site for reticulum cell sarcomas; the node may enlarge five to ten times its normal size. However, it often also involves the spleen (alone or with other abdominal organs), usually with a nodular growth pattern. The reticular cells develop within the white pulp and grossly form large white nodules which distort the enlarged germinal centers and cause irregularities in splenic morphology. In both spleen and liver, the neoplasm develops with a white nodular appearance in contrast with the smooth enlarged leukemic organs which are characteristic of thymic lymphoma and myeloid leukemia. Often, most, if not all, of the reticular tissues in the body will be involved with reticulum cell sarcoma as the disease becomes generalized. All of the lymph nodes, both superficial and deep, the Peyer's patches of the intestinal tract, the thymus, and the mediastinal lymph nodes may become affected.

Microscopically there is quite a variety of cell types which we have included in the general class of reticulum cell sarcoma. A great variation may exist within a single animal, as well as within a single tumor mass, as to the type of cell which is neoplastic, and the type of cell can vary depending upon the tissue in which it is found. In this general category of reticulum cell sarcoma, the neoplastic cells are most often very pleomorphic and range from rather typical reticular cells with large pale nuclei and a peripheral distribution of chromatin to rather large cells with small hyperchromatic nuclei and abundant eosinophilic cytoplasm. Each of these cell types may be seen in almost any reticulum cell sarcoma. A rather common morphological variant is a spindle-shaped cell whose tumor mass closely resembles a fibrosacroma with whorl formations which could possibly be mistaken for a solid tumor of mesodermal origin.

There does not appear to be a correlation, as might be expected, between the sites of involvement and the cell type which one observes. Rather than being able to group these into categories, our experience has been that there is great difficulty in "pigeonholing" these by cell types. It is possible that the information which was obtained from the strains described by Dunn[5] may be better able to be categorized than the ones in the strains with which we have primarily been working (RF, BALB/c).

Because of the relative ease for study (earlier occurrence with few other causes of mortality) of radiogenic thymic lymphoma and myeloid leukemia, reticulum cell sarcomas have received less experimental attention. Earlier occurring diseases are "cleaner" to work with, plus animal costs are lower as are other costly time and labor factors. Because reticulum cell sarcoma is a late occurring disease, many other disease relationships enter into the evaluation of its dose response to any particular insult, either chemical or physical. If animals are treated with increasing doses of radiation without correction for other intercurrent diseases, it is generally observed that there is a decline in incidences of reticulum cell sarcomas with increasing doses through a sub-LD_{50} dose range (Figure 3). However, when corrections are made to consider only animals that are at risk at these ages, the early reduced incidence is followed by a general plateauing of effect at doses of 100 to 300 rads.[13] In addition, the mean survival times of animals dying with reticulum cell sarcoma are not markedly influenced by increasing radiation dose. The disease still occurs very late in life and is shortened from 659 in control RF females to 599 at 300 rads [a temporal advancement of only 2 to 3 months (Table 1)].

Nonthymic Lymphoma

Nonthymic lymphoma (or lymphosarcoma) is a neoplastic disease primarily of the lymph nodes and spleen, and occasionally of the liver, in which the proliferating neoplastic cell closely resembles the mature lymphocyte. This disease has not been well-characterized or described in most previous studies. Spontaneous incidences are in the 6 to 7% range for female RF mice (Table 1). This slowly developing disease is accelerated temporally with increasing dose of irradiation but does not occur at the very early ages (9 to 12 months) as does thymic lymphoma (Table 1). Like reticulum cell sarcoma, nonthymic lymphoma occurs very late in life with mean survival times that approximate 700 days in control animals. While mean survival times were shortened by radiation (a maximum of 230 days at 300 rads), incidences were not affected and showed no dose dependence (Figure 4).

The leukemic cell types generally are relatively mature lymphocytes in contrast with thymic lymphoma which is composed of more immature lymphocytic forms; the course

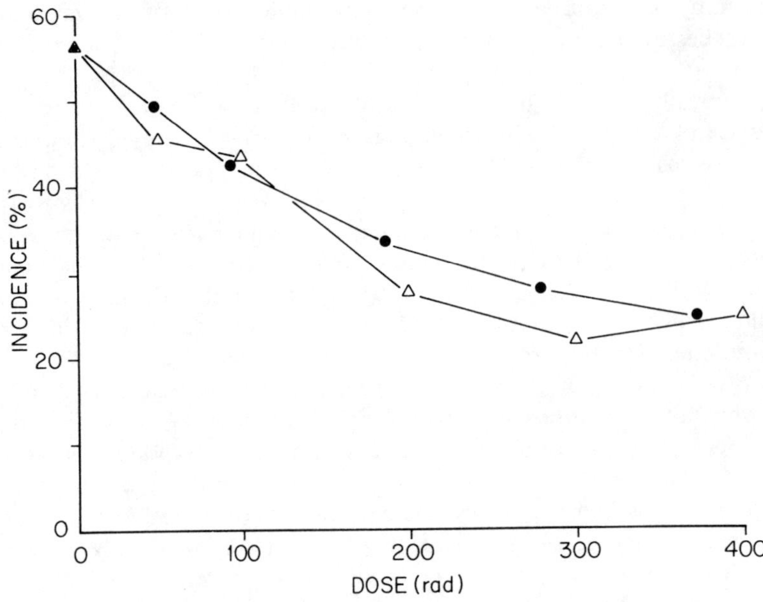

FIGURE 3. Incidences of reticulum cell sarcomas in female RF mice as a function of radiation dose after 60-Mev protons (●) or 300 kVp X-rays (△). (From Clapp, N. K., Darden, E. B., Jr., and Jernigan, M. C., *Radiat. Res.*, 57, 158, 1974. With permission.)

for this disease does not appear to be fulminating but a very slow-growing chronic one. Mitotic figures are relatively rare. Like reticulum cell sarcoma, it develops primarily in the white pulp of the spleen, in contrast with the metastasizing thymic lymphoma and myeloid leukemia which appear in the splenic red pulp, and in the lymph nodes, and occasionally in the Peyer's patches and liver. The leukemia may be either generalized in several organs or relatively confined to a single or perhaps two or three organs. A number of cases were incidental findings that did not contribute to the cause of death.

Shifts in Leukemia Incidence and Mean Survival Time After a Leukemogenic Dose of X-rays

A schematic drawing of the effects of 300 rads of ionizing radiation upon the quantitative and temporal relationships of leukemias in RF female mice is demonstrated in Figure 5. Radiation increased incidences of thymic lymphoma and myeloid leukemia, with a concomitant decrease in incidences of reticulum cell sarcoma; nonthymic lymphoma incidences were not altered. A similar temporal advancement (5 to 7 months) occurred in thymic lymphomas, myeloid leukemias, and nonthymic lymphomas, but reticulum cell sarcomas were only slightly advanced. The total percentage of leukemic mice (60 to 70%) was not significantly altered despite shifts in the numbers of individual leukemias and changes in times of occurrence.

Differential Diagnosis of Reticular Neoplasms

The leukemoid reaction is one of the responses of the mouse hemopoietic system which may add some difficulty to the differential diagnosis of leukemias. The myeloproliferative tissues respond to a variety of stimuli (e.g., hemorrhage or inflammation) to produce the specific cells needed in each situation, and this normal physiological response must be differentiated from leukemia. Particularly in infectious processes,

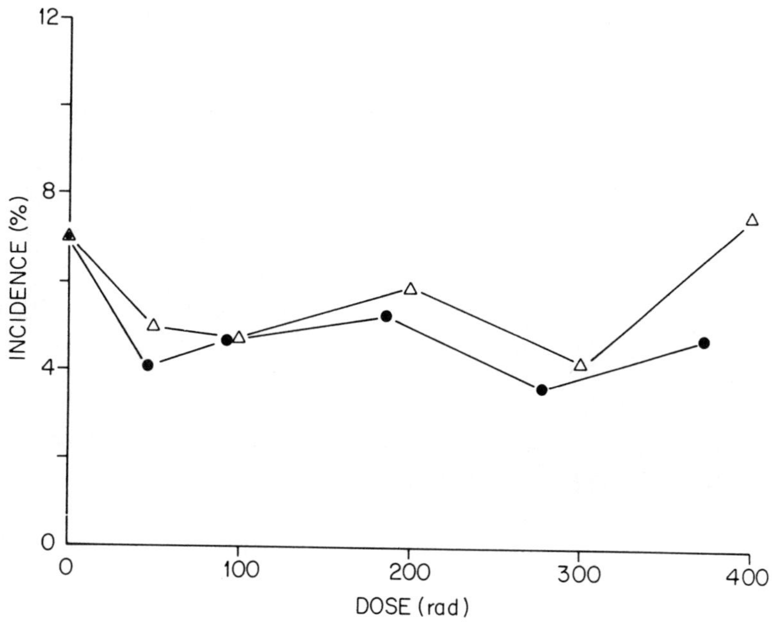

FIGURE 4. Incidences of nonthymic lymphomas in female RF mice as a function of radiation dose after 60-Mev protons (●) or 300 kVp X-rays (Δ). (From Clapp, N. K., Darden, E. B., Jr., and Jernigan, M. C., *Radiat. Res.*, 57, 158, 1974. With permission.)

marked granulocytopoiesis may occur in the red pulp of the spleen and the portal triad of the liver, as well as in lymph nodes and even the adrenal cortex. While the spleen is grossly enlarged (two to three times), each of the three developing cell lines (erythrocyte, granulocyte, and megakaryocyte) are present; despite a hypercellularity, the normal architecture of the spleen remains recognizable. All of the various stages in maturation of granulocytes are present, in contrast with the preponderance of only one developmental stage which is characteristic of myeloid leukemia.

In Table 2, the type of organ involvement and locations of leukemias in the RF mouse are compared. As in most disease processes, all of the involvements may not be found in each case, but the general frequency of occurrence and distribution within an organ are aids in diagnosis. Some of the organ distribution is probably related to the site of origin while other distributions possibly relate to the inherent mannerisms of the leukemia in question.

INDUCTION OF RETICULAR NEOPLASIA IN HUMANS

Since the ultimate concern of the researcher is to project and extrapolate his experimental findings either to predict the outcome of or to correlate with known radiation effects on humans, we will only briefly discuss reticular neoplasia in humans since the experimental data are quite comparable in relating to the relatively few observations made in humans.

The evaluation of leukemogenesis in certain human subpopulations who have been exposed to ionizing radiation shows a similarity in radiation effect upon reticular tissues in humans and laboratory animals. Prior to our learning about the severe effects caused by treating persons with X-rays, medical X-rays were used somewhat promiscuously for diagnostic and therapeutic reasons, with numerous patients being exposed to ionizing radiation for therapy of ankylosing spondylitis of the spine and other dis-

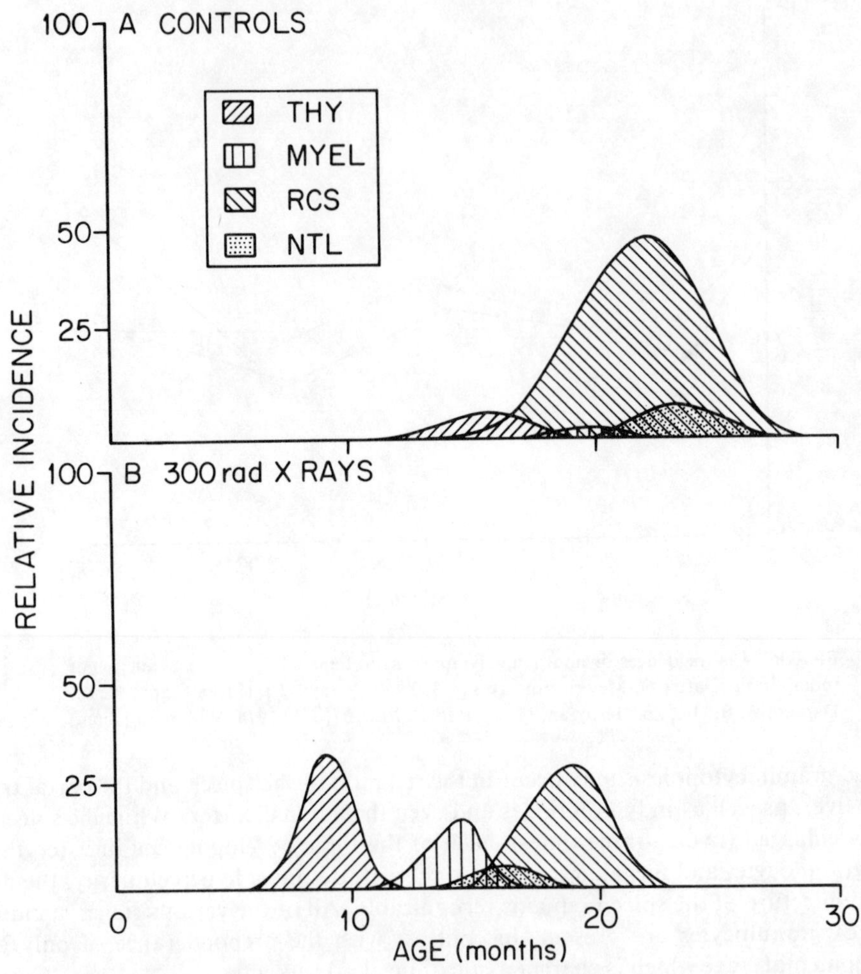

FIGURE 5. Relative incidences and times of occurrence of various types of leukemias in RF female mice with and without 300 rads of X-rays.[1] Areas under curves are relative times of occurrence. THY = thymic lymphoma; MYEL = myeloid leukemia; RCS = reticulum cell sarcoma; NTL = nonthymic lymphoma. Numbers are mean survival times for particular disease.

eases. Pelvimetry X-ray examination of pregnant women has exposed both the mother and the unborn fetus. At the same time, radiologists received large partial and whole-body doses while examining patients for various conditions, especially those which required fluoroscopic examination. Fortunately, such high exposures have since been drastically lowered through education and training of personnel using X-ray units. Another group of humans was exposed to varying doses of radiation when the atomic detonations occurred at Hiroshima and Nagasaki in Japan during World War II. While the doses in patients may be reasonably well calculated and determinations can be made relative to the portion(s) of the body which were exposed, the estimations of radiation dose to the Japanese survivors are very difficult to accurately determine due to shielding, unknown distances from hypocenter, etc. In addition, adequate matching controls are also very difficult to obtain for all of these groups from the heterogenous human population. This contrasts with the genetically well-defined mouse lines used experimentally.

Despite the interspecies and situation differences between human and experimental

Table 2
ORGAN INVOLVEMENT AND LOCATION OF LEUKEMIAS IN THE RF MOUSE. SUGGESTED AIDS FOR DIFFERENTIAL DIAGNOSIS

Organ	Thymic lymphoma	Myeloid leukemia	Reticulum cell sarcoma	Nonthymic lymphomas
Lung	Peribronchial, perivascular, atelectasis	Emboli, thrombi, petechiae	Occasional, nodular, may be perivascular	Rare
Liver	Perivascular, smooth surface	Perivascular, sinusoids involved, diffuse, smooth surface	Nodular	Perivascular, especially central veins
Thymus	Primary	Rarely, secondary	Secondary	Rare
Spleen	Metastatic to red pulp, smooth surface	Begins in red pulp, smooth surface	Begins in lymphatic nodule and enlarges outwardly, nodular surface	Begins in white pulp, smooth surface
Heart	Routinely in basal area, also pericardium	Rarely except within vessels	Rare	Rare
Sternum	Secondary invasion, pleura — cheese-like appearance	Necrosis of bone marrow	Rare in bone marrow	Rare
Lymph node	Common when generalized and slow growing, secondary	Secondary	Very common, often a primary site in a single node (e.g., mesenteric)	Common, primary
Blood	Approximately 50%	Near 100%	Rare, except in monocytic form	Occasional
Adrenal cortex	Occasional	High percentage	Occasional	Rare
Ovary and uterus	Common (50%)	Common	Occasional	Occasional
Kidney	Common	Common	Common	Occasional

From Clapp, N. K., TID-26373, 1973, National Technical Information Service, U.S. Department of Commerce, Springfield, Va. With permission.

data, we find that exposure to ionizing radiation increases the leukemia incidences in human populations as in laboratory animals. These increases have been greatest in those individuals exposed in utero or in early childhood, and less with increasing age at time of exposure.[16] Ohkita and Kamada[17] recently reported a marked increase in chronic granulocytic leukemia (which is simlar to murine myeloid leukemia) among proximally exposed survivors, especially in Hiroshima. The Hiroshima atomic bomb had a higher neutron component of radiation than did the one at Nagasaki, and this variation in radiation quality and the difference in induced leukemias suggest the need for further experimental work to elucidate the effect of radiation quality on leukemogenesis and other possible risk determinations. Another interesting observation which is now surfacing in analyzing the populations exposed at Hiroshima and Nagasaki is that the leukemogenic effects appear to be subsiding in these two populations. While genetic effects may still remain to be determined in current and subsequent generations, it would appear that the leukemogenic effect from the ionizing radiation may now be returning to near-normal levels. In addition, other late somatic effects such as solid (nonreticular) tumors of the thyroid gland, breast, and lung (and other organs) may be increased, but these appear to be unrelated to the reticular tissue responses which we are considering in this chapter.

We conclude from these observations in limited human exposure situations that the experimental models, while not duplicating exactly the reticular diseases in humans, are reasonably valid for risk estimates and for elucidating the mechanisms of ionizing radiation effects in leukemogenesis.

MODIFYING FACTORS AFFECTING RETICULAR TISSUE RESPONSE TO RADIATION

The response of the immune system (primarily reticular tissues) to ionizing radiation (with resulting leukemogenesis and associated tissue changes) has been studied extensively by numerous investigators during the past several years.[1,3,7-14,16,18-22] Numerous variables have been observed which alter the tissue response and, consequently, the production of leukemias. Some of these modifying factors are total dose, dose rate, radiation quality, and numerous host factors (i.e., sex, age, mouse strain, microbial flora, etc.). In order to determine the contribution of each parameter, experiments must be designed in which all variables are stabilized except the one to be evaluated.

The relationships of the variables are extremely complex and interrelated, but we will attempt to generalize the current status of our knowledge. Most of the earlier investigations were conducted using X- or gamma rays given at relatively high whole-body doses (50 to 500 rads) and at relatively high dose rates ($\sim$50 to 100 rads/min); andas a result, much of the experimental data which is needed for the inferential extrapolation to humans is either minimal or lacking at very low total doses ($\leqslant$25 rads) and at very low dose rates ($\leqslant$ a few rads/day). To experimentally determine significant changes at these low doses or at low dose rates requires a very large number of animals which must be extremely clean to minimize the effect of intercurrent disease (especially infectious diseases) in order to detect rather small changes in incidences (response to the treatment in question). Practically, it is very difficult to isolate only one variable at a time for experimental purposes, and this limitation further complicates the interpretation of results.

The dose-response curve (comparing the incidences of various diseases at different quantitative levels of radiation treatment) is perhaps the simplest variable to evaluate, but this end point is also modified, even given the same host factors, by changes in dose rate and the type of radiation used. We have shown some of the dose-response

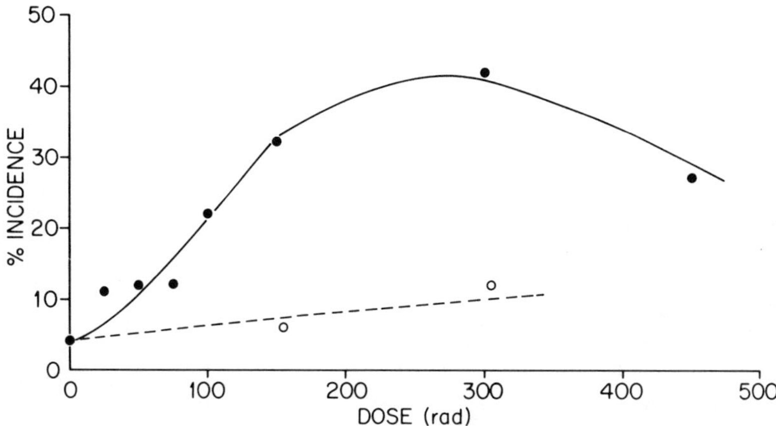

FIGURE 6. Incidence of myeloid leukemia in male RF mice after single (●) or daily (○) X- or γ-ray irradiation. (From Ullrich, R. L., *Radiation Biology in Cancer Research,* Meyn, R. E. and Withers, H. R., Eds., Raven Press, New York, 1980, 309. With permission.)

curves for the various leukemias (Figures 1—4) which demonstrate that the leukemogenic response is very complex and even varies from one type of leukemia to another. For myeloid leukemia in RF mice, Upton[12] observed an increased incidence from 25 to 300 rads (radiation given in the high dose-rate range) with a subsequent decline above 300 rads which was attributed to the influence of cell killing at higher doses (Figure 6); the expression of transformed cells was thus overwhelmed by the increase in dying cells. This data is similar to ours (Figure 2) except that the highest incidence was at 300 rads (Upton) vs. ∿200 rads (Clapp). Thus a simple mathematical expression could not describe the relationship between leukemia incidence and dose of radiation at all dose levels. Over the dose range of 0 to 100 rads (lowest dose was 25 rads), the incidence appeared to vary with the square of the dose, but a linear response could not be rejected.[13] Major and Mole[20] also suggested a similar relationship with dose for myeloid leukemia induction in CBA mice.

In a very extensive study in our laboratory (∿40,000 mice; RF and BALB/c strains), thymic lymphoma has also been studied using doses from 10 to 300 rads with very large numbers of mice (Figure 7). The dose response for thymic lymphoma differs from meyloid leukemia in that no decline in incidences was seen through 300 rads,[13] although a plateau was observed previously at 300 to 400 rads.[1,16] Cell killing did not appear to offer a significant contribution to the dose-response curve. In the high dose rate group (comparable to Upton's), the 0 to 25 rad range increased with the square of the dose, while over the 50 to 300 rad range a linear response was seen.[13] Since these mice were housed in barrier conditions, this factor may explain some of the differences in dose response. Generally, at lower doses the radiation appears to be more efficient (% of incidence change/rad) in causing leukemogenesis (both myeloid and thymic lymphoma).

As can be seen in Figures 6 and 7, the rate at which the animal is exposed to ionizing radiation dramatically affects the incidence of leukemia induced. By changing from a single acute exposure to a prolonged chronic exposure (same total dose) whereby the dose was given over several days rather than in a few minutes, the incidences were significantly reduced at all doses. Most of these response curves appear to be more linear or linear dose-squared or some other single relationship. However, the incidences may also be too low to show subtle shifts in the response. Dose rate appears to

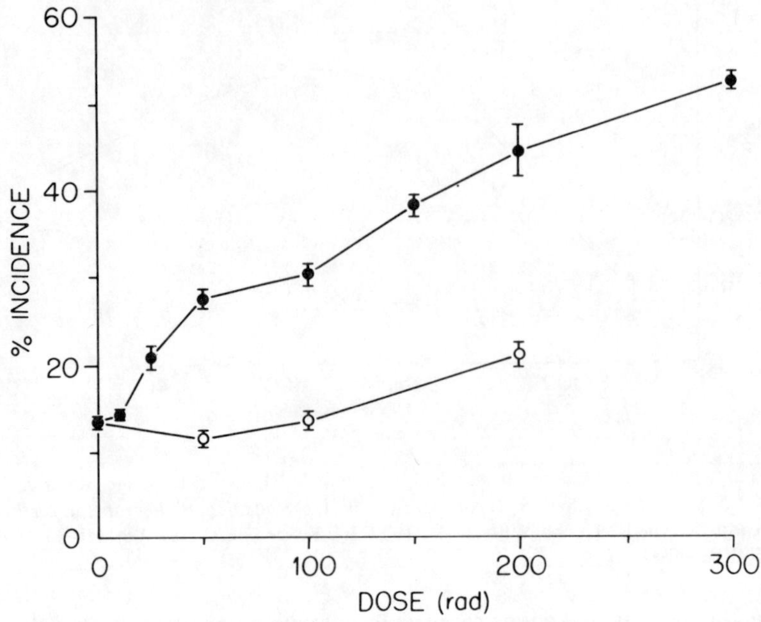

FIGURE 7. Incidence of thymic lymphoma in female RF mice after γ-ray irradiation at rates of 45 rads/min (●) or 8.3 rads/day (○). (From Ullrich, R. L. and Storer, J. B., *Late Biological Effects of Ionizing Radiation*, Vol. 2, International Atomic Energy Agency, Vienna, 1979, 101. With permission.)

be more significant in low linear energy transfer radiation (γ- or X-rays) than with high linear energy transfer particulate treatments such as neutrons. With neutrons, doses most often appear to be cumulative even when the radiation was given over longer periods of time.

The quality (physical characteristics) of ionizing radiation also dramatically affects the dose response. Most of the particulate radiations (protons, alphas, betas, and neutrons) have higher rates of energy deposit along a given length of tissue (linear energy transfer). For estimates of risk to populations, especially to humans, effects from each of these radiations are compared and expressed as relative biological effectiveness to the results from treatment with photon energies (gamma or X-rays), which both have a similar but relatively low linear energy transfer. This information is critical when determining maximum permissible levels for human exposures for both occupational personnel and the total population. In general, neutrons and other high linear energy transfer radiations are more effective and less dose-rate dependent than gamma rays with respect to life-shortening and the induction of neoplasms.[2,3,7,8,10] A linear relationship was reported for thymic lymphoma induction at both a higher and lower dose rate for neutrons in RFM mice with little dose-rate dependence at low doses while at the highest doses a low dose rate was more effective. The complexity of these responses and their interrelationships become obvious and also very difficult to isolate experimentally.

The response of the immune system to radiation is also dependent upon various host factors. Female mice are generally more susceptible to spontaneous thymic lymphoma and males to myeloid leukemia, and higher incidences of these neoplasms are generally induced in both sexes by radiation, especially in RFs. The age of the animal at the time of exposure may also alter the response; generally, the younger the animal the greater is its sensitivity to develop leukemia. One of the most interesting modifiers of leukemogenesis is that of microbial flora upon myeloid leukemogenesis. The female RF mouse develops maximally 20 to 25% incidence after 300 rads when raised in a conventional environment but does not develop myeloid leukemia if raised in a barrier condition.[14,15] Although the barrier-raised male develops an occasional case of myeloid leukemia, the numbers are drastically reduced as compared with conventionally reared mice.[14,15] In addition, both sexes develop higher incidences of thymic lymphomas after radiation when raised in a barrier as compared with being reared conventionally; thus the total numbers of leukemias remain about the same regardless of the environment, but the relative percentages of each leukemia are shifted. The cause of this effect is not known but may relate to cell turnover as a result of normal biological response to the microbes normally present.

SUMMARY

Neoplasia of the immune system is significant in the explanation of some life-shortening in aging animals as the induction of leukemias experimentally is the major contributing component to radiation-induced life-shortening. While exact duplicates of the human leukemias may not have been discovered by researchers at this point in time, many similarities exist which suggest that the experimental models are extremely helpful in studies of pathogenesis and mechanisms of action; this information may, in turn, aid in prognosis, prevention and/or therapy for these critical human diseases. In experimental models it is clear that interactions occur which can modify the responses of animals to leukemogenic insults. As our knowledge continues to grow and information blanks are filled, we anticipate an ever increasing understanding of the physiology and pathology of these tissues and their responses to stimuli which will aid in improving the health and longevity of man.

REFERENCES

1. **Clapp, N. K., Darden, E. B., Jr., and Jernigan, M. C.,** Relative effects of whole-body sublethal doses of 60-MeV protons and 300-kVp X-rays on disease incidences in RF mice, *Radiat. Res.*, 57, 158, 1974.
2. **Storer, J. B., Serrano, L. J., Darden, E. B., Jr., Jernigan, M. C., and Ullrich, R. L.,** Life shortening in RFM and BALB/c mice as a function of radiation quality, dose, and dose rate, *Radiat. Res.*, 78, 122, 1979.
3. **Upton, A. C., Randolph, M. L., and Conklin, J. W.,** Late effects of fast neutrons and gamma rays in mice as influenced by the dose rate of irradiation: life shortening, *Radiat. Res.*, 32, 493, 1967.
4. **Clapp, N. K.,** *An Atlas of RF Mouse Pathology: Disease Descriptions and Incidences,* TID-26373, 1973, National Technical Information Service, U.S. Department of Commerce, Springfield, Va.
5. **Dunn, T. B.,** Normal and pathologic anatomy of the reticular tissue in laboratory mice, *J. Natl. Cancer Inst.*, 14, 1281, 1954.
6. **Cosgrove, G. E., Satterfield, L. C., Bowles, N. D., and Klima, W. C.,** Diseases of aging untreated virgin female RFM and BALB/c mice, *J. Gerontol.*, 33, 178, 1978.
7. **Ullrich, R. L., Jernigan, M. C., Cosgrove, G. E., Satterfield, L. C., Bowles, N. D., and Storer, J. B.,** The influence of dose and dose rate on the incidence of neoplastic disease in RFM mice after neutron irradiation, *Radiat. Res.*, 68, 115, 1976.
8. **Ullrich, R. L. and Storer, J. B.,** The influence of dose, dose rate, and radiation quality on radiation carcinogenesis and life shortening in RFM and BALB/c mice, in *Late Biological Effects of Ionizing Radiation,* Vol. 2, IAEA-SM 224/204, International Atomic Energy Agency, Vienna, 1979, 95.
9. **Upton, A. C., Jenkins, V. K., Walburg, H. E., Jr., Tyndall, R. L., Conklin, J. W., and Wald, N.,** Observations on viral, chemical, and radiation-induced myeloid and lymphoid leukemias in RF mice, *J. Natl. Cancer Inst. Monogr.*, 22, 329, 1966.

10. **Upton, A. C., Randolph, M. L., and Conklin, J. W.,** Late effects of fast neutrons, and gamma-rays in mice as influenced by the dose of rate of irradiation: induction of neoplasia, *Radiat. Res.*, 41, 467, 1970.
11. **Upton, A.C. and Furth, J.,** The effects of cortisone on the development of spontaneous leukemia in mice and on its induction by irradiation, *Blood*, 9, 686, 1954.
12. **Upton, A. C., Jenkins, V. K., and Conklin, J. W.,** Myeloid leukemia in the mouse, *Ann. N. Y. Acad. Sci.*, 114, 189, 1964.
13. **Ullrich, R. L.,** Carcinogenesis in mice after low doses and dose rates, in *Radiation Biology in Cancer Research*, Meyn, R. E. and Withers, H. R., Eds., Raven Press, New York, 1980, 309.
14. **Walburg, H. E., Jr., Cosgrove, G. E., and Upton, A. C.,** Influence of microbial environment on development of myeloid leukemia in X-irradiated RFM mice, *Int. J. Cancer*, 3, 150, 1968.
15. **Upton, A. C., Allen, R. C., Brown, R. C., Clapp, N. K., Conklin, J. W., Cosgrove, G. E., Darden, E. B., Jr., Kastenbaum, M. A., Odell, T. T., Jr., Serrano, L. J., Tyndall, R. L., and Walburg, H. E., Jr.,** Quantitative experimental study of low-level radiation carcinogenesis, in *Radiation-Induced Cancer*, Unipub, New York, 1969, 425.
16. **Upton, A. C.,** Comparative observations on radiation carcinogenesis in man and animals, in *Carcinogenesis: A Broad Critique*, Williams & Wilkins, Baltimore, 1967, 631.
17. **Ohkita, T. and Kamada, N.,** Leukemia Among Atomic Bomb Survivors, 6th Int. Cong. Radiation Research, Tokyo, May 1979, 2.
18. **Kaplan, H. S.,** The role of radiation in experimental leukemogenesis, *J. Natl. Cancer Inst. Monogr.*, 14, 207, 1964.
19. **Kaplan, H. S.,** On the natural history of the murine leukemias: presidential address, *Cancer Res*,. 27, 1325, 1967.
20. **Major, I. R. and Mole, R. H.,** Myeloid leukemia in X-ray irradiated CBA mice, *Nature*, 272, 455, 1978.
21. **Upton, A. C.,** The dose-response relation in radiation-induced cancer, *Cancer Res.*, 21, 717, 1961.
22. **Upton, A. C., Wolff, F. F., Furth, J., and Kimball, A. W.,** A comparison of the induction of myeloid and lymphoid leukemias in X-irradiated RF mice, *Cancer Res.*, 18, 842, 1958.

Methods for Measuring Immune Competence

ASSESSING CELLULAR IMMUNE FUNCTION

Conrad H. Casavant and Daniel P. Stites

INTRODUCTION

Cell-mediated immunity is involved in a variety of immunologic phenomena including resistance to infection with intracellular parasites (viral, bacterial, fungal and protozoal infections), contact allergy, graft rejection, tumor destruction, and autoimmune disorders. Studies in both man and animals suggest a relationship between the appearance of certain diseases in adult life and the decline in immune function. The increased incidence of cancer and autoimmunity in an aged population is of note. This is not to say that the critical events leading to aging are under direct control of the immune system, but only that the waning of immunocompetence may play a significant role in the development of some diseases.

There are few systematic studies of cellular immunity in human aging populations. Data generated from any study are meaningful only when reliable in vivo and/or in vitro assays for assessment of cellular immune function are applied to the question. This section discusses current methods used to study cellular immunity with emphasis on laboratory aspects of T-cell function in man. Our purpose here is not to discuss the detailed interpretation of data published in the literature, but to point out the approaches and results of studies on the effect of aging on cell mediated immunity in man utilizing in vivo and in vitro methods.

DELAYED CUTANEOUS HYPERSENSITIVITY

Despite the development of a multitude of complex in vitro assays for assessment of cellular immunity, the relatively simple intradermal test remains a useful tool. One approach is to study responsiveness to antigens which a subject has been previously exposed to in early life. The classical example of this is tuberculin hypersensitivity. It appears that the number of positive skin tests to tuberculin progressively falls throughout life, especially after the age of 50-60 years.[1-6] A more comprehensive approach involves testing hypersensitivity to more ubiquitous antigens. Positive skin tests to Candida, mumps, trichophyton, and streptokinase-streptodornase progressively decline throughout life.[4-6] Another approach is to attempt primary sensitization to antigens to which individuals have had no previous exposure. The ability to develop contact hypersensitivity to dinitrochlorobenzene (DNCB) is diminished in subjects more than 70 years of age.[2,5] The biological events which occur following local injection of antigens are extremely complex and involve antigen processing, antigenic stimulation of lymphocytes, release of soluble mediators, and migration of macrophages to the dermal site. A defect in any one of these components may result in a diminished cellular immune response. The use of several concentrations of test antigens is important since aging individuals might show a diminished response with one concentration but a positive one when they are tested with a higher strength of antigen. The failure of aging subjects to respond to intradermal testing does not necessarily reflect diminished cellular immunity, but may be a result of loss of generalized skin reactivity.

LYMPHOCYTE SURFACE MARKERS

Identification of T-cells

Identification of T-cells has been made possible by two different laboratory approaches. Specific surface markers such as the presence of sheep red blood cell receptors (E rosettes) or human T-cell antigens facilitate the enumeration of T lymphocytes in peripheral blood and other lymphoid tissues. Functional assays such as lymphocyte activation or lymphocytotoxicity measure the immunocompetence of lymphocytes in vitro. Tables 1 and 2 list the selected in vitro assays currently used for quantitation and measuring T-cell function in man. In considering the use of assays for assessing cellular immune function either in normal, diseased, or aging populations, the limitations of these assays must be recognized. The interpretation of results of T-cell testing are complicated by inherent biological variation within lymphocyte populations and by lack of standardization of many of these methods. Despite these limitations, it is still possible to make important inferences regarding the cellular immune status of aging subjects.

Table 3 illustrates a summation of T-cell quantitation of aging individuals as compared to young adults. There are considerable discrepancies among studies of T-cell surface markers with advancing age. Some investigators have reported that the percent and absolute number of T-cells decrease with increasing age.[5,51-54] Others reported no significant differences between young adults and aging adults.[49,55,56] Additional studies have indicated that the percent and absolute number of T-cells may increase with advancing age.[49,50] It appears that increases in T-cell numbers were noted primarily in the eighth and ninth decade of life whereas these difference were not as common in the sixth and seventh decades. These conflicting findings could be explained by several possibilities: (a) variation in E rosette methods (b) difference in age and condition of health of subjects selected for study, (c) age related changes in the receptor on human lymphocytes responsible for rosette formation with sheep red blood cells (SRBC), and (d) age related changes in subpopulations of T-cells.

LYMPHOCYTE FUNCTION ASSAYS

Mitogen and Antigen Induced Transformation

Studies in man using in vitro T-cell assays clearly suggest that changes in immunocompetence with advancing age are a reflection of T-cell function (Table 4). The majority of studies indicate an age-associated decrease in blast transformation following mitogen stimulation of lymphocytes with Concanavalin A (Con A) and Phytohemagglutinin (PHA).[1,5,49,50,55,56] These mitogens selectively activate various populations of T-cells. A similar decrease in blast transformation was observed when lymphocytes from aging individuals were cultured in the presence of purified protein derivative (PPD),[5,62,65] streptolysin O or influenza vaccine,[62] Aspergillus,[5] or *Candida albicans* and SK-SD.[5,62] The need for optimizing culture conditions when performing lymphocyte transformation studies is essential. Varying concentrations of mitogens and culture duration can affect the degree of lymphocyte transformation. Depressed proliferative responses to PHA and Con A were reported in individuals over 50-years-old when lymphocytes were cultured in the presence of mitogens for 3 days. However, when these same cultures were prolonged for 5 days, lymphocytes from aged subjects showed an increased response.[67] Dose response curves are also essential since significant differences in lymphocyte responses from young and aging individuals can be missed if one concentration of mitogen is used.[67] Confusion may also result from a nonstandardized format for presentation of lymphocyte stimulation data. Results should be expressed as total counts per minute of isotope incorporation and as a stimulation index: a ratio of counts per minute in stimulated cultures to those in control cultures. High background proliferation of lymphocytes from aging subjects has been observed.[66] Thus, when stimulation data was expressed as a stimulation index, peripheral lymphocytes

Table 1
T-CELL ASSAYS IN MAN

Marker	Assay employed	Synonyms	Representative method	Results	Ref.
A. Sheep red blood cell (SRBC) receptor	1. SRBC rosettes (total)	T-cell rosette R-rosette E-rosette (erythrocyte) RFC E-RFC	Lymphocytes purified from blood by Ficoll Hypaque density gradient centrifugation; SRBC + Lymphocytes incubated at ratio 100:1 briefly at 37°C then overnight at 4°C; rosettes scored by counting lymphocytes surrounded by at least 3 SRBC	Mean = 62.5% From 20 studies[a] Range 47—82% Total subjects = 471	7—26
	2. "Active"-SRBC rosettes	Rapid rosette High affinity rosette A-RFC	Similar to Total E-RFC but SRBC exposed to lymphocytes for 5 min at 20°C; number of RFC after this brief incubation designated active rosettes	Mean = 26.8% From 4 studies Range 24—28% Total subjects = 223	16, 21, 27, 28
B. Human T-cell antigen	1. Surface membrane Immunofluorescence	Hu T-LA Anti T-cell test	Animal immunized with thymocytes of T-cells; antiserum absorbed to specificity with B-cells (CLL or cell lines); T-cells detected by surface immunofluorescent labeled antiserum or by double antibody (Sandwich) technique	Mean = 66% From 7 studies Range = 53—78% Total subjects = 92	29—35
	2. Cytoxicity	—	Anti-T serum and complement used to kill T cells; viability assessed by supravital dye or ^{51}Cr release		

[a] A number of studies excluded because of clearly suboptimal conditions.

Table 2
T-CELL ASSAYS IN MAN

Lymphocyte Function Assays

Assay	Stimulant	Synonyms	Representative method	Results	Ref.
Lymphocyte activation[a]	Mitogens—Phytohemagglutinin (PHA), Concanavalin A (Con A)	Lymphocyte transformation Lymphocyte stimulation Blastogenesis Blast transformation	Purified blood lymphocytes cultured with mitogen for 72 hr; DNA synthesis measured by incorporation of radioactive thymidine and detected by scintillation counting	10- to 250-fold[b] increase in DNA synthesis; compared to control with no added mitogen	
	Antigens—Microbial, e.g., candid, PPD, coccidioidin histoplasmin mumps, streptodornase, tetanus toxoid	Antigen transformation	Purified blood lymphocytes cultured with individual antigens and DNA synthesis assayed as above; cultures grown 5—7 days.		36—48
	Allogeneic cells—Mitomycin or X-irradiated lymphocytes	Mixed leukocyte culture (MLC) Mixed lymphocyte reaction (MLR) One way MLC or MLR	Lymphocytes from one individual cultured with mitomycin or X-irradiated stimulator cells for 5—7 days; DNA synthesis assayed as above	5- to 50-fold[b] control	
Lymphoctoxicity	Allogeneic cells (stimulator and target cells)	Cell mediated lympholysis (CML), cell mediated cytotoxicity (CMC)	Two stage test: (1)MLR performed (2)^{51}Cr labeled target cells added and specific T cell cytotoxicity induced by in vitro sensitization measured by ^{51}Cr release	10—70%[b] killing of target cells	

[a] All of these assays are relatively specific for T-cells. Accessory cells (macrophages, null cells) may also be required for maximal responses.
[b] Degree of responses varies widely due to culture conditions and other variables.

Table 3
EFFECT OF AGING ON T-CELL ASSAYS IN MAN

Lymphocyte Surface Markers

Marker	Assay employed	Total subjects	Age of subjects (years)		Results T-cells	Ref.
			Control	Aged		
Sheep red blood cell (SRBC) receptor	SRBC rosettes (total)	96	20—39	80—99	Increased in aged group	49
		46	60—69	90—98		50
		32	19—50	67—83	Decreased in aged group	51
		51	16—49	50—69		52
		106	18—41	70—87		53
		98	20—40	60—96		54
		107	20—50	50—>65		5
		48	25—40	75—96	No difference between aged and control group	55
		36	<40	>65		56
		204	20—39	40—79		49
Human T-cell antigen (HuTLA)	Antibody mediated cytotxicity	46	60—69	90—98	Increased in aged group	50
		96	20—39	80—99		49
		204	20—39	40—79	No difference between aged and control group	49

Table 4
EFFECT OF AGING ON T-CELL ASSAYS IN MAN

Lymphocyte Function Assays

Assay	Stimulant	Total subjects	Age of subjects (years)		Results	Ref.
			Control	Aged		
Lymphocyte activation	Mitogens — Phytohemagglutinin (PHA)	46	60—69	90—98	PHA response decreased in aged	50
		48	25—40	75—96		55
		146[a]	20—40	50—80		57
		172	20—35	60—101		58
		293[b]	1—50	60—98		59
		N.G.[c]	<40	>70		60
		59	20—40	70—83		61
		30	21—40	71—95		62
		20	25—35	72—86		63
		36	<40	>65		56
		40	<25	>60		1
		83	16—60	60—100		64
		88	18—40	>60		65
		244	20—39	40—99		49
		178	15—40	40—>65		5
		37[d]	18—43	60—92	No difference in response between aged and control subjects	66
	Concanavalin A (CON A)	244	20—59	60—99	Response decrease in aged subjects	49
		60	20—40	70—83		61
		37	18—43	60—92		66
		N.G.[c]	<40	>70		60
		20	25—35	72—82	No difference in response between aged and control subjects	63
		88	18—40	>60		65

	PPD	30	21—40	71—95	Response decreased in aged subjects	62
		88	18—40	>60		65
		185	20—65	>65		5
	Streptolysin O, influenza vaccine	30	21—40	71—95	Response decreased in aged subjects	62
	C. albicans, SK-SD	30	21—40	71—95	Response decreased in aged subjects	62
		185	20—65	>65		5
		88	18—40	>60	No difference in response between aged and control subjects	65
	Aspergillus	185	20—65	>65	Response decreased in aged subjects	5
	Mixed leukocyte culture (MLC)	48	25—40	75—96	Response decreased in aged subjects	55
		N.G.[c]	<40	>70		60
		60	20—30	40—99		49
		30	21—40	71—95	No difference in response between aged and control subjects	62
Lymphocytotoxicity	Cell mediated cytotoxicity (CMC)	79	20—40	70—83	Response decreased in aged subjects	61

[a] Progressively decreasing response with increasing age.
[b] PHA response measured as mitotic index.
[c] Not given.
[d] High spontaneous proliferation of lymphocytes from aged subjects.

from aging subjects appeared to be less responsive to PHA and Con A than those from young adult controls. However, total counts per minute of stimulated culture from lymphocytes from aging and control subjects were not significantly different.

ALLOGENIC CELL STIMULATION IN MIXED LYMPHOCYTE REACTION (MLR)

Standard reproducible assays for studying the allogenic MLR in man are not well-defined due primarily to difficulties in obtaining a line of standard stimulating cells. Three studies suggest a decline in responder activity of lymphocytes from aging individuals,[49,55,60] while one study reported no difference between aging individuals and young adult controls.[62] Nevertheless, lymphocytes from aging individuals were capable of acting as stimulating cells.

Information on the effect of aging on result of cell mediated cytotoxicity (CMC) is almost nonexistent. This test detects a population of cytotoxic cells generated during an allogenic MLR. However, results of one study suggest that CMC responses to allogenic cells of lymphocytes from aging donors were depressed when compared to the response of lymphocytes from young adults.[61]

Despite some discrepancies in studies assessing T-cell immunity in man, there appears to be a waning of the T-cell component of the immune system with advancing age. Whether this diminished immunological competence is a result of alterations in numbers or subpopulations of T-cells remains unclear. For example, increase in T suppressor cell function could result in T-cell (and B-cell) deficiencies. The nature of T-cell populations responsible for decreased immunocompetence needs to be elucidated. A deficiency of helper T-cells could affect immune surveillance or differentiation of B-cells into antibody producing cells. Two studies suggest that supressor activity of T-cells is decreased in aging individuals.[68,69] More refined assays to identify T-cell subpopulations will no doubt provide infomation in the future. Development of techniques that allow separation of lymphocytes into responder, helper, and supressor populations will provide information as to the key role each plays in the decline of T-cell immunity with aging. Only then will the precise role of this important class of immunocytes in production of disease associated with aging be fully appreciated.

REFERENCES

1. **Roberts-Thomson, I. C., Whittingham, S., Youngchaiyud, U., and Mackay, I. R.,** Ageing, immune response, and mortality, *Lancet,* 2, 368, 1974.
2. **Waldorf, D. S., Willkens, R. F., and Decker, J. L.,** Impaired delayed hypersensitivity in an aging population, *JAMA,* 203, 831, 1968.
3. **Giannini, D. and Sloan, R. S.,** A tuberculin survey of 1285 adults with special reference to the elderly, *Lancet,* 1, 525, 1957.
4. **Mackay, I. R.,** Ageing and immunological function in man, *Gerontologia,* 18, 285, 1972.
5. **Girard, J. P., Paychere, M., Cuevas, M., and Fernandes, B.,** Cell-mediated immunity in an ageing population, *Clin. Exp. Immunol.,* 27, 85, 1977.
6. **Forbes, I. J.,** Measurement of immunological function in clinical medicine, *Austr. N. Z. J. Med.,* 1, 160, 1971.
7. **Jondal, M., Holm, G., and Wigzell, H.,** Surface markers on human T and B lymphocytes, *J. Exp. Med.,* 136, 207, 1972.

8. **Greaves, M., Janossy, G., and Doenhoff, M.**, Selective triggering of human T and B lymphocytes in vitro by polyclonal mitogens, *J. Exp. Med.*, 140, 1, 1974.
9. **Mellstedt, H.**, *In vitro* activation of human T and B lymphocytes by pokeweed mitogen, *Clin. Exp. Immunol.*, 19, 75, 1975.
10. **Nowell, P. C., Daniele, R. P., and Winger, L. A.**, Kinetics of human lymphocyte proliferation: proportion of cells responsive to PHA and corrective with E rosette formation, *J. Reticuendothelial Soc.*, 17, 47, 1975.
11. **Jonsson, V.**, Technical aspects of the rosette technique for detecting human circulating B and T lymphocytes, *Scand. J. Haemat.*, 13, 361, 1974.
12. **Sasaki, M., Sekizawa, T., Takahasi, H., Abo, T., and Kumagai, K.**, Heterogenecity of human T lymphocytes to bind sheep erythrocytes and mitogenic responses of their subpopulation, *J. Immunol.*, 115, 1509, 1975.
13. **Chiao, J. W., Pantic, V. S., and Good, R. A.**, Human lymphocytes bearing receptors to complement components and SRBC, *Clin. Immunol. and Immunopathol.*, 4, 454, 1975.
14. **Mendes, N. F., Miki, S. S., and Peixinho, Z. F.**, Combined detection of human T and B lymphocytes of rosette formation with sheep erythrocytes and zymosan-C_3 complexes, *J. Immunol.*, 113, 531, 1974.
15. **Borella, L. and Sen, L.**, The distribution of lymphocytes with T and B cell surface markers in human bone marrow, *J. Immunol.*, 112, 836, 1974.
16. **Felsburg, P. J., Edelman, R., and Gelman, R. H.**, The active rosette test: correlation with delayed cutaneous hypersensitivity, *J. Immunol.*, 116, 1110, 1976.
17. **Sternswärd, J., Jondal, M., Vanky, F., Wigzell, H., and Sealy, R.**, Lymphopenia and change in distribution of human B and T lymphocytes in peripheral blood induced by irradiation for mammary carcinoma, *Lancet*, 1, 1352, 1972.
18. **Ross, G. D., Rabellino, E. M., Polley, M. O., and Grey, H. M.**, Combined studies of complement receptor and surface Ig-bearing cells and sheep erythrocyte rosette-forming cells in normal and leukemia human lymphocytes, *J. Clin. Invest.*, 52, 377, 1973.
19. **Smith, M. A., Evans, J., and Steel, C. M.**, Age related variation in proportion of circulating T cells, *Lancet*, 2, 922, 1974.
20. **Gross, R. L., Latty, A., William, E. A., and Newberne, P. M.**, Abnormal spontaneous rosette formation and rosette inhibition in lung carcinoma, *N. Engl. J. Med.*, 292, 439, 1975.
21. **Horowitz, S., Groshong, T., Albrecht, R., and Hong, A.**, The "active" rosette test in immunodeficiency diseases, *Clin. Immunol. and Immunopathol.*, 4, 405, 1975.
22. **Zeylemaker, W. P., Roos, M. T. L., Meyer, C. J. L. M., Schellekens, P. T. A., and Eijsvoogel, V. P.**, Separation of human lymphocyte subpopulations, *Cell. Immunol.*, 14, 346, 1974.
23. **Birnbaum, G.**, Numbers of rosette forming cells in human peripheral blood, *Cell. Immunol.*, 21, 371, 1976.
24. **Robinson, J. A. and Lertratanakul, Y.**, A simultaneous method for detection of T and B lymphocytes, *J. Immunol. Methods*, 8, 53, 1975.
25. **Stobo, J. D., Paul, S., Van Scoy, R. E., and Hermans, P. E.**, Suppressor thymic derived cells in fungal infection, *J. Clin. Invest.*, 57, 319, 1976.
26. **Aiuti, F., Lacava, V., Garofalo, J. A., D'Amelio, L., and D'Asero, C.**, Surface markers on human lymphocytes of normal subjects and of patients with primary immunodeficiencies, *Clin. Exp. Immunol.*, 15, 43, 1973.
27. **Gupta, S., Grieco, M. H., and Cushman, P.**, Impairment of rosette forming T lymphocytes in chronic marihuana smokers, *N. Engl. J. Med.*, 291, 874, 1974.
28. **Wybran, J. and Fudenberg, H. H.**, Thymus derived rosette forming cells in various human disease states: cancer, lymphoma, bacterial and viral infections and other diseases, *J. Clin. Invest.*, 52, 1026, 1973.
29. **Williams, R. C., DeBoard, J. S., Mellbye, O. J., Messner, R. P., and Lindstrom, F. D.**, Studies of T and B lymphocytes in patients with connective tissue diseases, *J. Clin. Invest.*, 52, 283, 1973.
30. **Owen, F. L. and Fanger, M. W.**, Studies on human T lymphocyte population, *J. Immunol.*, 113, 1128, 1974.
31. **Bobrove, A. M., Strober, S., Herzenberg, L. A., and DePamphilis, J. D.**, Identification and quantitation of thymus derived lymphocytes in human peripheral blood, *J. Immunol.*, 112, 520, 1974.
32. **Brouet, J. C. and Toben, H.**, Characterization of a subpopulation of human T lymphocytes reactive with a heteroantiserum to human brain, *J. Immunol.*, 116, 1041, 1976.
33. **Touraine, J. L., Touraine, F., Kiszkiss, D. F., Choi, Y. S., and Good, R. A.**, Heterologous specific antiserum for identification of human T lymphocytes, *Clin. Exp. Immunol.*, 16, 503, 1974.
34. **Rodt, H., Thierfelder, S., Thiel, E., Goetze, D., Netzel, B., Huhn, D., and Eulitz, M.**, Identification and quantitation of human T cell antigen by antisera purified from antibodies cross reacting with hemopoetic progenitors and other blood cells, *Immunogenetics*, 2, 411, 1975.

35. **Aiuti, F. and Wigzell, H.,** Function and distribution pattern of human T lymphocytes, *Clin. Exp. Immunol.,* 13, 183, 1973.
36. **Oppenheim, J. J., Doughtery, S., Chan, S. P., and Baker, J.,** Use of lymphocyte transformation to assess clinical disorders, in, *Laboratory Diagnosis of Immunologic Disorders,* Vyas, G. N., Stites, D. P., and Brecher, G., Eds., Grune & Stratton, New York, 1975, 87.
37. **Oppenheim, J. J. and Rosenstreich, D. L.,** *Mitogens in Immunobiology,* Academic Press, New York, 1976.
38. **Sondel, P. M., Chess, L., MacDermott, R. P., and Schlossman, S. F.,** Immunologic functions of isolated human lymphocyte subpopulations. III. Specific allogeneic lympholysis mediated by human T cell alone, *J. Immunol.,* 114, 982, 1975.
39. **Sondel, P. M., Chess, L., and Schlossman, S. F.,** Immunologic functions of isolated human lymphocyte subpopulations. IV. Stimulation of LMC and CML by human T cells, *Cell. Immunol.,* 18, 351, 1975.
40. **Dean, J. H., Silva, J. S., McCoy, J. L., Leonard, C. M., Cannon, G. B., and Herberman, R. B.,** Functional activities of rosette separated human peripheral blood lymphocytes, *J. Immunol.,* 115, 1449, 1975.
41. **Schmidtke, J. R. and Hatfield, S.,** Activation of pumped human thymus derived cells by mitogen. II. Monocyte macrophages potentiation of mitogen-induced DNA synthesis, *J. Immunol.,* 116, 357, 1976.
42. **Chess, L., MacDermott, R. P., and Schlossman, S. F.,** Immunologic functions of isolated human lymphocytes subpopulations. I. Quantitative isolation of human T and B cells and response to mitogens, *J. Immunol.,* 113, 1113, 1974.
43. **Chess, L., MacDermott, R. P., and Schlossman, S. F.,** Immunologic functions of isolated human lymphocytes subpopulations. II. Antigen triggering of T and B cells in vitro, *J. Immunol.,* 113, 1122, 1974.
44. **Bonnard, J. D., Lemos, L., and Chappuis, M.,** Cell-mediated lympholysis after sensitization in undirectional mixed lymphocyte culture in man, *Scand. J. Immunol.,* 3, 97, 1974.
45. **Wybran, J., Chantler, S., and Fudenberg, H. H.,** Human blood T cells: response to phytohemagglutinin, *J. Immunol.,* 110, 1157, 1973.
46. **Bach, F. M.,** *Serologic and Leukocyte Defined Approaches to Histocompatibility Testing in Laboratory Diagnosis of Immunologic Disorders,* Vyas, G. N., Stites, D. P., and Brecher, G., Eds., Grune & Stratton, New York, 1975, 185.
47. **Festenstein, H. and Démant, P., Eds.,** The genetic determinants and mechanisms of cell mediated immune reactions, *Transplant. Proc.,* 5, 1, 1973.
48. **Kirkpatrick, C. H.,** Mitogen and antigen induced lymphocyte responses in patients with infectious diseases, in, *Mitogens in Immunobiology,* Oppenheim, J. J. and Rosenstreich, D. H., Eds., Academic Press, New York, 1976, 639.
49. **Hallgren, H. M., Kersey, J. H., Dubey, D. P., and Yunis, E. J.,** Lymphocyte subsets and integrated immune function in aging humans, *Clin. Immunol. Immunopathol.,* 10, 65, 1978.
50. **Hallgren, H. M., Kersey, J. H., Gajl-Peczalska, K. J., Greenberg, L. J., and Yunis, E. J.,** T and B cells in aging humans, *Fed. Proc.,* 33, 646, 1974.
51. **Augener, W., Cohnen, G., Reuter, A., and Brittinger, G.,** Decrease of T lymphocytes during ageing, *Lancet,* 1, 1164, 1974.
52. **Carosella, E. D., Mochanko, K., and Braun, M.,** Rosette-forming T cells in human peripheral blood at different ages, *Cell. Immunol.,* 12, 323, 1974.
53. **Smith, M. A., Evans, J., and Steel, C. M.,** Age-related variation in proportion of circulating T cells, *Lancet,* 2, 922, 1974.
54. **Reddy, M. M. and Goh, K.,** B and T lymphocytes in man. IV. Circulating B, T and "null" lymphocytes in aging population, *J. Gerontol.,* 34, 5, 1979.
55. **Weksler, M. E. and Hutteroth, T. H.,** Impaired lymphocyte function in aged humans, *J. Clin. Invest.,* 53, 99, 1974.
56. **Fernandez, L. A., MacSween, J. M., and Langley, G. R.,** Lymphocyte responses to phytohaemagglutinin: Age-related effects, *Immunology,* 31: 583, 1976.
57. **Conard, R. A., Demoise, C. F., Scott, W. A., and Makar, M.,** Immunohematological studies of Marshall Islanders sixteen years after fallout radiation exposure, *J. Gerontol.,* 26, 28, 1971.
58. **Hallgren, H. M., Buckley, C. E., III, Gilbertsen, V. A., and Yunis, E. J.,** Lymphocyte phytohemagglutinin responsiveness, immunoglobulins and autoantibodies in aging humans, *J. Immunol.,* 111, 1101, 1973.
59. **Pisciotta, A. V., Westring, D. W., DePrey, C., and Walsh, B.,** Mitogenic effect of phytohaemagglutinin at different ages, *Nature,* 215, 193, 1967.
60. **Govaerts, A., Delespesse, G., and Duchateau, J.,** Alterations lymphocytaires au cours du vieillissement, *Ann. Immunol. (Inst. Pasteur),* 128C, 95, 1977.

61. **Kishimoto, S., Tomino, S., Inomata, K., Kotegawa, S., Saito, T., Kuroki, M., Mitsuya, H., and Hisamitsu, S.,** Age-related changes in the subsets and functions of human T lymphocytes, *J. Immunol.,* 121, 1773, 1978.
62. **Heine, K. M., Stobbe, H., Klatt, R., Sahi, J., and Herrmann, H.,** Lymphocyte function in the aged, *Helv. Med. Acta,* 35, 484, 1969—1970.
63. **Weiner, H. L., Scribner, D. J., Schocket, A. L., and Moorehead, J. W.,** Increased proliferative response of human peripheral blood lymphocytes to anti-immunoglobulin antibodies in elderly people, *Clin. Immunol. Immunopathol.,* 9, 356, 1978.
64. **Krzeminska-Lawkowiczowa, I., Lawkowicz, W., Traczyk, Z., Kraj, M., Arczynska, E., Ciesluk, S., and Krotochwil, L.,** Lymphocyte response in in vitro cultures to some mitogens, and serum immunoglobulin levels in aged subjects, *Arch. Immunol. Ther. Exp.,* 25, 87, 1977.
65. **Czlonkowska, A. and Korlak, J.,** The immune response during aging, *J. Gerontol.,* 34, 9, 1979.
66. **Ben-Zwi, A., Galili, U., Russell, A., and Schlesinger, M.,** Age-associated changes in subpopulations of human lymphocytes, *Clin. Immunol. Immunopathol.,* 7, 139, 1977.
67. **Foad, B. S. I., Adams, L. E., Yamauchi, Y., and Litwin, A.,** Phytomitogen responses of peripheral blood lymphocytes in young and older subjects, *Clin. Exp. Immunol.,* 17, 657, 1974.
68. **Hallgren, H. M. and Yunis, E. J.,** Suppressor lymphocytes in young and aged humans, *J. Immunol.,* 118, 2004, 1977.
69. **Antel, J. P., Weinrich, M., and Arnason, B. G. W.,** Circulating suppressor cells in man as a function of age, *Clin. Immunol. and Immunopathol.,* 9, 134, 1978.

METHODOLOGY: ASSESSING HUMORAL IMMUNE FUNCTION

Justine S. Garvey

INTRODUCTION

The immune response can conveniently be regarded as having three major effectors: the globular proteins known as either immunoglobulins or antibodies* that are released into the blood stream, certain cells that require or act more effectively in conjunction with antibodies, and other cells that are effective in the absence of antibody. Those functions for which antibody alone is responsible are called humoral responses, hence the collective term for these functions is "humoral immunity".

Tests for humoral immune function described below will be discussed in three main categories: (1) those for the detection and measurement of immunoglobulin in serum, (2) those for the determination of serum antibody activity, and (3) those for the quantitation of B-cells and the secretion of antibody. Some results will be selected from the literature, demonstrating the application of the assays in assessing the effect of age on the immune response.

DETECTION AND MEASUREMENT OF IMMUNOGLOBULIN IN SERUM

Cellulose Acetate Electrophoresis

The principles of electrophoresis together with a detailed procedure have been discussed.[1] Electrophoresis on a cellulose acetate membrane provides a simple and rapid method for qualitative and, to some extent, quantitative evaluation of serum proteins. Direct staining of the membrane permits visual observation of separated components immediately after completing the electrophoretic run. The membrane can be made transparent for quantitation of the components with a densitometer or it may be completely dissolved for quantitative recovery of the fractions. As seen in Figure 1, the resolution of this technique is limited to five or six major peaks. When an abnormality is apparent in one of them, e.g., the gamma peak, one of two techniques may be used as the next step in identification; either specific immunoelectrophoresis (IEP) for a qualitative analysis or radial immunodiffusion (RID) for a quantitative determination of an abnormality in one class of immunoglobulin, i.e., IgG, IgM, or IgA. Cellulose acetate electrophoresis has been applied to studies of monoclonal and polyclonal gammopathies as well as heavy and light chain disease. Characteristic results from these studies can be found in technical literature available from equipment suppliers (e.g., Millipore®, Gelman, Beckman).

Immunoelectrophoresis[1]

This two-step procedure combining electrophoresis and immunoprecipitation has several applications including a more defined analysis of serum components. The first step is the electrophoresis of a serum sample from a well cut in the center of an agarose coated slide. The second step is a diffusion of specific antisera from each of two troughs cut parallel to each other and on both sides of the well. Generally one of the troughs contains a polyvalent serum (i.e., antihuman immunoglobulins) while the sec-

* The two terms are often used interchangeably. However, in the ensuing methodology, "immunoglobulin" will describe a general class of molecules, whereas "antibody" will refer to a particular immunoglobulin with antigenic specificity.

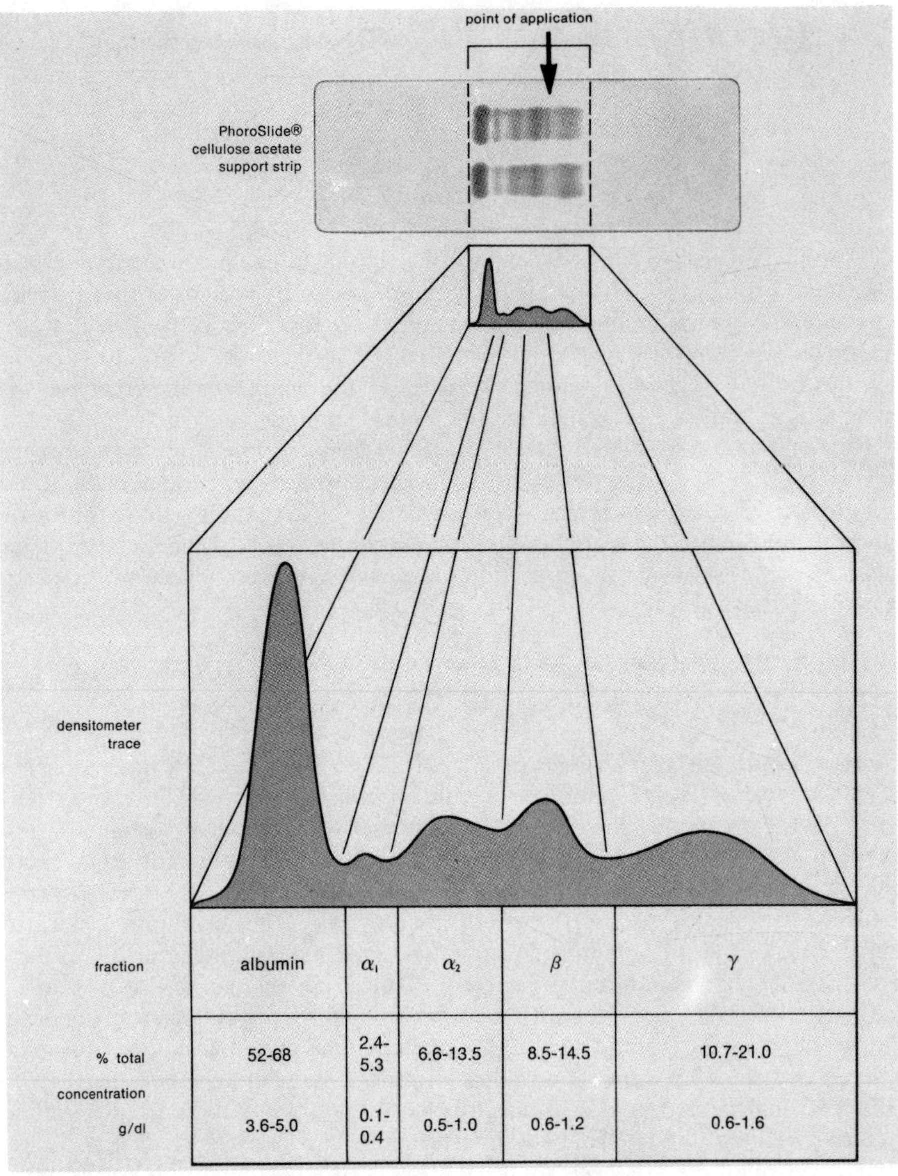

FIGURE 1. Electrophoretic separation of a normal human serum on cellulose acetate support. (From Millipore Technical Bulletin, AR 710, 1974, 2. Reprinted with permission of Millipore Corporation, Bedford, Mass.)

ond trough contains a monovalent serum (i.e., antihuman IgG). Shown in Figure 2 are the results that were obtained for normal rabbit serum. Under similar assay conditions, normal human serum would show a similar pattern. Various abnormalities in human immunoglobulin classes are identified by well-characterized patterns printed in technical literature and published reports.

Radial Immunodiffusion (RID)[1]

This immunoassay can provide an accurate measurement of a small amount of an antigen, e.g., an immunoglobulin in a mixture of diverse antigens such as serum. A monospecific serum prepared against an Ig class of protein, e.g., IgG, is added to fluid

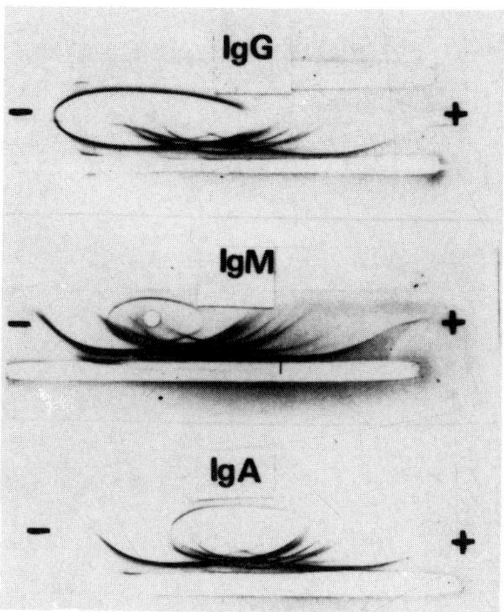

FIGURE 2. Multiple and single immunoelectrophoretic arcs obtained with polyvalent and monovalent antisera. Following electrophoresis of normal rabbit serum (central wells), polyvalent goat antiserum against rabbit serum was added to all three lower troughs. The upper troughs received goat antisera specific for three immunoglobulin heavy chains — i.e., anti-γ chain (top), anti-μ chain (center), and anti-α chain (bottom). Note the reactions of identity between each single upper arc and the homologous γ globulin in the polyvalent pattern below. (Reproduced from *Methods in Immunology,* 3rd ed., 1977, 331, written by Justine S. Garvey, Natalie E. Cremer, and Dieter H. Sussdorf, with permission of publishers, Benjamin/Cummings Inc., Reading, Mass.)

agar that is used to coat a slide, and at least four wells are punched in the agar. To three of them are added a known but different concentration of an IgG reference standard and to the fourth is added the unknown serum. The standards and the unknown diffuse radially from the wells into the gel and a halo of precipitation forms around each well. Certain quantitative relationships exist between the halo diameter and the concentration of the antigen. A quick result can be obtained while the halo is still expanding ("timed" diffusion) by making a linear plot of the log of the standard antigen concentration (x) vs. halo diameter (y).[3] The more accurate determination takes longer and is read after the halo stops expanding ("limit" diffusion). Here, one makes a linear plot of the standard antigen concentration vs. the square of the halo diameter.[4] The halo diameter of the unknown is then used to determine the unknown concentration from the standard curve. It is of great importance, especially in "limit" diffusion, to be aware of the fact that the size of the halo varies inversely with antibody concentration. There are commercially available prepared slides for RID and it is imperative that they be used according to the manufacturer's specifications, since they are usually designated for "timed" diffusion.

When this assay was used in observing the serum concentration of IgG, IgA, and IgM throughout the lifetime of humans, results were obtained as shown in Figure 3

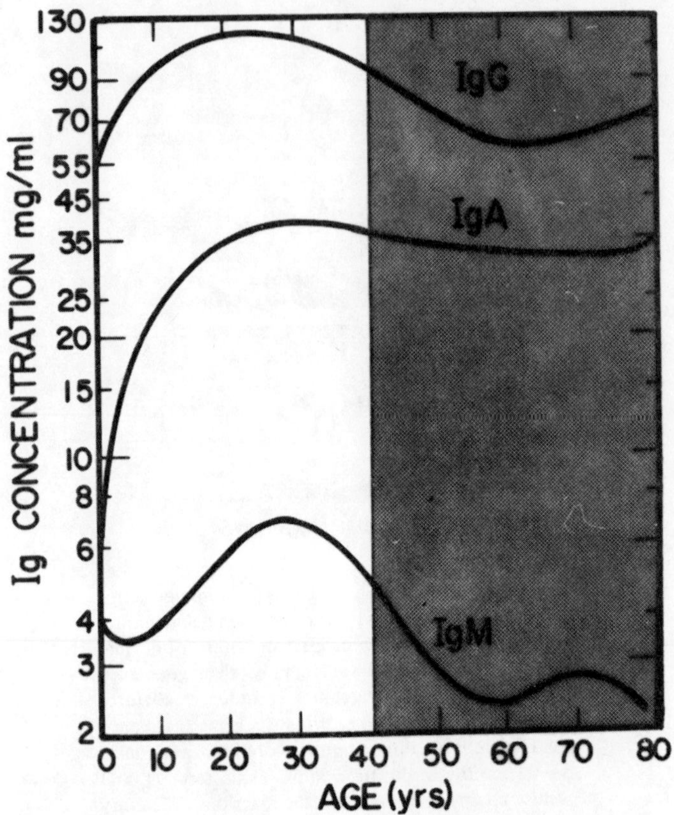

FIGURE 3. Geometric mean serum immunoglobulin levels decline in apparently healthy subjects beyond early adult life. The older subjects sampled in this study were beyond the period of maximum change (shaded area). Note the relative elevation of geometric mean levels of IgG and IgM in older persons at the extremes of life. Levels are expressed in mg/mℓ in relation to a particular laboratory secondary reference standard. (From Buckley, C. E., III, Buckley, E. C., and Dorsey, F. C., *Fed. Proc.*, 33, 2036, 1974. With permission.)

from a longitudinal study[5] and in Table 1 from a nonlongitudinal study in which significant bias was absent.[6] These findings fail to agree, and a more recent report of survivors and nonsurvivors in a late life study led to the conclusion that immunoglobulin levels are predictors of survival, i.e., IgG levels were lower in nonsurvivors than in survivor peers.[7] These discrepancies stress the importance of minimizing variations between laboratories by using the reference standard prepared by the Immunology Branch of the World Health Organization, referred to as 67/95, and a related preparation 67/86 that is obtained by writing to: Director, Immunoglobulin Reference Center, 6715 Electronic Drive, Springfield, VA 22151. An immunoglobulin concentration is provisionally stated in terms of International Units (IU) until reliability can be given to mg/mℓ.[8]

Electroimmunoassay (EIA, also known as Rocket Immunoassay)

Wells are cut side by side at one end of an antibody-containing gel and filled with antigen. As in RID there are at least three standards of different known concentration that are assayed together with the unknown. Conditions are chosen so that the anti-

TABLE 1
CONCENTRATIONS OF IgG, IgA, AND IgM IN HUMAN SERA DURING AGING

Age		IgG geometric mean value (range ± 1.96 s.d.)			IgA geometric mean value (range ± 1.96 s.d.)			IgM geometric mean value (range ± 1.96 s.d.)		
(years)	n	mg/mℓ	i.u.	Difference[a]	mg/mℓ	i.u.	Difference[a]	mg/mℓ	i.u.	Difference[a]
20—30	23	10.86 (7.20—16.37)	135 (90—204)	P<0.02	1.93 (1.18—3.23)	136 (84—227)	P<0.01	1.06 (0.61—1.82)	125 (72—215)	n.s.
41—50	40	11.09 (7.13 —17.23)	138 (89—214)	P<0.02	1.45 (0.63—3.36)	102 (44—237)	P<0.001	1.13 (0.52—2.48)	134 (61—293)	n.s.
51—65	49	11.60 (7.66—17.57)	144 (95—219)	n.s.	1.65 (0.76—3.56)	124 (57—269)	P<0.001	1.18 (0.61—2.30)	140 (72—272)	P<0.01
>95	59	12.48 (7.64—20.40)	155 (95—253)		2.54 (1.16—5.54)	179 (82—390)		1.05 (0.34—3.24)	124 (40—383)	

Note: n.s. = not significant.

[a] Significance of difference between the given age group and the over 95 years group.

From Radl, J., Sepers, J. M., Skvaril, F., Morell, A., and Hijmans, W., *Clin. Exp. Immunol.*, 22, 86, 1975. With permission.

Table 2
COMPARISON OF IgG SUBCLASS LEVELS BETWEEN YOUNG ADULTS AND AGED PERSONS

	Young adults—geometric mean value (range ± 1.96 s.d.) (mg/mℓ)	Aged persons (>95) geometric mean value (range ± 1.96 s.d.) (mg/mℓ)	Significance of difference between the two groups
n	108	57	
IgGl	6.4	7.3	P <0.02
	(3.8—10.7)	(3.4—15.4)	
IgG2	3.0	3.3	n.s.
	(1.5—6.0)	(1.2—9.4)	
IgG3	0.5	0.8	P<0.001
	(0.2—1.3)	(0.2—3.1)	
IgG4	0.3	0.3	n.s.
	(0.04—2.1)	(0.04—3.5)	

Note: n.s. = not significant.

From Radl, J., Sepers, J. M., Skvaril, F., Morell, A., and Hijmans, W., *Clin. Exp. Immunol.*, 28, 87, 1975. With permission.

body in the gel will not migrate during electrophoresis, whereas antigen molecules migrate according to their differing electrophoretic mobilities. (Chemical methods have been used to modify either the antigen or antibody when both are immunoglobulins.[8]) Antigen migrates from the well and encounters the antibody molecules in the gel, forming antigen-antibody complexes that precipitate. At the leading boundary of the antigen migration, antigen is in excess so that there is a continual dissolving of the precipitate and a reforming of it further along the path of migration. Eventually a point in migration is reached when there is a stable line of precipitate that persists along the outer edges and the moving front of the antigen migration. This has a rocket-like shape and remains stationary regardless of continued electrophoresis. The height of the rocket is directly proportional to the antigen concentration and indirectly proportional to the antibody concentration. Reference standards electrophoresed in the same gel as the unknown allow a standard curve to be plotted for use in determining the unknown concentration.

Radioimmunosorbent Test (RIST)

This radioimmunoassay can provide precise quantitation of serum components at very low concentrations, and has been used to study serum immunoglobulins. For instance, subclass variations in IgG with aging have been reported using the RIST (Table 2). An important application has been in the study of IgE, an immunoglobulin involved in immediate hypersensitivity reactions and also found in increasing serum concentrations during parasitic (particularly helminthic) infections. Unfortunately, IgE represents only 0.002% of the total serum immunoglobulin, and a very sensitive assay is needed for its detection.

In the RIST (Figure 4), reference and unknown sera are incubated with antibody to IgE (A-IgE in Figure 4)[9] which has been insolubilized by attachment to the walls of polystyrene test tubes, paper disk, cellulose, or Sephadex® microspheres. A second incubation is then performed with ^{125}I antibody to IgE. The amount of bound radioisotope-labeled antibody is directly related to the IgE content of the original serum.

Recent investigations have shown that immediate type hypersensitivity reactions are

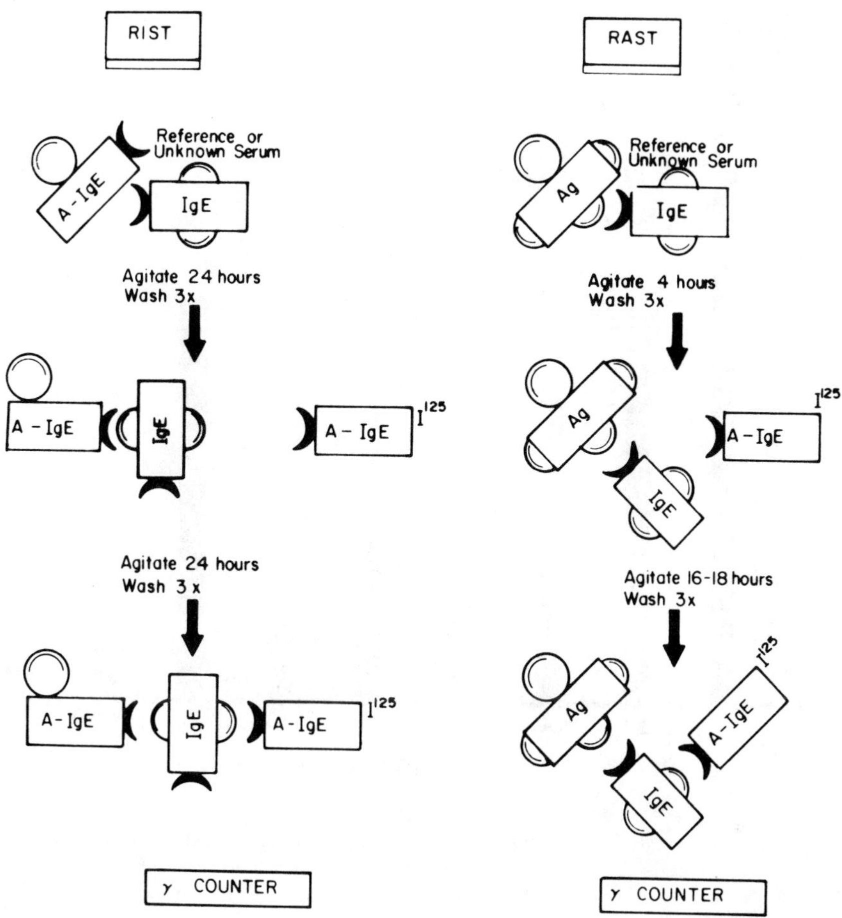

FIGURE 4. Schematic diagram of radioimmunosorbent test (RIST) and the radioallergosorbent test (RAST). RIST is used to detect IgE immunoglobulin and RAST is used to detect anti-IgE antibody. (From Waldman, R. H., Brestel, E. P., Delafuente, J. D., Longley, S., and Panush, R. S., *Clinical Concepts of Immunology*, Williams & Wilkins, Baltimore©, 1979, 249. With permission.)

less frequent in aged humans.[10] These findings as well as observations in the same study of decreased total IgE (Figure 5) and IgE specific antibodies (assayed by RAST, also Figure 4) are in accord with the existence of an age-associated natural desensitization of atopic patients. Related to the human findings are results in a rat model[11] (also assayed by RIST) that shows serum IgE levels which parallel human IgE levels (Figure 6).

SERUM ANTIBODY ACTIVITY

Quantitative Precipitation

This assay, developed in 1923 by Michael Heidelberger, was one of the first to give quantitative data about serum antibody titers. Although currently not in general use, this test provides basic information essential to the understanding of most antigen-antibody reactions. Thus, it is logical to have a thorough knowledge of this assay although not with the idea that one would actually perform the assay or read a citation of it in the literature on aging.

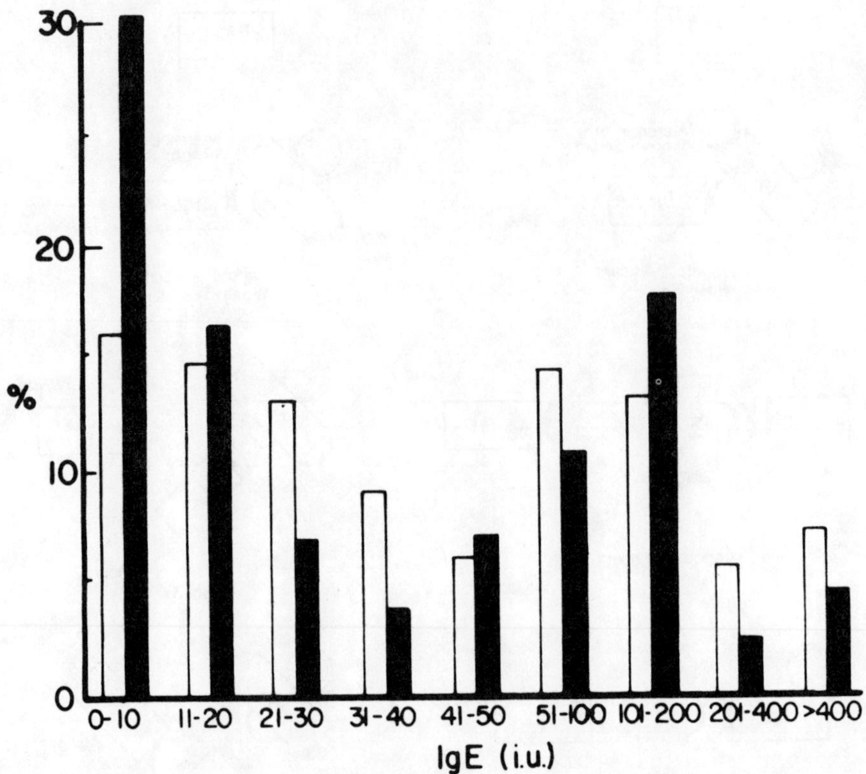

FIGURE 5. Serum IgE concentration in young (□) and old subjects (■). The young subjects were less than 60 years (mean age 37.9). The old subjects were more than 70 years (mean age 80.1). (From Delespeese, G., DeMauberge, J., Kennes, B., Nicaise, R. and Govaerts, A., *Clin. Allergy*, 7, 15. 1977. With permission.)

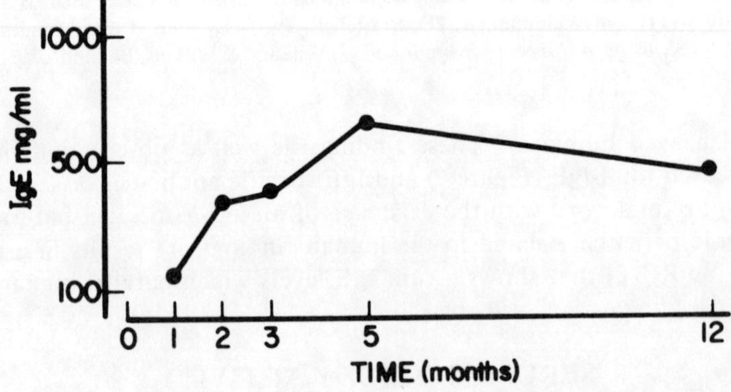

FIGURE 6. Influence of age on total serum IgE levels (median values) in inbred BN-rats. (From Pauwels, R., Bazin, H., Platteau, B., and Vander Straeten, J., *Immunology*, 36, 147, 1979. With permission.)

The precipitation test is performed in tubes to which both the antigen and antibody are added in solution; the specific antiserum is kept constant in both volume and concentration while the antigen is added in varying concentrations at constant volume.

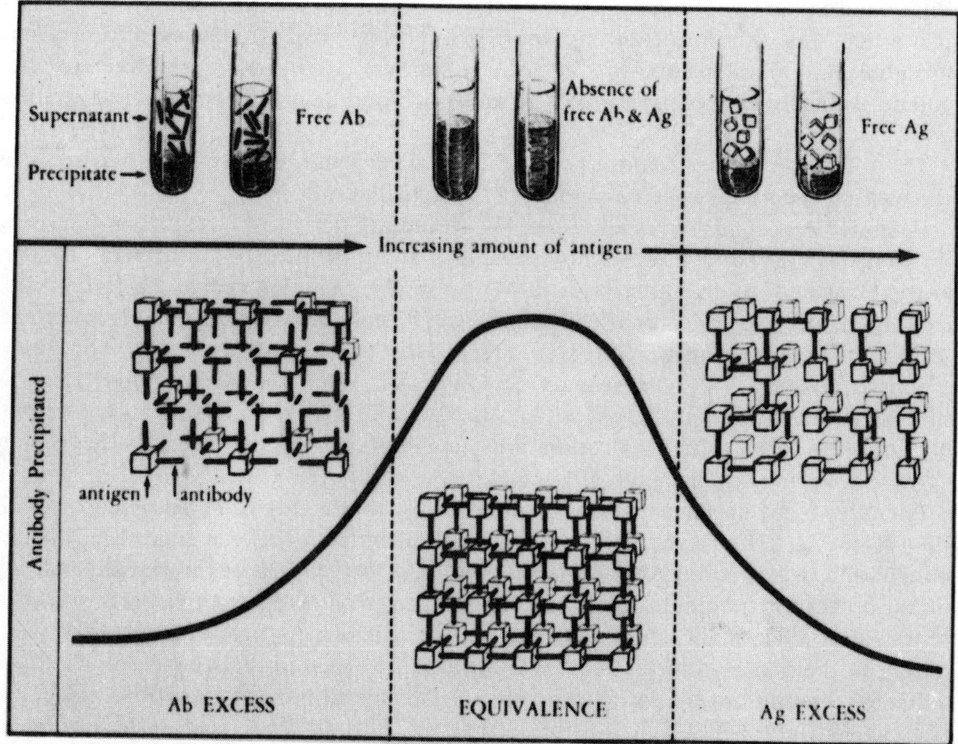

FIGURE 7. Schematic representation of the quantitative precipitation curve. (From Zmijeweski, C. M., Hubscher, T. T., and Bellanti, J. A., *Immunology: Basic Processes,* Bellanti, J. A., Ed., W. B. Saunders, Philadelphia, 1979, 215. With permission).

The reaction of precipitation occurs in two stages. The first is the specific combination of antigen and antibody which requires seconds or minutes and the second is the aggregation of complexes to a visible size which may require hours or days. The precipitates are then collected by centrifugation and the decanted supernates are tested for the presence of antigen or antibody by the *interfacial ring test.*

Care is taken to identify the tube in the reaction sequence having only antigen-antibody complexes (as determined by a negative interfacial test for both excess free antigen and antibody in the supernate). This tube is the *equivalence* tube which defines one region, the equivalence region, of a typical precipitation reaction as shown in Figure 7. (Also shown in Figure 7 are the regions of antibody or antigen excess as determined by interfacial assays and the compositions of the insoluble and soluble complexes found in the precipitates and supernates, respectively.)

The concentration of antibody protein is determined indirectly by measuring the nitrogen content of the precipitate. The amount of added antigen-nitrogen is subtracted from the total precipitated nitrogen to give the amount of precipitated antibody-nitrogen. In the equivalence tube, all available antibody has been precipitated, and thus the calculation of antibody-nitrogen in the precipitate will measure the serum concentration of the antibody.

Nephelometry[13] — This technique uses the light scattering properties of small antigen-antibody complexes (found in the antibody-excess region of the precipitation curve) to quantitate serum immunoglobulins. An intense monochromatic beam generated by a helium-neon laser is scattered by the sample mixture and an electronic detector measures the degree of scatter. Recent technological advances indicate a high sensitivity and capability for this technique whose routine application to clinical problems such as the quantitation of an immunoglobulin seems likely (replacing measurement by radial immunodiffusion, etc., mentioned earlier). However, the requirement for potent, optically clear antisera may be an insurmountable problem in some applications.[14]

The following are basic concepts of a humoral response that reflect on the previous text and are generally observed in most of the tests that follow.

Primary vs. secondary responses — The serum antibody response differs following the first (primary) and subsequent (secondary) administrations of antigen. Generally, in the primary response, there is a slower antibody induction time (seen as a greater lag time before the appearance of antibody); the peak antibody response is lower and the decline of the response is faster (see Figure 8).

Switch in Ig class — The primary response to a T-cell dependent antigen such as sheep erythrocytes is mainly IgM with a small amount of IgG appearing later. Depending upon the dose, route of injection, and time interval between injections the secondary response may be predominantly IgG, (see Figure 8).

Affinity — An important property of antibody that is discussed below under DNP fluorescence is *affinity,* defined as the strength of binding between an antigenic determinant and its antibody. Another term, *avidity,* is used to denote the overall tendency of antibodies to combine with multivalent antigen, while the term affinity is restricted to univalent antigen for which common terms are hapten or ligand. High affinity antibody to the hapten dinitrophenyl was synthesized when both a low dose of antigen and a long immunization period were used.[15] This maturation of an antibody response is dependent upon cellular cooperation between T- and B-cells and an expansion of clones of B-cells. The latter differentiate into plasma cells with membrane proteins (see Figure 8 and the next section) having the same affinity properties as the antibody that circulates during the course of the response.

Classification of antigen-antibody reactions — The different reactions between antigen and antibody are shown in Figure 9. Primary reactions are simply a binding of antigen and antibody into soluble complexes that remain invisible to the unaided eye; these reactions will be discussed in some detail below. Secondary reactions are usually, but not necessarily, the consequence of primary binding, e.g., precipitation in which cross-linking occurs between the soluble complexes formed in the primary reaction. These small complexes become large complexes that fall out of solution as visible aggregates (see Figure 7). Tertiary reactions involve an additional parameter which is biological. Insofar as they are reactions that occur in vivo or are in vitro cellular assays to aid in assessing in vivo activities, they are considered in the section "Assessing Cellular Immune Function".

Sensitivity — The choice and interpretation of an assay to assess the humoral response will depend upon the sensitivity of various assays given in Table 3.

Primary Binding Assays

DNP Fluorescence

Primary binding is the formation of complexes by the monovalent hapten, DNP, and the antibodies in a specific antiserum obtained from immunization with a DNP-protein conjugate. At any single hapten concentration, a reversible chemical equilibrium is established where $K = [Ab \cdot DNP] \div [Ab][DNP]$. The term K_o is commonly used and has the special meaning of the reciprocal of "the free hapten concentration at which one half the total number of antibody sites are occupied." K_o has the dimensions of liters $mole^{-1}$ and the calculation comes from a series of determinations of K at different hapten concentrations. The higher the value of K_o, the stronger the attraction

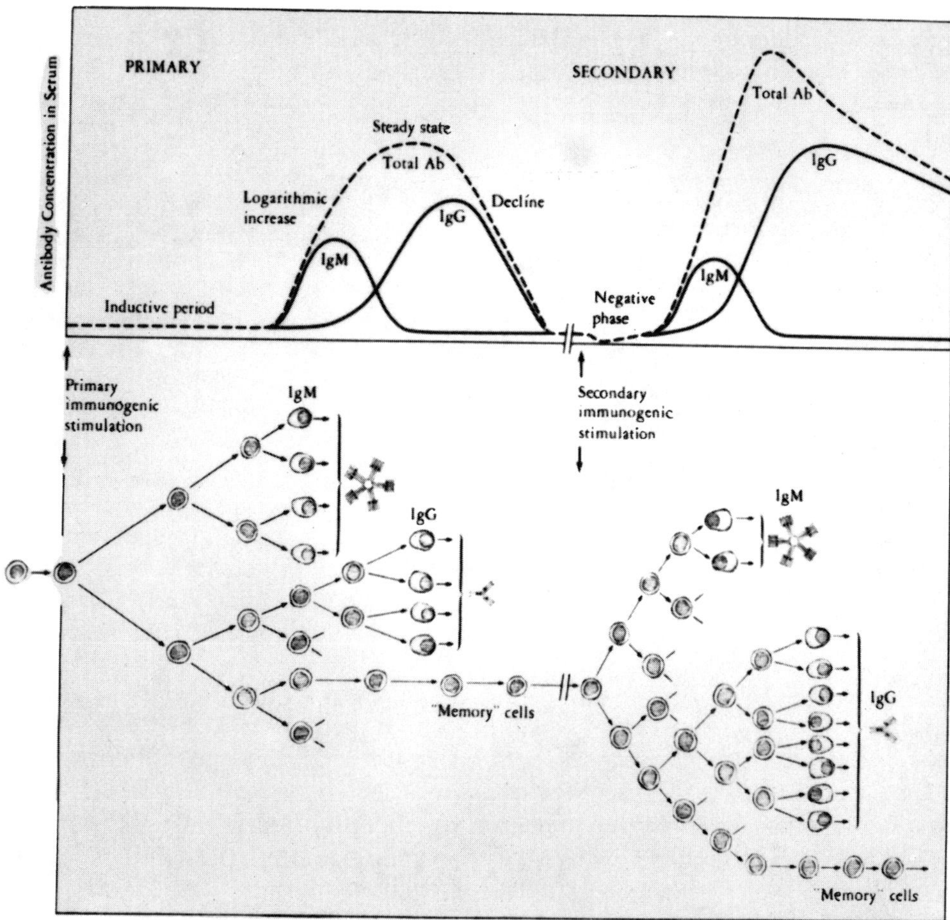

FIGURE 8. Schematic representation of humoral and cellular events in the primary and secondary (anamnestic) antibody responses. (●), lymphocyte; ◑, plasma cell. (From Herscowitz, H. B., *Immunology: Basic Processes*, Ballanti, J. A., Ed., W. B. Saunders, Philadelphia, 1979, 155. With permission.)

between hapten and antibody. For example, two antibodies with K_o values of 1×10^{-9} liters mole^{-1} and 1×10^{-6} liters mole^{-1} have a 1000-fold difference in binding; thus 1 $\mu\ell$ of the former will give the same binding as 1 mℓ of the latter, or the higher affinity antibody may be diluted 1000-fold to obtain equivalent binding in the same reaction volume. When the hapten has the unique spectral properties for fluorescence measurement and the requirement for pure antibody is also satisfied, fluorescence offers a rapid, sensitive method for obtaining a K_o value and other thermodynamic data from hapten-antibody reactions.

Equilibrium Dialysis

This method finds more general application than fluorescence because of less rigorous requirements and high sensitivity when the hapten is radio-labeled. A range of labeled hapten concentrations are prepared and placed in a series of containers, in each of which are immersed a dialysis bag that contains a given amount of specific antibody (as IgG) and another bag that contain normal IgG. The hapten passes freely through the dialysis membrane until equilibrium is reached, i.e., the free hapten concentration is the same inside and outside the bag. Samples are removed from the antibody com-

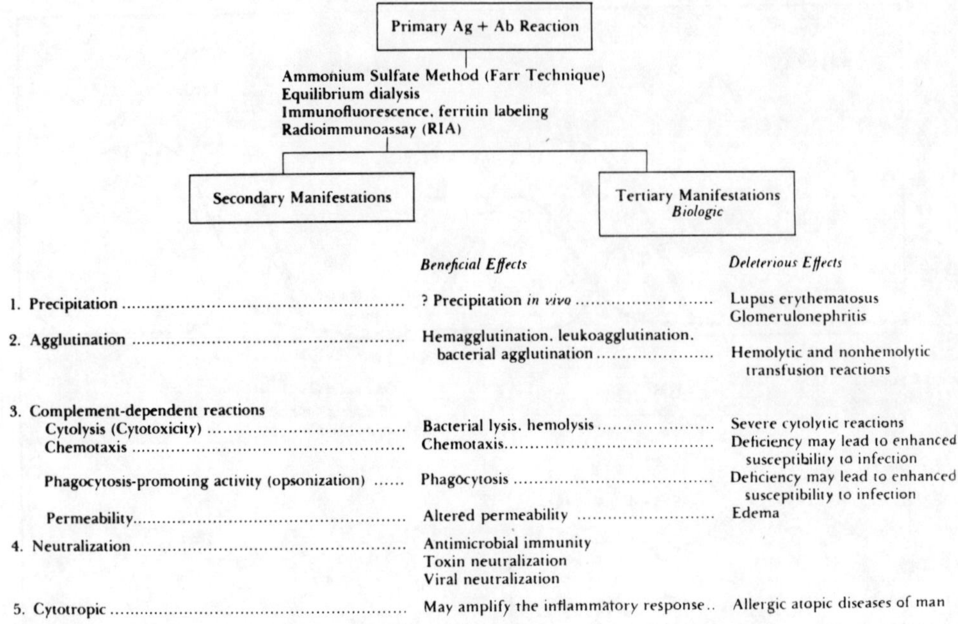

FIGURE 9. Schematic representation of antigen-antibody reactions. (From Zmijewski, C. M., Hubscher, T. T., and Bellanti, J. A., *Immunology: Basic Processes,* Bellanti, J. A., Ed., W. B. Saunders, Philadelphia, 1979, 204. With permission.

Table 3
SENSITIVITY OF QUANTITATIVE TESTS MEASURING ANTIBODY NITROGEN OF HIGH-AVIDITY ANTIBODY

Test	mg Ab N/mℓ or test
Precipitin reactions	3—20
Immunoelectrophoresis	3—20
Double diffusion in agar gel	0.2—1.0
Complement fixation	0.01—0.1
Radial immunodiffusion	0.008—0.025
Bacterial agglutination	0.01
Hemolysis	0.001—0.03
Passive hemagglutination	0.005
Passive cutaneous anaphylaxis	0.003
Antitoxin neutralization	0.003
Antigen-combining globulin technique (Farr)	0.0001—0.001
Radioimmunoassay	0.0001—0.001
Enzyme-linked assays	0.0001—0.001
Virus neutralization	0.00001—0.0001
Bactericidal test	0.00001—0.0001

From Zmijewski, C. M., Hubscher, T. T., and Belanti, J. A., *Immunology: Basic Processes,* Belanti, J. A., Ed., W. B. Saunders, Philadelphia, 1979, 214. With permission.

partment (inside the bag), normal IgG compartment (inside bag), and the free hapten compartment (outside the bag), and the radioactivity is measured in each. The determination of bound (b) hapten is obtained by subtraction of the hapten found with the

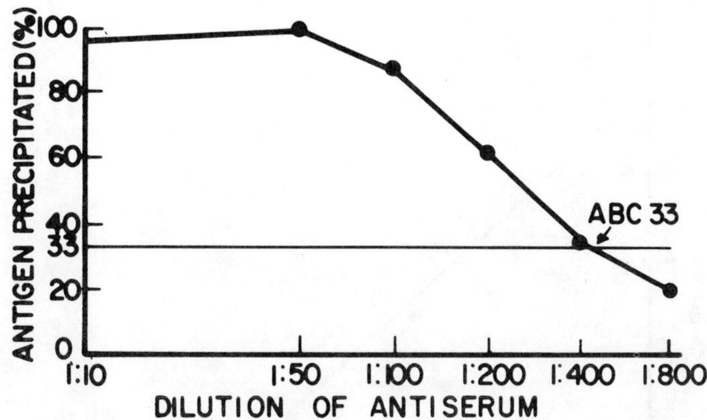

FIGURE 10. Percent of I*BSA antigen precipitated after the addition of SAS by a number of dilutions of a single antiserum. Curve indicates that the ABC-33 end-point or the dilution of antiserum that would precipitate 33% of the antigen added is 1:420. (From Minden, P. and Farr, R. S., *Handbook of Experimental Immunology,* Vol. 1, 3rd ed., Weir, D. M., Ed., Blackwell Scientific, Oxford, 1978, 13. With permission.)

normal immunoglobulin from that found with the antibody. The free hapten (c) is the measurement in solution outside the bag. A plot of 1/b vs. 1/c results in a curve whose x intercept gives the reciprocal of the total antibody binding sites.[16] The details for the assay and calculations of affinity are referenced.[1]

Farr Assay[17]

The ABC (antigen binding capacity)-33 assay was developed by Richard S. Farr for the purpose of measuring all the antibody sites that could bind specific antigen. The assay resulted from the realization that some serum antibody, although specific for the antigen, failed to form precipitable complexes. The prototype BSA-anti BSA reaction makes use of ammonium sulfate at a final concentration of 50% saturation to precipitate the complexes from the free uncombined antigen. Substitution of ^{125}I-BSA for BSA and use of a range of antiserum dilutions that results in 33% antigen binding are standard conditions (see Figure 10). Although 33% antigen binding is arbitrary, a lower (but not higher) value is suggested so that antigen is present in sufficient excess to avoid spontaneous precipitation. Separation by centrifugation of bound (complexed) ^{125}I from the ^{125}I-BSA which remains free in solution and γ-counting of either the bound or free ^{125}I (usually the bound for convenience in data analysis) provides an assay that has gained wide use. The procedure, modified in whole or in part, has been adapted to other antigen-antibody measurements. The use of ammonium sulfate is one means for separation of complexes from free labeled antigen in the competitive type of radioimmunoassay that follows.

Competitive-Type Radioimmunoassay

Most radioimmunoassays that are performed clinically are available from pharmaceutical vendors as kits with all reagents supplied along with fully described procedures. There are variations in the assay particularly when one reagent is in solid phase as described in Figure 4 for RIST (total IgE in a serum) or RAST (anti-IgE) in which case the bound complexes are separated from free antigen by centrifugation. Other common methods of separation are precipitation by ammonium sulfate, e.g., an assay for DNA,[18] absorption and removal of the free antigen by charcoal, or precipitation

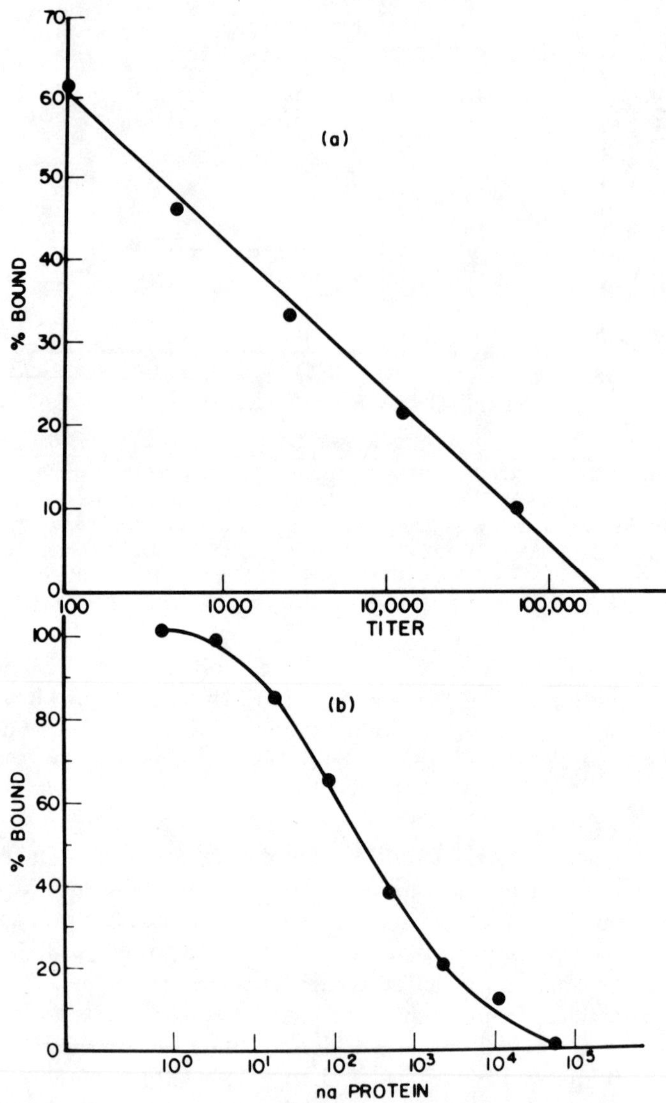

FIGURE 11. (a) Antibody titration curve of antiserum used in the standard curve drawn in (b) for a competitive binding assay. (Reprinted with permission from *Immunochemistry,* 15, 866, Van Vander Mallie, R. J. and Garvey, J. S., Production and Study of Antibody, Produced against rat cadmium thionein, © 1978, Pergamon Press, Ltd.)

of the complexes by a double antibody reagent, i.e., antibody against the immunoglobulin of the species in which the specific antibody was produced, or use of protein A. (Both reagents bind to the Fc region of immunoglobulin. Protein A is a membrane protein of most strains of *Staphylococcus aureus* and binds to the subclasses IgG1, IgG2, IgG4, and to some but not all preparations of IgA and IgM.) The first phase of the assay involves the determination of the conditions of complex formation at equilibrium. A series of antibody dilutions and a constant concentration of labeled antigen are used to optimize parameters for sensitive measurement of bound antigen, i.e., at a level of radioactivity for rapid but accurate reproducibility (see dilution curve, Figure 11). The dilution of antibody that results in precipitation of 30 to 60% of the precipitable labeled antigen under the optimized conditions is used to establish a standard reference curve. Then a series of assay tubes, each prepared with a different, but known concentration of nonlabeled antigen is allowed to incubate with the antibody. In a second incubation a constant amount of ^{125}I antigen is added to each assay tube. The third step involves introduction of a reagent, such as a second antibody (anti-immunoglobulin), that will allow separation of bound from free complexes. The final step is separation of bound antigen from free antigen; usually the bound phase is counted. In the actual assay of competitor, tubes for the standard curve are redetermined along with varying amounts of competitor assumed to be in the range of the standard curve. The standard curve is drawn with 100% bound defined as the binding of noninhibited radioactive complex corrected for background binding of diluent. The known amounts of competitor allow a standard curve to be drawn as shown in Figure 11. From the percent binding, the amount of competitor, i.e., unknown, can be determined from interpolation of the standard curve as shown in Figure 11. The sensitivity of the standard curve with respect to the slope and range of antigen readings is largely determined by the affinity of the antibody.

Enzyme-Linked-Immunosorbent Assay (ELISA)[20]

This assay is likely to find use as either an alternate or substitute for many present radioimmunoassays. A simplified version of the assay depends upon adsorption of antigen to wells of a microtiter plate. After vigorous washing to remove unadsorbed antigen, specific antibody in physiologic buffer is added and allowed to complex with the adsorbed antigen. The third incubation is with an enzyme-coupled second antibody (antibody agains the species of immunoglobulin used for production of the first antibody or Protein A). The final incubation is with enzyme substrate, following which a colored reaction product is measured with a spectrophotometer. If the sensitivity can equal that of the radioimmunoassay, the main advantages of the assay will be reduced costs for reagents and equipment, decreased reaction times, elimination of radioisotopes, and the capability of complete automation with computerized data reduction.

Secondary Binding Assays

Gel Diffusion

Unlike the quantitative precipitation assay that is performed with both reagents (antigen and antibody) in solution, gel diffusion reactions are usually performed by having one reagent, e.g., *Oudin* tube assay, or both reagents, e.g., *Ouchterlony* plate or slide assay, in solution but the precipitate is always stabilized in the gel. The Ouchterlony assay is now the most commonly used version. A template for cutting wells is usually adjusted in dimensions for use on a microscope slide in which case the volumes of required reagents are $\sim 5\ \mu\ell$. This method is qualitative and gives information about the minimal number of antigen-antibody reactions occurring in a mixture of antigens and antibodies and distinguishes those which have complete identity, partial identity, or nonidentity with each other. For quantitation by gel diffusion, see the earlier description of RID.

Crossed Immunoelectrophoresis[21]

Gel diffusion is combined with electrophoresis in the sensitive but qualitative separation known as immunoelectrophoresis described earlier. In crossed-immunoelectrophoresis, quantitation is achieved. Electrophoresis occurs in two dimensions in which the first is achieved in plain agarose and the components of an antigen mixture, e.g., human serum along with a marker substance; such as carbamylated transferrin in known concentration, are resolved into electrophoretically distinct components. In the second electrophoresis, which is perpendicular to the first but carried out in an agarose that contains antibody, e.g., an antiserum vs. human serum, the components are separated as peaks. The varying areas of these correspond to the relative concentrations of the components. Accurate quantitation can be derived using the reference standard.

Hemagglutination

Direct

Agglutination takes place when particulate antigens are exposed to their appropriate antibodies under suitable conditions. Like precipitation, the reaction is secondary, involving binding, then cross-linkage to form coarse aggregates that are easily distinguished by a rough "settling out" pattern in the reaction tube or microtiter well in which the cells and antibody are mixed. If there is no reaction the cells settle as a discrete button.

Human red blood cells are classified as A, B, AB, or O type to denote which antigen of the major blood group types is present on the cells. Humans also possess in their serum, anti-A or anti-B agglutinin, depending upon which antigen type is on their erythrocytes, i.e., an A individual has anti-B antibody. When humans provide antibodies for characterizing the cell antigens of other humans, such antibodies are referred to as *isoagglutinins* and the antigens are isoantigens (or alloantigens). Since humans have isohemagglutinins without being immunized, the likely explanation for their appearance is that bacterial substances are ingested and/or inhaled that are antigenically similar to A and B substances. Of interest with respect to aging studies, is the finding that isoagglutinin titer decreases with age[22] (see Figure 12).

Indirect (or Passive)[1]

Agglutination is more sensitive than precipitation as an assay for antibody (see Table 3). In order to take advantage of this sensitivity, soluble antigen is adsorbed onto particles (latex or bentonite), or onto tannic acid, or chromium chloride treated erythrocytes to form antigen "coated" cells. "Conjugated" cells are prepared by chemical reactions with glutaraldehyde, bisdiazobenzidine, carbodiimide reagent, or Fast black B that cause covalent linkage of the antigen to the cell. Formalinized cell antigen conjugates are convenient for routine use when proven to be as satisfactory as fresh cells in a particular assay.

Antiglobulin Test

This is the most commonly used passive hemagglutination test because of its clinical application in detecting autoimmune diseases and drug sensitivity in which antibody has been produced against the altered erythrocyte membrane. The antierythrocyte antibody of IgG class, although adsorbed to the erythrocyte, fails to cause agglutination. The antiglobulin reagent, also known as "Coombs reagent", "cross-links" the IgG, resulting in agglutination.

Complement-Mediated Hemolysis[1]

When fresh serum (guinea pig, unless another species is specified) is added to antibody-coated, i.e., sensitized erythrocytes (EA), the cells (EAC) are lyzed. A group of at least 13 serum proteins collectively referred to as complement (C) that attach, when activated, to the erythrocyte membrane are responsible for this phenomenon. The initial activation phase involves C1 (a trimolecular complex of $\overline{\text{C1q}}$, C1r, and C1s), C4 and C2 and requires Ca^{++} and Mg^{++} ions. The enzyme product, $\overline{\text{C42}}$, cleaves C3, resulting in activated $\overline{\text{C3b}}$ which binds to the membrane. C3 is the central component of C and when excessive amounts are formed the breakdown products C3b and C3d may

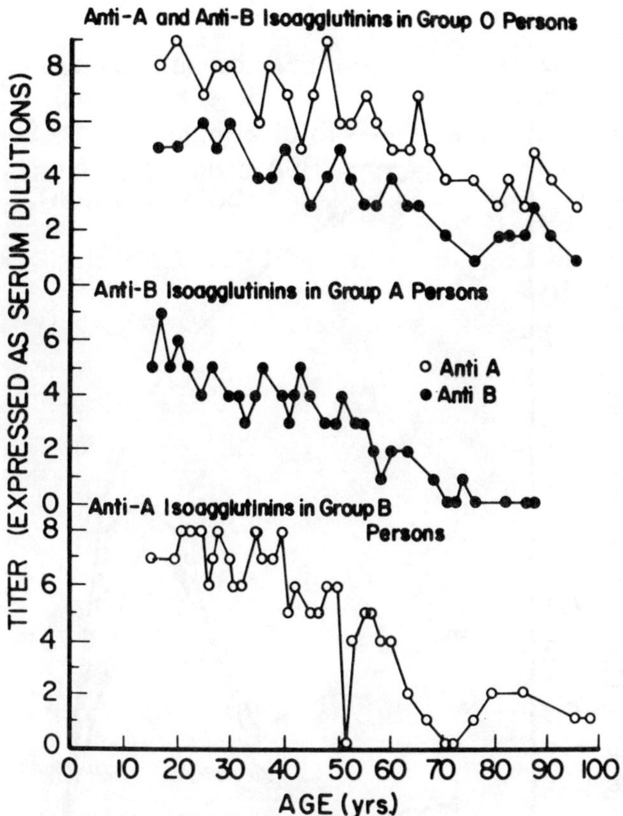

FIGURE 12. The results are plotted as a summary of 734 titers of anti-A and anti-B antibodies carried out on blood specimens from 378 persons who ranged in age from 15 to 98 years. Of this series, 174 patients were group 0, 150 group A, and 54 group B. Each point on each graph depicts an average titration value from sera derived from individuals of the same age belonging to the corresponding blood group (a number from 0 to 9 is assigned to indicate serial dilutions). (From Somers, H. and Kuhns, W. J., *Proc. Soc. Exp. Biol. Med.*, 141, 1104, 1972. With permission.)

be detected in electrophoretic patterns of human plasma. The sequence of complement activation continues with a second or lytic phase involving membrane attachment of the trimolecular complex $\overline{C567}$. Reaction of C8 produces a membrane lesion and activation of C9, a release of hemoglobulin that is measured spectrophotometrically to quantitate the amount of hemolysin antibody. The assay may be modified to titrate hemolytic complement in the serum, a constant concentration of sensitized erythrocytes being reacted with dilutions of the complement. A varying degree of hemolysis results that is related to the amount of complement. The serum dilution that lyses 50% of the sensitized erythrocytes is the CH_{50} value. A study of an individual complement component can be performed if it is titrated with all the other components being present in excess. For example, to measure C4, purified C1 is added to sensitized erythrocytes (EAC1). Dilutions of the C4 source are incubated with EAC1. After this, C2 and then C3-9 are added in excess and the mixture incubated for a standard interval of time. The degree of hemolysis is measured spectrophotometrically by detection of hemoglobin in the supernatant. Some complement components, e.g., C3 and C4, may

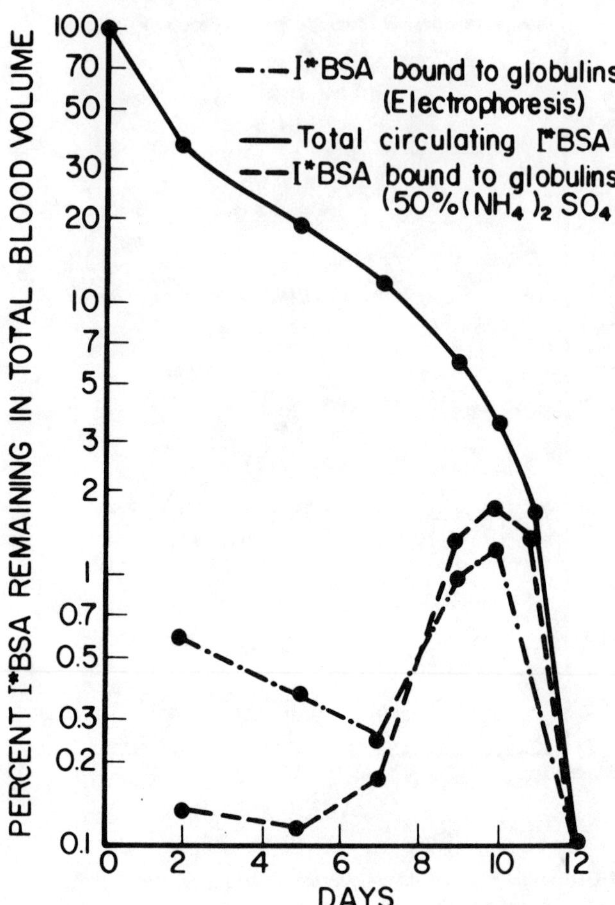

FIGURE 13. Behavior of I*BSA in a rabbit #6958 injected with 250 mg I*BSA/kg. This rabbit showed an immune elimination of the antigen with an appearance of a fair amount of I* BSA-anti-BSA complexes, as represented by ammonium sulfate precipitated I* activity, both prior to and during the immune elimination of I*BSA. Two days after the injection 0.3-0.6% of the total I* activity which was injected, migrated electrophoretically as a globulin component that represented 1.3-2.0% of the total radioactivity which was in the blood at that time. (From Weigle, W. O. and Deichmiller, M. P., *J. Immunol.*, 84, 435, ©1960, Williams & Wilkins, Baltimore. With permission.)

be determined by radial immunodiffusion (described earlier). RIA provides a less sensitive measurement than the hemolytic assay but the latter has drawbacks in long assay time, expensive reagents, and a more demanding training than for most assays.

Immune Complexes (IC)

The immune response to a foreign antigen that circulates, produced the findings shown in Figure 13. This figure is similar to a reversed plotting of Figure 7. The part of the curve showing complexes at an early time in antibody formation is in antigen excess, switching to antibody excess and finally, as antibody begins to circulate in abundance, antigen is completely eliminated and antibody exists free. IC can persist from chronic antigen stimulation and lead to pathological conditions. Animal models to simulate clinical cases have been studied; and, because the antigen is known and is exogenous, the composition of the complexes can be studied. The reversibility of IC at acid pH can provide dissociation of their constituents for recovery by ultracentrifugation on sucrose gradients[23] and study of their size and other characteristics. This methodology can lead to reproducible isolation of the complexes that have clinical importance and for which current methods of detection will be discussed. In general, neither antigen specificity nor precise information about the antibody can be established for IC, and substances such as C-reactive protein, endotoxin, nucleic acids, or polyanions may interfere with the accuracy of the assays by which they are quantitated.

The antigen of IC deposits is normally sequestered or hidden; but, when released into the circulation, it is available to cause a switch from tolerance to sensitization. Alternatively auto (self) antigens may be altered and acquire new antigenic determinants due to drug treatment, viral infection, or exposure to miscellaneous compounds of exogenous origin. As humans age, they have more disease of an autoimmune nature (See chapters entitled "Aging Theories and Immunological Senescence: Perspects and Prospects" and "Immunosuppression, Autoimmunity and Precocious Aging: Observations and Speculations".) and thus, aging studies require the methodology for detecting IC present in tissues and in serum and other biological fluids.

Detection in Tissues

In general, immunocytochemical techniques are used that involve fluorescence or peroxidase staining. In the former, a fluorescein (yellow-green) or rhodamine (red) conjugate of anti-Ig or anticomplement is applied to frozen tissue sections that are examined with an ultraviolet microscope, equipped with suitable filters for the fluorochrome and preferably with incident (epi-) illumination. Background staining and nonspecificity can be troublesome, so precautions in preparation of the conjugate and its use with proper controls are extremely important. High titer antibody of high specificity must be used for preparation of the conjugate. Antigen should be pure for immunization and the antibody be absorbed until rendered specific for the class of Ig to be detected. The conjugate is absorbed with tissue powder or purified by chromatography to reduce background staining. It is evaluated further in order to avoid nonspecificity by determining its protein to dye ratio (100:1 or greater usually being optimal). Its staining is optimized by use of varying dilutions on normal and test tissue sections to determine conditions for bright, specific fluorescence. Granular deposits of immunoglobulin accompanied by complement staining are considered indicative of IC. It is therefore useful to apply a different fluorochrome, e.g., fluorescein to detect Ig and rhodamine to detect complement.

The advantage of peroxidase staining is the capability for both electronmicroscopy as well as light microscopy. Horseradish peroxidase may be coupled to antibody using glutaraldehyde as a cross-linker. Tissue sections are then exposed to this antibody-enzyme conjugate. Addition of diaminobenzidine and H_2O_2 initiates an enzymatic oxidation of the dye, resulting in staining in local areas around the enzyme molecules. Technical aspects of both fluorescence and peroxidase staining are fully described.[24]

Detection in Serum or in Other Biologic Fluids[25,26]

There are a multiplicity of methods available for the detection of IC of which the principal ones are given in Table 4. Since no single method is preferred, it is conventional to use more than one; accordingly, only basic information and guidelines will be presented.

Tests for IC are dependent upon *standardization* with a uniform, stable material that performs comparably with the test sample under the assay conditions. The most reliable standard is aggregated human globulin (AHG) that is prepared by each individual laboratory under standard conditions that consist essentially of the following

Table 4
SENSITIVITY OF TESTS FOR DETECTION OF IMMUNE COMPLEXES (IC)[a]

Principle of test	Nature of test	μg/mℓ[24]	μg/mℓ[25]
Complement dependent	Assay of anticomplement activity	0.1	
	Reaction with Clq		
	Precipitation (gel diffusion)	500	100
	RIA (polyethylene glycol pptd)	100	50
	Deviation	5	5
	ELISA	0.1	
Complement independent	Rheumatoid factor		
	Precipitation (mRF)		100 (gel diffusion) 1 (quant pptn)
	RIA		25 mRF 0.35[b]pRF
	Fab fragment, RIA	13	
Alteration in cell adhesiveness	Platelet aggregation (human only)	1	1
Binding to B-cell membrane receptors	RIA with Raji cells		6[26]

Note: Abbreviations — RIA, radioimmunoassay; ELISA, enzyme linked immunosorbent assay; mRF, monoclonal rheumatoid factor; and pRF, polyclonal rheumatoid factor.

[a] Minimal concentration of soluble heat-aggregated Ig, AHG, detected.
[b] Soluble tetanus toxoid-antitoxoid complexes; no data for AHG.

steps:[25] (1) preparation of Cohn fraction II human IgG, 100 mℓ, 1% in 0.15 *M* saline, (2) heating in a water bath for 12 min at 63°C, (3) cooling, (4) addition of 6.7 g sodium sulfate in 1 g increments with dissolving after each addition of the salt, (5) incubation at 4°C for 1 hr, (6) centrifugation to pellet the precipitate, (7) discard of supernate and redissolving of pellet in 10 mℓ of assay buffer, (8) dialysis overnight against fresh buffer, (9) centrifugation, (10) storage of the supernate, AHG, in ampoules at −20°C, and (11) thawing and dilution of an ampoule of AHG for standardization of respective assay.

Complement-Dependent Assays

These form one of the two general groups of assays; that is to say, conventional assays for IC depend upon their reaction with either complement (i.e., C1q, the recognition component of the classical complement system, see earlier discussion on complement) or with an anti-IgG (e.g., rheumatoid factor) reagent. Binding of IC in which the antibody is IgM or IgG (especially IgG1 and IgG3) to C1q, leads to activation of the complement system, thereby depressing its hemolytic activity. C1q binding cannot be considered specific for IC. It binds to DNA (which is the basis of C1q separation by precipitation as C1q-DNA from serum, DNAase treatment and Sephadex® G200 chromatography with EDTA elution) and also to C-reactive protein, heparin, protamine, and bacterial lipopolysaccharide.

The *anticomplementary activity assay* is very sensitive and is the only IC assay read as hemolysis. In order that sensitivity not be reduced by C1q already bound to IC, the sample is freed from autologous complement activity by heat inactivation.* Then it is mixed in various dilutions with fresh normal serum which serves as a source of normal complement activity. The hemolytic activity, CH_{50} (described earlier) of the fresh normal serum is measured with and without the addition of the IC sample. The anticomplementary activity of the sample is expressed as the percentage reduction of the CH_{50} value of the serum.

The reaction of IC with C1q may be made visible in a *gel diffusion precipitation* test (see previous description of gel diffusion) in which AHG (see standardization) and test samples are placed in peripheral wells to diffuse and react with C1q diffusing from a central well cut in the agar.

Sensitivity is improved over gel diffusion precipitation by using a radioassay in which ^{125}I-labeled C1q is reacted with test samples and with AHG, and the radioactivity that is precipitated with polyethylene glycol is measured. The test has the drawbacks inherent in the use of C1q that were mentioned earlier. Nevertheless the test has usefulness in its simplicity for following sequential titers of SLE patients.

The *C1q deviation test* is a radioimmunoassay providing higher sensitivity than the previous one. IC are quantitated by their ability to inhibit binding of ^{125}I-C1q to sensitized erythrocytes, EA, so this is basically a competitive binding assay. The diluted, heated-inactivated test serum and ^{125}I-C1q are incubated 15 min, 20°C. (Heating reverses binding of endogenous complement to complexes and renders them accessible to C1q; whereas dilution prior to heating reduces aggregation.) EA are added and incubation is continued an additional 15 min, 20°C. A portion of the reaction mixture is layered onto high density sucrose and centrifuged. The ^{125}I in both the supernate and pellet are measured. From a simultaneous determination of the uptake of ^{125}I-C1q by EA in the presence of normal serum it is possible to determine the inhibition of uptake (or percent deviation of C1q) by the test sample. The diminished binding as compared to that of AHG is then used to calculate the amount of IC in the test sample.

Complement-Independent Assays

Cryoglobulin and rheumatoid factor are two special types of protein which may have considerable importance in human diseases. A cryoprotein is any serum protein or protein complex that precipitates from solution on cooling and redissolves on warming, but, a cryoglobulin is usually a mixture of immunoglobulins having rheumatoid activity. Cryoglobulins have importance in clinical diagnosis of IC disease and also in investigations of unknown antigen. They may contain all the constituents of circulating IC and thus provide a means of concentrating, purifying, and identifying the components of IC.

Rheumatoid factor (RF) denotes any antibody that has a specificity for IgG, thus it is an anti-immunoglobulin antibody. Although the name is derived from a close association with rheumatoid arthritis, RF is present in many nonrheumatoid diseases. The classical RF is a 19S IgM molecule but other molecules have anti-IgG activity, e.g., 7S-8S IgM, IgG, and IgA. RF is directed against the Fc portion of the IgG molecule. Questions are highly relevant about the precise form of IgG that provides the stimulus for production of RF; specificities that different RF possess; and the role that antigen-antibody ratios may have on the exposure or reaction of unique determinants; yet, discussion must focus on the use of RF in the detection and quantitation of IC.

As noted in Table 4, the use of monoclonal RF (mRF) offers a more sensitive assay

* Recent studies with a nonhuman IC model have failed to show that heating unmasks C1q-blocked complexes to better reactivity with added, i.e., extrinsic C1q. Accordingly, more information is needed on the effective removal of endogenous/autologous C1q from IC that are subsequently exposed to added C1q. These comments also apply to the C1q deviation test described below.[23a]

in liquid than in gel precipitation of AHG used for standardization of the assay. RIA uses either a polyclonal RF (pRF) or mRF and as shown in the table the sensitivity is extremely high for the pRF assay. Its drawback is the assay time of 4 days. Day 1: pRF (primary antibody) in IgM carrier + IC sample (competing source of altered IgG) are incubated. Day 2: ^{125}I-IC or ^{125}I-AHG (standard) is added for a second incubation. Day 3: Anti-IgM (second antibody) is used to precipitate the complexes formed in the previous two steps. Day 4: Complexes are pelleted by centrifugation and the tubes are counted.

At the present time the *^{125}I-Fab assay* is considered too complicated for routine clinical use. The Fab fragment of an animal antihuman IgG is prepared by methods utilizing affinity chromatography (for isolation of pure anti-IgG), papain digestion (for preparation of Fab), and iodination (for radiolabeling of ^{125}I-Fab) that is subsequently used to precipitate IC.

Platelet Aggregation Test

The mechanism of IC induced platelet aggregation is unclear. Human blood is the only satisfactory source of platelets for assay and use of AHG as an internal standard is necessary. There is the disadvantage that many agents other than IC cause platelet aggregation.

Raji Cell Radioimmunoassay[27]

The Raji cell line is of human lymphoblastoid origin, is maintained in continuous culture, has B-cell characteristics, and is used in an in vitro assay to detect and to quantitate IC in human biological fluids. Membrane bound Ig is absent from these cells but they have a large number of Fc receptors of low avidity and receptors for C3-C3b, C3d, and C1q (terms discussed in complement-mediated hemolysis) are present. At first Raji cells were used in a qualitative immunofluorescence assay for the detection of complement-fixing IC. A modified test quantitates IC by measuring the uptake of radioactive antibody by IgG in the IC bound to the cells. The required materials are AHG for standardization (prepared as noted previously); antiserum to human IgG prepared in a rabbit, purified on DEAE and radioiodinated; and standardized Raji cells. The test consists of reacting the serum to be tested for IC with Raji cells. After an incubation followed by washing, rabbit ^{125}I anti-human IgG is added; the uptake of ^{125}I is determined and referred to a standard curve of radioactive antibody uptake by cells previously incubated with varying amounts of AHG in serum. Experiments have shown that the radioactive antibody is proportional to AHG bound to cells and this is proportional to the quantity of AHG present in the serum. In the Raji cell test, in order to differentiate between normal human serum and serum containing IgG complexes, one must add radioactive antibody in excess to saturate the monomeric 7S IgG bound to cells via Fc receptors. The assay is based on the ability of the Raji cells to bind much more IgG from a serum containing IgG type IC with fixed complement than from normal human serum. This higher binding is explained by postulating that the complement receptors are in greater number or of higher affinity for their ligand molecules than the Fc receptors.

A disadvantage with the Raji cell assay is the need for cell culture maintenance. Although antilymphocyte antibodies in some sera may interfere with the assay, there can be less concern about errors in measurement from numerous interfering materials than in the C1q assays. Apart from the ability of Raji cells to detect IC in vitro, there is the possibility of their providing a tool by which antigens involved in IC disease may be identified and sera against these antigens be made available for research on the genesis of IC diseases.

Table 5
ENUMERATION OF HUMAN
T AND B LYMPHOCYTES[a]

Assay	Specificity	
	T cell	B cell
Surface Ig (SIg)	±	+
Fc receptor	±	+
C1q receptor	+	+
C4b receptor	−	+
C3b receptor	−	+
C3d receptor	−	+
E rosettes	+	−
EA rosettes	+	+
EAC rosettes	−	+
Anti-T cell antiserum	+	−
Anti-B cell antiserum	−	+

[a] Rearranged from Reference 9.

QUANTITATION OF B-CELLS AND SECRETION OF ANTIBODY

In this concluding part, attention will be given to cell assays, but only as they serve to evaluate humoral immunity. The assessment of other roles of cells of the immune system is fully discussed in the section entitled "Assessing Cellular Immune Function", where it will be pointed out that the induction of immunity, as well as its regulation and maintenance in a steady state, requires the collaboration between different classes of cells: T, B, and macrophage. Nevertheless, it is the B-cell that is indispensible to the humoral response (see Figure 8). Some B-cells secrete antibody, while others undergo terminal differentiation to form plasma cells that have abundant rough endoplasmic reticulum and are highly specialized in the secretion of antibody.

In pyogenic bacterial infections, antibodies are responsible for both recruitment of phagocytic cells to sites of bacterial multiplication and for opsonization of the bacteria for phagocytosis.[28] Furthermore, in vivo phagocytosis, that invokes the killing of bacteria, is more efficient with IgM than with IgG,[29] thus resembling in vitro hemolysis and hemagglutination. However, for the reason that phagocytes are not cells that are committed to antibody secretion, any of the following methodologies will involve them only indirectly.

Lymphocyte Separation

Human lymphocytes are obtained from leukocyte-rich human plasma using a Ficoll-Hypaque gradient.[1,30] Peripheral blood cells of other species than human, and also the lymphocytes of lymphoid organs (tonsil, spleen, lymph node), may be obtained similarly, but with modification for optimalization, e.g., change in gradient density and cell load. Criteria that will assure representative cell evaluations are a greater than 70% yield and a viability approaching 100%. It is obvious from Table 5 that there are unique receptors for both B-cells and T-cells that may be used in obtaining subpopulations. B-cells, by virtue of their surface Ig, bind to covalently-linked columns of anti-$(Fab)_2$; whereas, non-Ig cells pass through the column without binding. The Ig positive cells can be quantitatively recovered from the column by competitive inhibition with free IG or, under special conditions, by enzyme digestion of the insoluble immunoabsorbent. Both the Ig^+ and Ig− cells are subsequently rosetted as EAC and E rosettes, respectively, allowing an isolation of three distinct cell populations.[31]

Receptor Recognition

It is the presence of membrane or surface immunoglobulin, SIg, that is the single, most important criterion in distinguishing a B from a T-cell (see Table 5). B-cells, macrophages, and some null cells (lymphocytes that lack SIgG and fail to react with anti-T cell serum) have Fc receptors whereas B-cells, monocytes, and neutrophils have complement receptors. The presence of a similar receptor on more than one cell type emphasizes the care that must be taken in using receptors to distinguish cell types. Furthermore, not all B-cells possess the three markers, SIg, C3, and Fc. Single and double receptor-bearing cells are sometimes identified.

Surface Immunoglobulin (SIg)

A fluorochrome anti-immunoglobulin is prepared as discussed in earlier procedures; but with the important consideration that the Fc portion of the immunoglobulin may cause an aberrantly high enumeration of cells because of the presence of Fc receptors and Ig on the same cell.[32] Precaution can be taken to remove complexes from the antiserum by adsorption to insolubilized antigen and by high speed centrifugation or the unwanted staining can be circumvented by labeling $(Fab')_2$ instead of the immunoglobulin.[33] The cells must also be handled gently to maintain high viability while removing surface proteins that may interfere with staining. When this is accomplished, the viable, stained cell may show a series of changes in fluorescence. Initially, rather uniform labeling is apparent, followed by "patching" of the complex as it spreads over the cell surface, then a localization of "capping" at one pole of the cell, and finally interiorization of the complex. Polyvalent anti-immunoglobulin class serum should detect the total number of B-cells whereas specific monovalent class serum will show that IgM and IgD are the predominant classes of SIg. Fluorescence microscopy provides visual detection whereas a fluorescence activated cell sorter (FACS) equipped with laser beams can be employed to separate these subpopulations. An instrument description of FACS, its capability in sorting and analyzing cell subpopulations, and examples of quantitative data are well described.[34]

A quantitative estimate of the amount of Ig on a cell surface can be obtained by the antigen binding capacity (ABC) inhibition assay. A known number of cells compete with the binding of radiolabeled antigen to an antiserum of known ABC.[35] Cells may also be radiolabeled by lactoperoxidase,[1] their membranes solubilized by detergent and sonication, the ^{125}I membrane immunoglobulin precipitated with antiserum and the specific complex electrophoresed on an SDS-polyacrylamide gel to provide an initial separation of the immunoglobulin that can be quantitated and characterized biochemically.[36]

Fc Receptor

Binding to this B-cell receptor occurs via the Fc region of immunoglobulin in either immune complexes (IC) or in heat-aggregated human immunoglobulin (AHG) but not with Fc of native immunoglobulin. Either radiolabeled or fluorescein-labeled IC or AHG is used with scintillation counting or fluorescent microscopy, respectively, for detection. For accurate enumeration of B-cells, correction must be made for the presence of other cells (T, null, and macrophage) that may also be counted because of their Fc receptor.

Complement Receptors C14 and C3d

Human lymphocytes contain two different types of complement receptors: the immune adherance receptor detected by EAC14 (formed by sequential addition of C1 and C4 to EA) and the C3d receptor detected by EAC3d (prepared by addition of C5

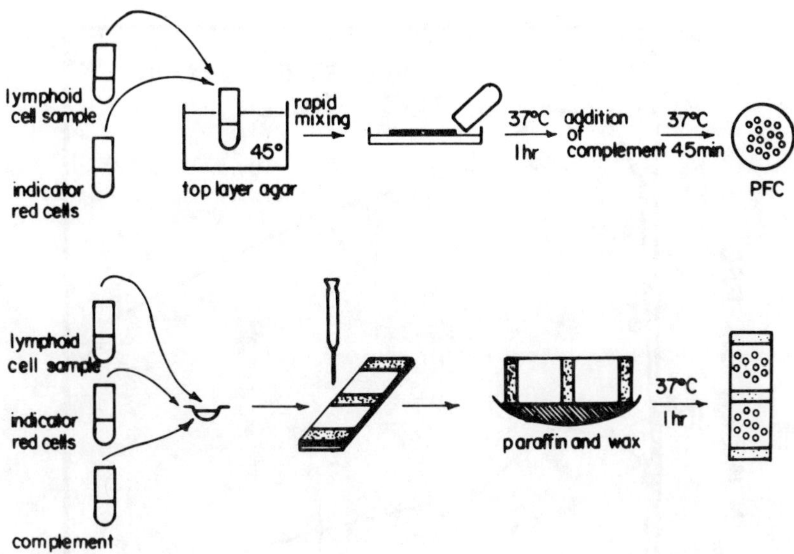

FIGURE 14. Flow diagram of the plaque-forming cell assay. The standard Jerne-Nordin method (top) and Cunningham-Szenberg modification (bottom) are shown. (From Lefkovits, I. and Cosenza, H., *Immunological Methods,* Lefkovits, I. and Pernis, B., Eds., Academic Press, New York, 1979, 278. With permission.)

deficient mouse serum to EA with subsequent cleavage of C4 and C3b so that only C3d is present).[37] The two complement receptors are antigenically distinct but located on different molecules. Normal lymphocytes may have one or the other of the two receptors or both. Neutrophils and monocytes rosette also. Two techniques that are used to distinguish the non-B cells take advantage of endogenous peroxidase staining by neutrophils and monocytes and latex particle ingestion by phagocytes.[38] Other methods used to remove phagocytes are carbonyl iron uptake and plastic/nylon adherance, but cell depletion methods have the general disadvantage of some degree of nonselectivity.

Anti-B Cell Antibody

Antiserum prepared against lymphocytes from patients with the B-cell form of chronic lymphocytic leukemia is also used to detect B-cells. In 98% of chronic lymphocytic leukemia the lymphocyte is a B-cell of monoclonal origin.[39]

Hemolytic Plaque Assay

This assay detects single antibody-forming cells (lymphoid cells). In its original form lymph node cells from a rabbit injected with sheep red cell stromata or splenic cells from mice injected with sheep erythrocytes were mixed with sheep erythrocytes and agar that solidified into a shallow layer in a Petri plate.[40] After a 1 hr incubation at 37°C, guinea pig serum was added as a source of complement and reincubation was continued for 30 to 45 min. Plaques, or zones of hemolysis appeared, each with a centralized cell that was presumably responsible for the secreted antibody that complexed with the red cell membrane antigen and caused complement-mediated lysis (see Figure 14). The plaques that developed by addition of complement alone are "direct" and attributed to antibody of IgM class, whereas those requiring a developing antiserum, i.e., anti-immunoglobulin, are of IgG class. A modified procedure uses a slide rather than plate surface on which the mixture of cells in agar is allowed to solidify.[1] Another form of the assay is performed in a liquid medium (see Figure 14) containing

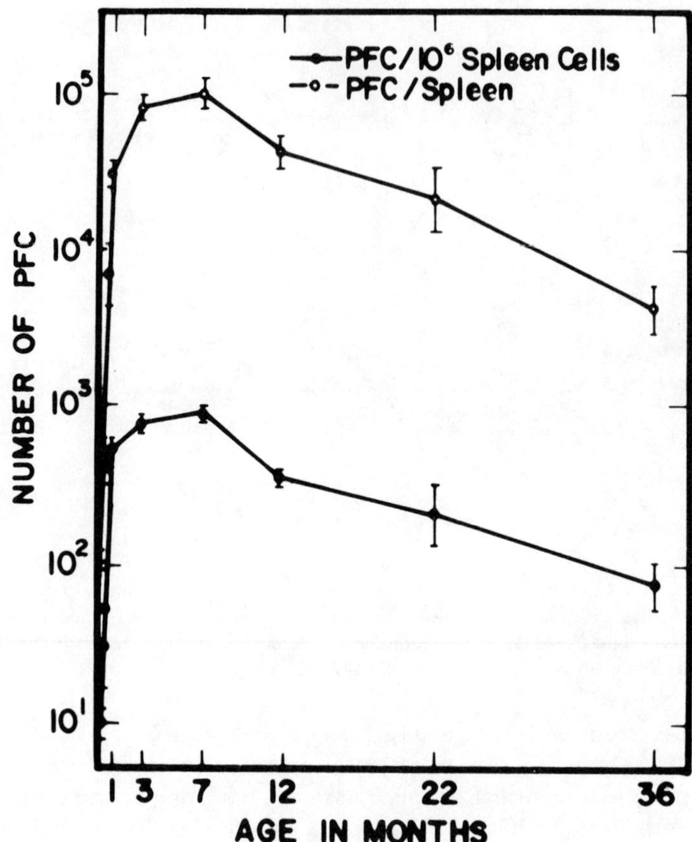

FIGURE 15. Assessment of humoral immune response as plaque-forming cells in CBA mice of various ages at 4 days after an intraperitoneal injection of 4 × 10^7 sheep erythrocytes l/g body weight. (From *J. Nat. Cancer Inst.*, 37, 513, 1966.)

a mixture of all reagents, added at one time to a chamber that is sealed and incubated.[42] By a variety of methods, e.g., bisdiazobenzidine, chromium chloride, or carbodiimide conjugation, a soluble antigen (used also as immunogen) may be attached to the erythrocyte membrane; otherwise, the assay is performed unchanged. A recent modification uses methyl cellulose[43] to provide a medium from which the plaque-forming cells are easily removed and further manipulated. The assay has yielded data from several investigations on the humoral immune response in aged experimental animals. Examples from these studies are Figures 15 and 16 that demonstrate the findings from two laboratories in which a different strain of mouse was studied.

CONCLUSION

The information gained thus far about immunity with aging has come largely from studies of the effectors of immunity as isolated parameters whereas they are known to interlock with one another to form an intricate communicating system. Dysfunction may arise from either an increased or a decreased activity of an immune component with aging. Change must be observed on an individual basis, as the rate of aging differs among the subjects of a study regardless of species and an attempted uniformity by

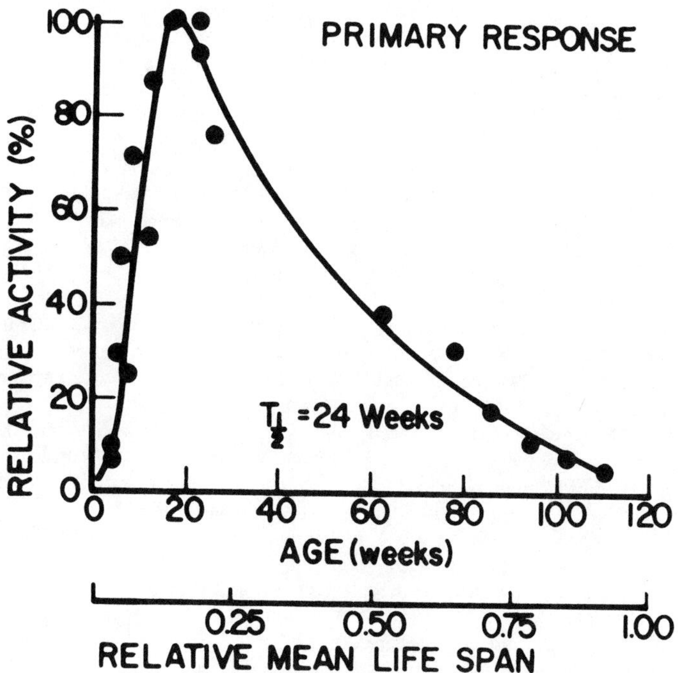

FIGURE 16. Assessment of humoral immune response in $BC3F_1$ (C57BL × C3H/He) mice at various ages after a single injection of sheep erythrocytes. The responsiveness of these mice was based on the determination of peak serum titer and peak number of plaque-forming cells in the spleens. (From Nordin, A. A. and Makinoden T., *Fed. Proc.*, 33, 2034, 1974. With permission.)

inbreeding. Amidst this complexity, discrimatory and careful use of existing and evolving methodology will quicken the pace with which progress is made in aging as a new area of immunological research.

ACKNOWLEDGMENT

Support by Grant No. AG0111 from the National Institutes of Health is acknowledged.

REFERENCES

1. Garvey, J. S., Cremer, N. E., and Sussdorf, D. H., *Methods in Immunology,* 3rd ed., Wm. A. Benjamin, Reading, Mass. 1977, 97, 178, 275, 293, 321, 328, 340, 360, 379, 411, 486.
2. Immunoglobulin Abnormality Detection, Millipore Technical Bulletin, AR 710, Millipore Corporation, Bedford, Mass. 1974, 2.
3. Fahey, J. L. and McKelvey, E. M., Quantitative determination of serum immunoglobulins in antibody-agar plates, *J. Immunology,* 94, 84, 1965.

4. **Mancini, G., Carbonara, A. O., and Heremans, J. F.,** Immunochemical quantitation of antigens by single radial immunodiffusion, *Immunochemistry,* 2, 235, 1965.
5. **Buckley, C. E., III, Buckley, E. C., and Dorsey, F. C.,** Longitudinal changes in serum immunoglobulin levels in older humans, *Fed. Proc.,* 33, 2036, 1974.
6. **Radl, J., Sepers, J. M., Skvaril, F., Morell, A., and Hijmans, W.,** Immunoglobulin patterns in humans over 95 years of age, *Clin. Exp. Immunol.,* 22, 84, 1975.
7. **Buckley, C. E., III and Roseman, J. M.,** Immunity and survival, *J. Am. Geriatr. Soc.,* 6, 241, 1976.
8. **Davis, N. C. and Ho, M.,** Quantitation of immunoglobulins, in *Manual of Clinical Immunology,* Rose, N. R. and Friedman, H., Eds., Am. Soc. Microbiol., Washington, D.C., 1976, 4.
9. **Brestel, E. P., Delafuente, J. D., Longley, S., and Panush, R. S.,** Evaluation of patients with immunologic disease, in *Clinical Concepts of Immunology,* Waldman, R. H., Ed., Williams & Wilkins, Baltimore, 1979, 227.
10. **Delespesse, G., DeMaubeuge, J., Kennes, B., Nicaise, R., and Govaerts, A.,** IgE mediated hypersensitivity in aging, *Clin. Allergy,* 7, 155, 1977.
11. **Pauwels, R., Bazin, H., Platteau, B., and Vander Straeten, M.,** The effect of age on IgE production in rats, *Immunology,* 36, 145, 1979.
12a. **Zmijewski, C. M., Hubscher, T. T., and Bellanti, J. A.,** Antigen-antibody interactions, in *Immunology: Basic Processes,* Bellanti, J. A., Ed., W. B. Saunders, Philadelphia, 1979, 203.
12b. **Herscowitz, H. B.,** Immunophysiology: Cell function and cellular interactions, in *Immunology: Basic Processes,* Bellanti, J. A., Ed., W. B. Saunders, Philadelphia, 1979, 151.
13. **Benacerraf, B. and Unanue, E. R.,** *Textbook of Immunology,* Williams & Wilkins, Baltimore, 1979, 56.
14. **Stites, D. P.,** Clinical laboratory methods for detection of antigens and antibodies, in *Basic and Clinical Immunology,* 2nd ed., Fudenberg, H. H., Stites, D. P., Caldwell, J. L., and Wells, J. V., Eds., Lange, Los Altos, Calif., 1978, chap. 27.
15. **Eisen, H. N. and Siskind, G. W.,** Variations in affinities of antibodies during the immune response, *Biochemistry,* 3, 996, 1964.
16. **Nisonoff, A. and Pressman, D.,** Heterogeneity and average combining constants of antibodies from individual rabbits, *J. Immunol.,* 80, 417, 1958.
17. **Minden, P. and Farr, R. S.,** Ammonium sulphate method to measure antigen-binding capacity, in *Handbook of Experimental Immunology,* Vol. 1, 3rd ed., Weir, D. M., Ed., Blackwell Scientific, Oxford, 1978, chap. 13.
18. **Reeves, W. G. and Marriott, D. W.,** Radioisotope techniques, in *Techniques in Clinical Immunology,* Thompson, R. A., Ed., Blackwell Scientific, Oxford, 1977, 116.
19. **Vander Mallie, R. J. and Garvey, J. S.,** Production and study of antibody produced against rat cadmium thionein, *Immunochemistry,* 15, 857, 1978.
20. **Engvall, E.,** Enzyme-linked immunosorbent assay, ELISA, in *Biomedical Applications of Immobilized Enzymes and Proteins,* Vol. 2, Chang, T. M. S., Ed., Plenum Press, New York, 1977, chap. 30.
21. **Milford-Ward, A.,** Immunoprecipitation in the evaluation of the proteins in plasma and body fluids, in *Techniques in Clinical Immunology,* Thompson, R. A., Ed., Blackwell Scientific, Oxford, 1977, 1.
22. **Somers, H. and Kuhns, W. J.,** Blood group antibodies in old age, *Proc. Soc. Exp. Biol. Med.,* 141, 1104, 1972.
22a. **Weigle, W. O. and Deichmiller, M. P.,** The electrophoretic behavior of circulating antigen-antibody complexes, *J. Immunol.,* 84, 434, 1960.
23. **Benveniste, J. and Bruneau, C.,** Detection and characterization of circulating immune complexes by ultracentrifugation. Technical aspects, *J. Immunol. Methods,* 26, 99, 1979.
23a. **Teppo, A. M. and Wager, O.,** Heating at 56°C does not eliminate immune complex-bound C1q, *Scand. J. Immunol.,* 10, 431, 1979.
24. **Sternberger, L. A.,** *Immunocytochemistry,* 2nd ed., John Wiley & Sons, New York, 1979, 24 and 84.
25. **Jones, J. V. and Cumming, R. H.,** Tests for circulating immune complexes, in *Techniques in Clinical Immunology,* Thompson, R. A., Ed., Blackwell Scientific, Oxford, 1977, 136.
26. **Agnello, V.,** Detection of immune complexes, in *Manual of Clinical Immunology,* Rose, N. R. and Friedman, H., Eds., Am. Soc. Microbiol., Washington, D. C., 1976, 669.
27. **Theofilopoulos, A. N. and Dixon, F. J.,** Complement receptors on Raji cells as in vitro detectors of immune complexes in human sera, in *Manual of Clinical Immunology,* Rose, N. R. and Friedman, H., Eds., Am. Soc. Microbiol., Washington, D.C., 1976, 676.
28. **Allison, A. C.,** Interactions of antibodies, complement components and various cell types in immunity against viruses and pyogenic bacteria, *Transplantation Rev.,* 19, 3, 1974.
29. **Rowley, D. and Turner, K. J.,** Number of molecules of antibody required to promote phagocytosis of one bacterium, *Nature (London),* 210, 496, 1966.

30. **Oppenheim, J. J. and Schecter, B.,** Lymphocyte transformation, in *Manual of Clinical Immunology,* Rose, N. R. and Friedman, H., Eds., Am. Soc. Microbiol., Washington, D. C., 1976, 81.
31. **Chess, L. and Schlossman, S. F.,** Methods for the separation of unique human lymphocyte subpopulations, in *Manual of Clinical Immunology,* Rose, N. R. and Friedman, H., Eds., Am. Soc. Microbiol., Washington, D. C., 1976, 77.
32. **Winchester, R. K., Fu, S. M., Hoffman, T., and Kunkel, H. G.,** IgG on lymphocyte surfaces; technical problems and the significance of a third cell population, *J. Immunol.,* 114, 1210, 1975.
33. **Forni, L.,** Reagents for immunofluorescence and their use for studying lymphoid cell products, in *Immunological Methods,* Lefkovits, I. and Pernis, B., Eds., Academic Press, New York, 1979, 151.
34. **Herzenberg, L. A. and Herzenberg, L. A.,** Analysis and separation using the fluorescence activated cell sorter (FACS), in *Handbook of Experimental Immunology,* Vol. 2, 3rd ed., Weir, D. M., Ed., Blackwell Scientific, Oxford, 1978, chap. 22.
35. **Kennel, S. J., Del Villano, B. C., and Lerner, R. A.,** Approaches to the quantitation and isolation of immunoglobulins associated with plasma membranes, in *Immune Response at the Cellular Level,* Zacharia, T., Ed., Marcel Dekker, New York, 1973, 1.
36. **Vitetta, E. S. Baur, S., and Uhr, J. W.,** Cell surface immunoglobulin. II. Isolation and characterization of immunoglobulin from mouse splenic lymphocytes, *J. Exper. Med.,* 134, 242, 1971.
37. **Winchester, R. J. and Ross, G.,** Methods for enumerating lymphocyte populations, in *Manual of Clinical Immunology,* Rose, N. R. and Friedman, H., Eds., Am. Soc. Microbiol., Washington, D.C., 1976, 64.
38. **Waller, C. A. and MacLennan, I. C. M.,** Analysis of lymphocytes in blood and tissues, in *Techniques in Clinical Immunology,* Thompson, R. A., Ed., Blackwell Scientific, Oxford, 1977, 170.
39. **Billing, R., Rafizadeh, B, Drew, I., Hartman, G., Gale, R., and Terasaki, P.,** Human B-lymphocyte antigens expressed by lymphocytic and myelocytic leukemia cells. 1. Detection by rabbit antisera, *J. Exp. Med.,* 144, 167, 1976.
40. **Jerne, N. K. and Nordin, A. A.,** Plaque formation in agar by single antibody producing cells, *Science,* 140, 405, 1963.
41. **Cunningham, A. J. and Szenberg, A.,** Further improvements in the plaque techniques for detecting single antibody-forming cells, *Immunology,* 14, 599, 1968.
42. **Lefkovits, I. and Cosenza, H.,** Assay for plaque-forming cells, in *Immunological Methods,* Lefkovits, I. and Pernis, B., Eds., Academic Press, New York, 1979, 277.
43. **Shulman, M.,** Plaquing and recovering of individual antibody-producing cells, in *Immunological Methods,* Lefkovits, I. and Pernis, B., Eds., Academic Press, New York, 1979, 287.
44. **Wigzell, H. and Stjernswärd, J.,** Age-dependent rise and fall of immunological reactivity in the CBA mouse, *J. Natl. Cancer Inst.,* 37, 513, 1966.
45. **Nordin, A. A. and Makinodan, T.,** Humoral immunity in aging, *Fed. Proc.,* 33, 2033, 1974.

Maintenance of Animals for Aging Studies

DEVELOPMENT AND MAINTENANCE OF SPF COLONIES AND THEIR USE IN AGING STUDIES

Robert C. Allen and Chou C. Hong

INTRODUCTION

It has become increasingly evident that the indigenous or normal microflora of both man and animals exert profound and often little understood effects on the host. Organisms commonly found in the intestinal tract can produce pathogenic effects under certain conditions and conversely many of the organisms considered to be frank pathogens can persist in the host without producing any untoward reaction.

There is little reason to doubt that the variations in response in a given experiment may result from uncontrolled or undefined fluctuations in the microbial flora. Such variations on host response have been causally related to microbial changes or to microbial shifts in the so-called "normal flora". On the other hand, overt or subclinical infection from the introduction of or activation of pathogenic microorganisms such as *Salmonella, Pasteurella, Bartonella,* lymphocytic choriomeningitis virus, polyoma, Sendai virus, ectromelia virus, etc., may completely destroy whole experiments.

Changes in the indigenous microflora often become manifest when animals are placed in an environment removed from that in which their microflora was derived; thus leading to further potential variations in host response. While such variations may be tolerated in some short-term experiments, their magnification may greatly interfere or make impossible the accurate interpretation of long-term experiments such as aging effects on immunological response, tumor induction, and other life-shortening processes.

The various practices and procedures which may be employed to maintain healthy control animals for their expected life span are the subject of this chapter. Where possible, the most practical solution for a given type of experiment is set forth with a comparison of methods and examples wherever possible. These methods, procedures, and many of the precautions suggested, apply to the design of new facilities as well as any necessary alterations or renovations to existing facilities that may be required to provide the maximal protection of the colony from extraneous environmental influences. Unfortunately, only a partial presentation of facilities, design structure, and air handling design is within the scope of this chapter. However, a number of the pertinent considerations have been included covering this important area.

Fortunately, many of the lessons learned in the middle and late 1960s from long-term low level irradiation studies and on tumor induction and life-shortening processes, as well as the major microbiologic containment emphasis placed on the Apollo series manned moon landings, can be applied directly today to life span studies and the long-term effects on other physiological parameters.

FACILITY SUPPORT

Certain fundamental specifications must be established prior to the design and construction of a new facility for the maintenance of SPF or microbiologically defined mice for long term ontological geratology studies. These include a rodent- and vermin-proof masonry structure with a minimum of exterior openings: absolute regulation of the ambient environment, equipment for sterilization, pasteurization and sanitation of all materials admitted to the areas, provision for shower, locker area and secure entrance of personnel, procedures and equipment for ensuring the safe egress of animals and waste, an auxiliary source of electric power, and equipment for proper heating, cooling, humidifying, and ventilating. These same criteria apply to the renovation of existing facilities which require upgrading for this type of study.[1-3]

Interior walls should be vapor sealed, insulated, and finished with a smooth epoxy or urethane coating. Ceilings should be constructed following the same principles as for the walls; however, suspended ceilings should be free hanging and caulked at the wall joint with a two-component polysulfide material or equivalent. Reinforced concrete with a hardening compound provides good flooring with skid-proofing and should be coved at the wall junctures with an epoxy grout. The floor and coving should then be painted with an epoxy paint, thus, effectively providing monolithic room construction.

The proper control of temperature, humidity, air pressure, ventilation, and air filtration is of importance in the maintenance of environmental homeostasis for the mice in the long term ontological geratology study. The mice should be affected as little as possible by any variations in the external climatic conditions. An adequate method of air handling can be attained with a mechanical unit employing air filtration, heating, cooling, humidifying, and ventilaing. The heating ventilation, and air conditioning (HVAC) of a barrier facility should be controlled to provide 15 air changes per hour of freshly conditioned filtered air. The filter system should be at least 90% effective for the removal of 0.3 μm particles, which approaches 100% efficiency for larger particles. HEPA 99.9% effective filters for 0.3 micron particles may be used if sufficient funds for the heating and ventilation (HAV) system are available. The room circulation should be low velocity and draft free. A positive air pressure corridor should be included in the design and is designated as the "clean" corridor; similarly a negative air pressure corridor serves as the "dirty" corridor. The flow pattern of all personnel, equipment, and materials is always from "clean" to "dirty" corridors. Air pressure monitors located on a central panel are desirable to assure the integrity of the barrier and may be combined with remote damper controllers for optimal convenience.

A primary consideration in the design of the new facilities or in the renovation of old facilities is the integrity of the air handling system. An all too common engineering practice has been to filter the air, dry it, and then rehumidify it downstream from the absolute filters. This can lead to a major build of bacteria in the rehumidifier in the coil drain pans, particularly of *Pseudomonas aeruginosa,* which results in a continuous potential source of contamination. Contrary to the notion that filters downstream of the rehumidification coils will rapidly clog absolute filters, with proper prefiltering absolute filters have retained their efficiency under these conditions without clogging for several years.[4]

The animal room temperature should be maintained at 76°F ± 2° and the relative humidity 50 ± 10% with each animal room, including a temperature and humidity recorder attached to a central alarm system installed in the facility manager's office, in order that changes outside the allowable tolerances are noted and corrected promptly. This is done in most cases without the necessity of entering the animal areas. The lighting for all animal quarters should be automatically controlled with a dark-light ratio of 14:10 for most rodents.

Facilities may require uni- or bidirectional containment. The former in cases where only the protection of the animals is required and the latter where the use of slow viruses or other possibly infectious agents may be employed as part of a projected study. Such a design is described in Reference 5.

COLONY DEVELOPMENT

The choice of mouse strain, whether inbred or hybrid, is contingent upon the dictates

Table 1
MEAN LIFE SPANS OF INBRED AND HYBRID MICE[a]

Mean Life Span (Days)

	SPF		Conventional	
	Female	Male	Female	Male
Inbred strain				
A/He	—	—	520 ± 9.0	478 ± 7.0
A	558 ±[b] 19.7	512 ± 21.1	481 ± 8.0	503 ± 11.0
AKR	312 ± 9.4	350 ± 10.8	256 ± 3.0	272 ± 5.0
Balb/c	561 ± 30.3	509 ± 26.3	532 ± 15.0	485 ± 9.0
C_3H	676 ± 9.8	590 ± 18.6	398 ± 6.0	407 ± 7.0
$C_{57}Bl/6$	580 ± 35.8	645 ± 34.2	653 ± 13.0	539 ± 7.0
C57Br/cd	660 ± 22.7	577 ± 29.8	588 ± 14.0	475 ± 13.0
C57L	604 ± 27.6	473 ± 30.9	577 ± 19.0	532 ± 13.0
DBA/1	686 ± 33.3	487 ± 35.9	582 ± 11.0	438 ± 9.0
DBA/2	719 ± 35.4	629 ± 42.1	547 ± 9.0	415 ± 9.0
CBA	825 ± 32.5	486 ± 39.0	527 ± 15.0	527 ± 17.0
NZB	441 ± 12.1	459 ± 13.3	—	—
NZW	733 ± 42.8	802 ± 34.0	—	—
129	666 ± 23.2	699 ± 29.8	496 ± 21.0	616 ± 29.0
SWR	—	—	496 ± 21.0	616 ± 29.0
RFM/Un	—	785 ± 10.0[c]	605 ± 20.0	595 ± 20.0
Outbred strain				
LACA	664 ± 29.9	660 ± 38.5	—	—
LACG	617 ± 26.2	536 ± 38.9	—	—

[a] Virgins.
[b] Mean life span ± standard errors.
[c] Microbiologically defined.

of any particular study and will not be extensively covered here other than to provide a list of the more commonly used mouse strains in aging studies[6-9] and their expected life spans as shown in Table 1.

As may be noted in Table 1 where comparative data is provided for conventional and SPF animals, the microbial status of the animals plays a definite role which must be taken into consideration in any aging study. Therefore, the selection of the type of mouse; conventional, SPF, defined flora, or germfree, for a particular study will be a critical basic decision for a given study.

There are two prime methods to developing the colony for aging studies: (a) procurement of healthy SPF mice from the reputable breeder and (b) establishment of foundation stock and production colonies on-site, from either SPF or germfree animals. In the latter case, a defined microflora which is perhaps preferable may be employed.

1. If a small number of animals are to be used for the study, it may be more economically feasible and less time consuming for the investigator to procure the healthy SPF animals from the reputable breeder. However, it is necessary to carefully evaluate the animal vendor's quarantine and health maintenance procedures with this approach. Each breeder must be evaluated according to (a) the type of animal facility in which animals are bred and held, (b) the breeding system used, (c) the health status of the animals supplied, diagnostic routines, i.e., viral serology, microbiology, parasitology, and (d) the methods of transportation to

be employed, i.e., filtered cages, etc. Even though these considerations may be adequately satisfied, the newly received animals should be placed in quarantine until the health status has been completely evaluated. This period of isolation, besides giving the animals time to adjust to their new environment and to recover from the stress of shipmen, also allows the professional staff to observe the animals and perform necessary diagnostic tests to confirm that the animals meet the basic criteria required for the study. The more thorough the evaluation, the less likelihood of introducing any undesirable microorganisms into the colony with a possible resultant failure of the experiment.

There are varying suggestions as to how long newly arrived animals should be quarantined. Several reports[10] suggest a period of 6 days to 4 weeks as an appropriate period of acclimatization. However, as a general principle, the variable factors including age, weight, strain, sex, supplier of animals, mode and length of transportation, season of the year, and weather in which the animals were received, preclude a firm recommendation on an acceptable minimum length of quarantine.

2. Initially it may be necessary to establish germfree pedigreed breeding pairs of each strain of mice which will be used for the aging study. The establishment of germ free pedigreed animals has been described previously.[11,12]

   The animals must be microbiologically monitored prior to and after their receiving a defined microflora such as proposed by Schaedler[13] or Upton et. al.,[5] if such is to be employed. They are then transferred in specifically designed containers through the pass box into the barrier or alternatively contaminated in the barrier.

   If the required strains of animals can be acquired only from a source of questionable microbiological status, it may be caesarian-derived and placed in germ free isolators on foster mothers. Upon arrival from the source, the pedigreed pairs are placed in germ free environment. The technique for caesarian derivation and maintainance used is previously described.[1,14]

Once the germfree foundation stocks of each strain are established, offspring may be given an autochthonous microflora with the desired microbiological cocktail. Animals then may be transferred into the barrier. Since up to 12 weeks may be required for such a microflora to completely stabilize (see Figure 1),[15], it may be desirable to utilize such animals as the expansion breeding stock for the experiment itself and thus allow the offspring to be naturally contaminated by the parents. In which case, stabilization is more rapid and reproducible in regard to time frame (see Figure 2).

The foundation colonies will require approximately 6 to 8 months to reach peak production depending on the production efficiency index. If they were originally obtainable germfree, reproduction gains would be more rapid.

The breeding programs for a large colony of mice inbred strains consists of two to three steps.[16,17] All strains should have a foundation colony. Inbred strains which have a low production efficiency usually require an expansion step (pedigreed expansion colony). In the foundation colony and pedigree expansion colony all matings are between brother-sister. All foundation colony and pedigreed matings are thus pedigreed and all are monogamous, i.e., the male and female are left together through their breeding life span. The pedigreed expansion colony (PEC) breeders are brother-sister mated offspring from the foundation colony. This step is only necessary if the foundation colony is not able to produce sufficient offspring to maintain the breeder numbers in the production colony. The production colony matings may follow the out-

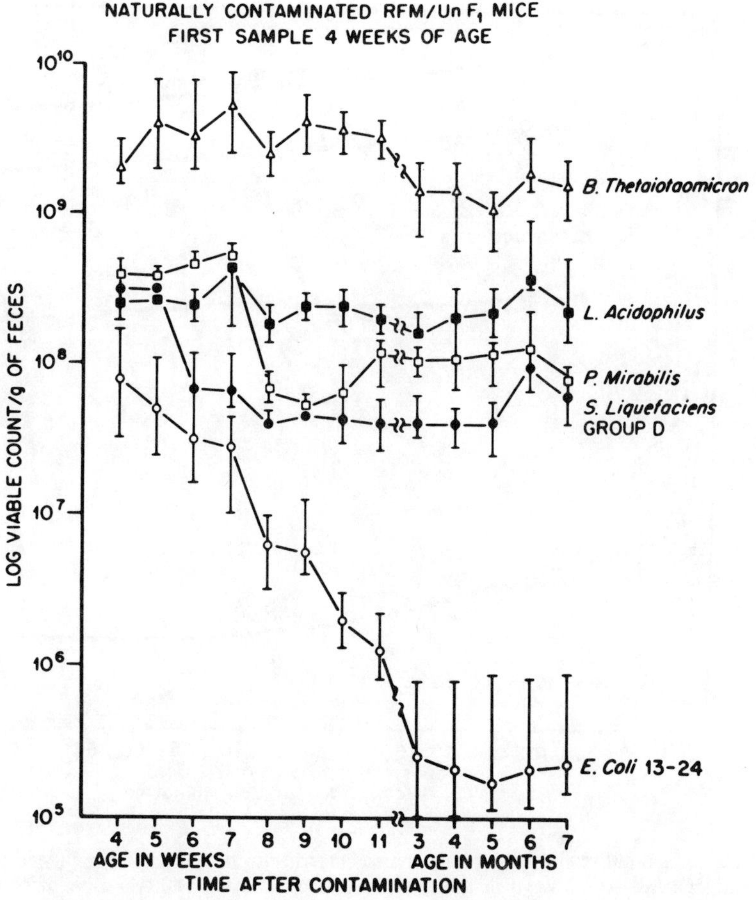

FIGURE 1. First generation offspring naturally contaminated from parental stock over a 7 month period. Parental stock was of germfree origin specifically contaminated through the feed at 4 weeks of age. *Staphylococcus albus* and *Clostridium* sp. also used to specifically contaminate the parents did not establish in the naturally contaminated offspring.

breeding pattern and breeding animals will not be pedigreed. Selection of a random breeding system in the production colony for long-term experiments may be desirable to eliminate line selection such as shown in Table 2. The procedure should also serve to allow comparative studies on the same strain of mice, but perhaps obtained from a different source and by investigators between laboratories.

On the other hand, circumstances may dictate that a strict inbreeding schedule be followed. This may be accomplished similarly by brother-sister matings and replacing the production stock from the pedigreed stock. Identifications will follow the mating unit system and production records will be kept accordingly. The breeder ratios may be four females with one male or at the ratio at which production efficiency is greatest. The mating unit should be maintained as an entity for its entire breeding life span. In general, the mice should be weaned at 21 days of age because of the pending parturition of the second litter which occurs in continuous matings (Figure 3).

The breeding programs for outbred and random bred matings should follow the random pattern and the random scheme will prevent inadvertant inbreeding.

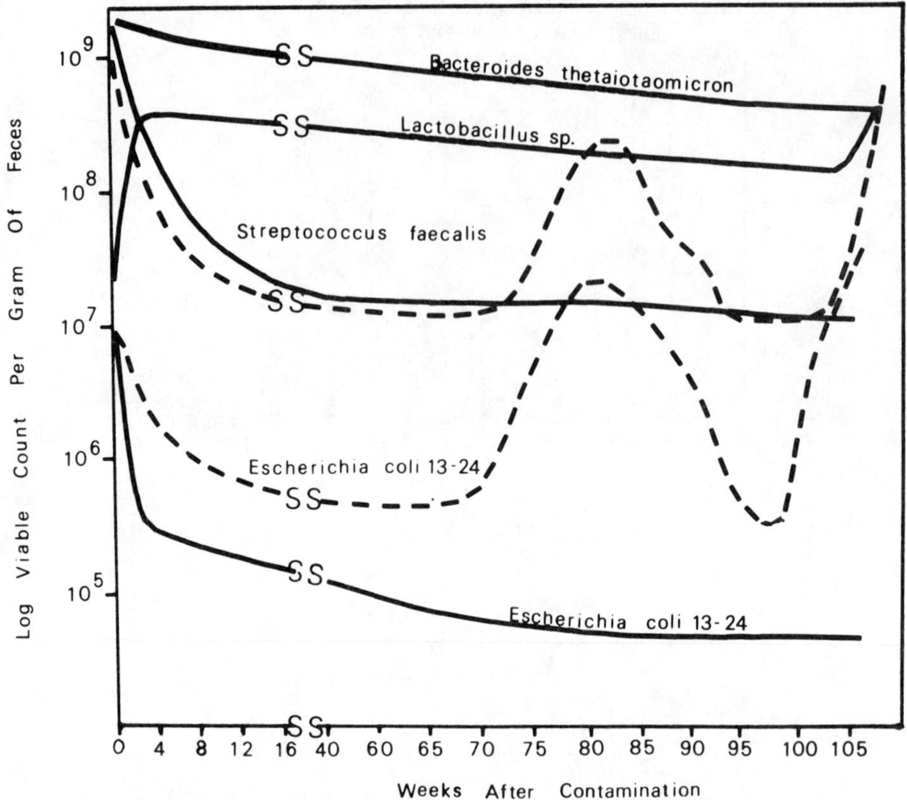

FIGURE 2. Quantitative and stability of a defined macroflora given to germfree animals at 4 weeks of age and studied weekly over their life span. Two cages of males and two cages of females with five animals per cage are shown; variations in the males (dashed lines). *Streptococcus faecalis*; and *Escherichia coli* were apparent after about 1½ years of age and fluctuated over the remaining life span of animals.

ANIMAL CARE

Husbandry

All animal care should be in accordance with the Guide for Laboratory Animal Facility and Care (PHS Publication No. 1024),[17] Care and Treatment of Laboratory Animal (NIH 4206), Policy NIH Guide for Grants and Contracts No. 7, and Laboratory Animal Welfare Act (P.L. 89-554), as amended by the Animal Welfare Act of 1970 and 1976 (P.L. 91-579 and 94-279).

Adult mice require 15 in.^{2} of cage floor space per animal. The commonly used clear polycarbonate cage of 7.5 in. wide by 10 in. long by 5 in. high will house five such mice.

Ideally only one strain of mice should be housed per room; however, where the number of mice is kept small, more than one strain may be housed on opposite sides of a room. To prevent accidental mixing of strains it is desirable that each strain has a uniquely different hair coat color. Once set up, the integrity of the room must be held intact until the termination of the aging study. No animals should be admitted directly into the holding rooms that are used for the study.

All animals must be observed daily and every effort made to prevent rodents from escaping from the cages. If there is an escape from a cage and the mouse becomes

Table 2
MAMMARY TUMOR INCIDENCE BY FAMILY LINE BETWEEN PEC[a] AND PRODUCTION OF C_3H/HeJ MICE

Family	Source	No tumor	Tumor	Incidence (%)
29166	PEC	35	15	30.00
29166	Prod	136	19	12.26
28964	PEC	27	23	46.00
28964	Prod	66	23	25.84
27999	PEC	48	25	34.25
27999	Prod	84	22	20.75
29735	PEC	41	14	25.45
29735	Prod	37	6	13.95
28962	PEC	22	11	33.33
28962	Prod	55	6	9.83
Total	PEC	173	88	33.72
Total	Prod	378	76	16.74

Note: Only line 29735 in PEC is significantly lower than the higher 28974 line; however, other lines are generally lower than this particular line. In production mice in the later generation there are significant differences between line 28964 and the low incidence lines 29166, 29735, and 28962. This was found to be due to the effect of trio-mating in the production colony as opposed to pair mating in the PEC colony. Other contributory factors were undoubtedly high incidence of infantile diarrhea in the trio-mated offspring and associated higher preweaning mortality. Thus, rather unexpected consequences may arise from a simple thing as a change in mating protocol.

[a] PEC = pedigreed expansion colony.

exposed to a noncontrolled environment, it should be destroyed, and noted in the protocol records, rather than to replace it and put the colony at risk.

A diet should be selected which contains balanced nutrients properly fortified for steam sterilization prior to use.[18,19] Water with approximately 18 ppm chlorine[20] should be provided in sterilized bottls which are changed three times per week. The bedding used should be sterilized preferably by a high pressure-high vacuum autoclave, as ethylene oxide sterilization, particularly of shaving bedding may produce toxic effects due to ethylene glycol formation[21-23] prior to use. The same diet and bedding should be used through the entire aging study to prevent adding any additional variables to the experiment.[24]

Animal Identification

All animals must be positively identified by a cage card. The cage card number, animal identification, and cage location should be recorded in a log book. The cage card will accompany the animal as it is transferred to clean caging. As the cards become soiled or torn, they are replaced by new cards bearing the original and subsequent pertinent information. Should the experiment comprise such a large number of animals that hand bookkeeping is unwieldy, computer programs may be desired for record keeping.

Personnel

During the aging experiment, the only people who should be allowed through the

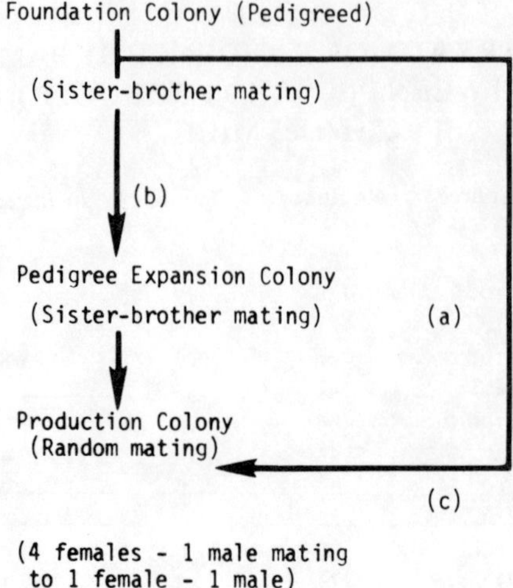

(a) Strains have the high production efficiency index

(b) The strains which have the low production efficiency index require the intermediate expansion step.

(c) 1:1; 1:2; 1:4 Rationale

FIGURE 3. Breeding scheme of producing inbred strain of mice.

showers into the barrier area and the animal rooms or facility, are the animal technicians and the scientists conducting the experiment. Maintenance staff may enter in an emergency in barrier facilities, but they should shower and don sterile clothes, caps, masks, boots, and gloves. However, most services can be maintained from outside the animal rooms with proper design. On entering the barrier area, personnel should remove their street clothes, shower and put on the sterile clothes listed above, as supplied by the "Institute". On leaving the barrier area, a shower is optimal before again donning street clothes. Sterile clothes (shift, pants, socks, pullover) are autoclaved weekly and a fresh supply stocked in the entry locker area. Disposable sterile gloves are most conveniently used within the barrier. A clear example of the rationale for sterile clothing is given under the section on health monitoring in Table 3.

Animal technicians should have a definite duty assignment and no contact with any other areas particularly those housing other animal colonies. Contact with any other activity in the building may be permitted only on instruction by the immediate supervisor. Personnel not assigned to the aging study should not be permitted to enter unless prior approval has been obtained from the scientists who conduct the experiment and this should be discouraged except for the most cogent reasons.

Visitors should not be permitted to enter the animal rooms and other barrier areas in the building at any time.

Sanitation

Cage racks should be chemically sterilized in place each week. The individual cages should be changed weekly or twice weekly depending on the number of mice present and cage size employed. Cage washing should be carried out in a mechanical cage washer effective in removing all bedding and debris. Bedding should be placed in each

Table 3
MICROBIOLOGICAL RESULTS OF PERSONNEL SAMPLING

Animal technician	Nose	Hand
A	*Staphylococcus albus*	*S. albus*
	Bacillus sp.	*Bacillus* sp.
B	*S. albus*	*S. albus*
C	*S. albus*	*S. albus*
	Pseudomonas aeruginosa	*S. aureus*
D	*S. albus*	*S. albus*
	Klebsiella-Aerobacter	Klebsiella-Aerobacter
		S. aureus
E	*S. albus*	*S. albus*
	Klebsiella-Aerobacter	Hemolytic streptococcus
	S. aureus	
F	*S. albus*	*S. albus*
	Hemolytic streptococcus	*Bacillus* sp.
	Klebsiella-Aerobacter	*S. aureus*
G	*S. albus*	*S. albus*
	Bacillus sp.	
	Hemolytic streptococcus	
H	*S. albus*	*S. albus*
I	*S. albus*	*S. albus*
	Klebsiella-Aerobacter	
	Proteus mirabilis	
J	*S. albus*	*S. albus*
	Bacillus sp.	
	Hemolytic streptococcus	

cage prior to sterilization into the animal quarters. High pressure, high vacuum autoclaving should be utilized rather than ethylene oxide due to its aforementioned toxic effects.[21-23]

Water bottles, stoppers, and sipper tubes should be changed three times a week following washing through the cagewash machine and sterilization prior to reentry into the animal quarters. Water bottles should be filled automatically with chlorinated water (18 ppm chlorine) within the barrier facility. Cage tops should be changed at least once a month. All feed should be sterilized into the barrier and stored in plastic containers with tight sealing lids. Alternatively, presterilized food in double sealed bags may be passed into the barrier through a dip tank.

The corridors and service areas should be cleaned and sanitized with quaternary ammonium compounds applied by either steam sterilized mops or if the barrier is of sufficient size to warrant, it may be scrubbed with a machine with sterile circular brush attached. The area should be rinsed and excessive water removed preferably by a wet vacuum. If drains are present in corridors, they should have airtight covers and a deep trap at least 12 in. into which disinfectant should be poured following use. Since drains as normally installed are prime sources of bacterial contamination in a barrier, particular attention should be paid to their proper installation and maintenance.

Health Monitoring

Health monitoring plays a vital role particularly in aging studies. Every effort must be made to assure that the animals are microbiologically unaltered and that genetic integrity has been maintained for inbred strains of animals. To assure this, the sampling procedure as described in the ILAR's Long-Term Holding of Laboratory Rodents,[2] ILAR's Standards and Guidelines for the Breeding, Care and Management of Laboratory Animals: Rodents,[17] and other procedures[3] may be used. This includes monitoring both the animal and environment[25,26] when parasitology, pathology, microbiology, and serology all must be employed.[27-48]

Pilot Animals

The aging study of laboratory mice must be carefully maintained for their full life span without any intercurrent interruption. Five to ten additional cages of animals from the stock colony should be added to each experimental room randomly among the other cages of aging mice. At regular intervals (every 1 to 2 months), one or more animals of each sex should be clinically examined, bled, then sacrificed and subjected to a complete necropsy, with full laboratory evaluation including bacterial isolation, endo- and ectoparasite examination and serology for detection of latent murine viruses. The purpose of this procedure is to make certain that the experimental animals in each room are not contaminated with any infectious or latent agents which could modify or invalidate the data obtained for various parameters which may be under investigation in the aging study itself.

Sick and Dead Animals from the Aging Study

If an animal becomes ill or dies unexpectedly during the study, a complete diagnostic workup is essential. Every effort must be made to determine whether the illness or death is due to disease, an unrecognized variable in the experimental procedure, or is due to solely natural factors. The complete work should include parasitologic, pathologic, microbiologic, hematologic, serologic examination, and clinical chemistry studies. If a pathogen or opportunistic bacteria or virus is found, the significance of that agent on the animals and its effect on the experiments must be carefully evaluated. Knowledge of the epidemiology of the particular disease is essential to its control and to predicting its effect on the outcome of the study. The diagnosis and examination of infectious diseases of mice are briefly described in Table 4.

Microbiologic Evaluation of Environment and Equipment

Routine weekly microbiologic examination of room floor, air vent, cages, racks, and water bottles is recommended to detect the presence of undesirable microorganisms, to document changes in the microbiologic environment, and to evaluate routine sanitation procedures as well as to assess the ventilation system's integrity. The Rodac grid plates (60 × 15 mm in size) filled with nutrient agar may be used for this procedure. The area and equipment are stamped by the plates. Those plates are labeled, dated, and incubated at 37°C overnight. The number of colonies are counted and recorded. Complete identification of all microorganisms is carried out routinely and entered in the experimental records. This assessment affords a secondary check on the performance of sterilization equipment and operations.

The following monitoring protocol (Table 5) which is modified from the suggested protocol of Laboratory Animal Management: Rodent (ILAR) is recommended as a guide for this purpose.

Qualitative and Quantitative Fecal Sampling

The autochthonous flora provided to the colony animals may be monitored both qualitatively and quantitatively from fresh fecal samples collected in a randomized fashion from one cage in each room per week.

While *Escherichia coli* is often included in the flora, it is difficult to assess any superimposition of additional variants of flora organisms to the system without employing rather tedious and expensive microbiological techniques. Thus, for such qualitative assessment, a genetically marked strain such as *E. coli* M13-24 may be employed.

Table 4
INFECTIOUS DISEASES OF MICE

Disease	Diagnosis	Examination
Virus		
Adenovirus infection	Serology; CF,[a] SN,[b] intranuclear inclusions; heart, kidney, adrenal	Focal necrosis; heart
K-Virus infection	Serology; HI,[c] SN; intranuclear inclusions; endothelial cells	Interstitial pneumonia with proliferation of endothelial cells
Lactic dehydrogenase (LDH) virus infection	Elevation of plasma LDH serology SN	None
Lymphocytic choriomeningitis infection	Guinea pig or LCM-free mouse inoculation; serology: CF,[d] SN	Lymphocytic chorimeningitis; necrosis; liver and lymphoid tissue
Mammary tumor virus	Lesions; serology:SN	Mammary adenocarcinomas, adrenocanthomas, carcinosarcomas
Minute virus of mice	Serology: SN, HI, CF	Encephalitis; choriomeningitis
Mouse (Theiler's) encephalomyelitis (GD VII)	Serology: HI, neonatal hamster inoculation	Necrosis: brain stem, spinal cord
Mouse hepatitis	Serology: CF, FA, SN mouse inoculation	Focal necrosis: liver, lymph nodes, brain
Mouse papule disease	Intracytoplasmic inclusions: epidermis, virus isolation	Papules in skin
Mouse pneumonitis (Nigg virus inf.)	CF; elementary bodies: bronchial epithelium	Interstitial and bronchopneumonia
Mouse thymic agent infection	Inoculation of newborn mice	Focal thymic necrosis
Murine leukemia	CF Mu L [e] and XC[f] tests	Lymphocytic granulocytic or erythrocytic leukemia
Pneumonia virus of mice infection	Serology: HI, SN, inoc. of PVM-free mice	Interstitial pneumonia pulmonary edema
Polyoma virus infection	Serology: HI, SN, CF, FA	Tumors in various sites
Reovirus infection (hepatoencephalomyelitis)	Serology: HI, FA, CF, SN	Necrosis: liver, myocardium, pancreas, neuronal degeneration; encephalitis
Epidemic diarrhea of infant mice (EDIM)	Serology: FA, diarrhea, intracytoplastic or intranuclear inclusions in small intestinal epithelium	Histopath. exam of sm. intestine
Ectromelia	Serology: HI, CF, FA, SN intracytoplastic inclusions in skin	Histopath. exam. of affected area

Table 4 (continued)
INFECTIOUS DISEASES OF MICE

Disease	Diagnosis	Examination
Salivary gland virus (cytomegalovirus) infection	Lesions	Intranuclear inclusions salivary-duct epithelium
Sendai virus infection	Serology: HI, CF, FA, SN	Interstitial pneumonia
Bacteria		
Streptobacillus moniliformis	Culture respiratory passages	Nelson test
Streptococci (pyogenic and viridans)	Culture organs and feces	Feces: mitis-salivarius agar plus tellurite, organs: blood agar
Micrococci spp.	Culture organs and feces	Feces: staph medium 110, organs: blood agar
Salmonella spp.	Culture organs and feces	Feces: selenite to McConkey, S-S or brilliant green agar to triple sugar iron agar; organ: McConkey agar
Bacillus piliformis (Tyzzer's disease)	Isolation of agent	Animal passage and culture in tissue cells or chick embryo
Shigella spp.	Culture organs and feces	Same as salmonella
Corynebacterium spp.	Culture organs and feces	Feces:dextrose proteose #3 agar plus tellurite blood solution. organs: blood agar
Pasteurella spp.	Culture organs	Blood agar and tryptose agar
Pseudomonas aeruginosa	Culture organs and feces	Feces: McConkey agar, organs: glycerol agar
Paracolobactrum spp.	Culture feces	EMB or McConkey agar
Enterococci spp.	Culture organs and feces	Feces: sodium azide blood agar, organs: blood agar
Proteus spp.	Culture feces	Selenite to urea broth
Bortedella bronchiseptica	Culture lungs	Blood agar
E. coli	Culture feces	EMB, McConkey agar
Anaerobes	Culture feces and organs	Feces: thioglycollate broth, organs: blood agar in N_2 anaerobic chamber
Leptospira ballum	Culture blood and kidney	Ellinghausen's
Erysipelothrix insidiosa	Culture organs	Blood agar and tellurite agar

Listeria monocytogenesis	Culture organs	Tryptose agar
Vibrio spp.	Culture feces	McConkey agar
Bartonella	Observe organism in blood	Splenectomize mice and make blood smears
Protozoa		
Giardia	Observe trophs or cysts in feces	Direct fecal smear in saline
Coccidia	Observe cysts in feces	Feces flotation
Toxoplasmosis	Observe cysts in brain, isolate or serology	Histopath exam of brain, inj. brain i/p, antibody test
Eperythrozoonosis	Observe organism in blood	Splenectomize and blood smear
Encephalitozoon	Observe pathology and organism	Histopath exam of brain and kidney
Endamoeba	Observe cysts in feces and culture	Direct fecal smear and culture
Parasites		
Endoparasites	Observe ova or adults	Examine intestinal contents and fecal flotation
Ectoparasites	Observe adults	Kill mice and collect
Fungi		
Fungi	Culture the affected tissues and organs	Sabouraud agar plus antibiotics

[a] Complement fixation.
[b] Serum neutralization.
[c] Hemagglutination inhibition.
[d] Immunofluorescence.
[e] Complement fixation for murine leukemia.
[f] XC cell cytopathogenicity test.

Table 5
RECOMMENDED MONITORING PROTOCOL

Specimen	Sample size	Frequency
Food and bedding[a]	Every newly arrived batch	On arrival
Cages, water bottles, racks (both used and clean)	1%	Weekly
Floor, air vent, and work spaces[b]	1 sample from the areas of each room	Weekly
Used water bottles (for *Pseudomonas aeruginosa* and proteus spp.)	1%[c]	Weekly
Cage fecal samples	1%[c]	Weekly
Pilot animals — pathologic, microbiologic, parasitologic, and serologic examinations	2—3	2 months

[a] Detect the number of G(−) bacteria present.
[b] Sample size may be reduced if no positive are found in a period of 6 months.
[c] Detect both the number of G(−) bacteria and pathogens.

CONCLUSION

Long-term studies of aging involve both environmental and other stress phenomena as an integral part of the study in addition to the genetic makeup of the animals. The information provided here gives an overview presently available on a number of the more controllable variables known to play an important role in long-term physiological response when conditions are controlled. The characteristics affected by the environmental stress depend on both external and internal variables. The internal variables, including the diet, water, and microflora have been covered more completely. The external factors include ambient temperature, humidity, light cycle, bedding, caging, air quality, and space provided for the animals. While we have perhaps overemphasized the more expensive barrier concept, it has been done because experience has shown that it works well in practice. Use of modified clean rooms with a vertical laminar flow of absolute filtered air or horizontal laminar flow of absolute filtered air, are viable alternatives also, but perhaps more difficult to control over extended periods. These along with filter cabinets may provide most reliable if placed in semibarrier rooms. That is, rooms isolated from other animal areas by a positive air pressure differential and with a separate air handling system.

In studies of this type, preplanning and strict observance of the health status and microbial status of the animals in conjunction with a vigorous and consistant monitoring program, are the keystones to a measure of assurance of success. Additionally, it should be emphasized that all personnel, particularly caretaker personnel, should be thoroughly trained and be cognizant of the fact that even minor deviations from established procedures and protocols may have disasterous effects on the outcome of long-term study.

Current feeling is that much of the experimental work done in the past may be invalid due to the neglect and inability of distinguishing between experimental effects and uncontrolled variables causing the high rate of natural morbidity found in most conventional colonies. Research investigators should no longer be hesitant about using both rigorously controlled environment barrier facilities and animals with a defined or semidefined microflora if reliable and reproducible studies of various factors on the aging process are to be concluded successfully.

REFERENCES

1. Standards and Guidelines for the Breeding, Care, and Management of Laboratory Animals: Gnotobiotes, Institute of Laboratory Animal Resources, Subcommittee on Standards for Gnotobiotes, Committee on Standards, National Research Council, National Academy of Sciences, Washington, D.C., 1970.
2. Laboratory Animal Management: Rodents, institute for Laboratory Animal Resources, National Academy of Sciences, Washington, D.C., 1977.
3. **Simmons, M. L. and Brick, J. O.,** *The Laboratory Mouse: selection and management,* Prentice-Hall, Englewood Cliffs, N.J., 1970.
4. **Walburg, H. E., Jr., Mynatt, E. I., Cosgrove, E. G., Tyndall, R. L., and Robie, D. M.,** Microbiological evaluation of an isolation facility for the production of specific-pathogen-free mice, *Lab. Anim. Care,* 15, 208, 1965.
5. **Upton, A. C., Allen, R. C., Borwn, R. C., Clapp, N. K., Conklin, J. W., Cosgrove, G. E., Darden, E. B., Jr., Kastenbaum, M. A., Odell, T. T., Jr., Serrano, L. J., Tyndall, R. L., and Walburg, H. E., Jr.,** Quantitative experimental study of low-level radiation carcinogenesis, in *Radiation Induced Cancer,* International Atomic Energy Agency, Vienna, 1969, 425.
6. **Russell, E. S.,** Lifespan and aging patterns, in *Biology of the Laboratory Mouse,* 2nd ed., Green, E. L., Ed., McGraw-Hill, New York, 1966, 511.
7. **Festing, M. and Blackman, D. K.,** Lifespan of specified-pathogen free mice and rats, *Lab. Anim.,* 5, 179, 1971.
8. **Crispens, C. G., Jr.,** *Handbook on the Laboratory Mouse,* Charles C Thomas, Springfield, Ill., 1975.
9. **Storer, J. B.,** Longevity and gross pathology at death in 22 inbred mouse strain, *J. Gerontol.,* 21, 404, 1966.
10. **Grant, L., Hopkinson, P., Jennings, G., and Jenner, F. A.,** Period of adjustment of rats used for experimental studies, *Nature (London),* 232, 135, 1971.
11. **Davey, D. G.,** Establishing and maintaining a colony of specific pathogen free mice, rats, and guinea pigs, collected papers, *Lab. Anim. Center,* 8, 17, 1959.
12. **Nelson, J. B. and Collins, G. R.,** The establishment and maintenance of a specific pathogen-free colony of swiss mice, *Proc. Anim. Care Panel,* 11, 65, 1961.
13. **Dubos, F. P. and Schaedler, R. W.,** The effect of the intestinal flora on the growth rate of mice, and on their susceptibility to experimental infections, *J. Exp. Med.,* 111, 407, 1960.
14. **Heneghan, J. B., Ed.,** *Germfree Research: Biological Effect on Gnotobiotic Environments,* Academic Press, New York, 1973.
15. **Allen, R. C.,** unpublished data.
16. Standards and Guidelines for the Breeding, Care, and Management of Laboratory Animals: Rodents, Institute of Laboratory Animal Resources, Subcommittee on Rodent Standards, Committee on Standards, National Research Council, National Academy of Sciences, Washington, D.C., 1969.
17. Institute of Laboratory Animal Resources, Committee on Revision of the Guide for Laboratory Animal Facilities and Care, National Research Council, Guide for the Care and Use of Laboratory Animals, Publ. No. National Institute of Health 74-23, U.S. Government Printing Office, Washington, D.C., 1974.
18. **Foster, H. L., Black, C. O., and Pfau, E. S.,** A pasteurization process for pelleted diets, *Lab Anim. Care,* 14, 373, 1964.
19. **Williams, F. P., Christie, R. J., Johnson, D. J., and Whitney, R. A., Jr.,** A new autoclave system for sterilizing vitamin-fortified commercial rodent diets with lower nutrient loss, *Lab Anim. Care,* 18, 195, 1968.
20. **McPherson, C. W.,** Reduction of pseudomonas aeruginosa and coliform bacteria in mouse drinking water following treatment with hydrochloric acid or chlorine, *Lab. Anim. Care,* 13, 737, 1963.
21. **Meier, H., Allen, R. C., and Hoag, W. G.,** Spontaneous hemorrhagic diathesis in inbred mice due to single or multiple "prothrombin-complex" deficiencies, *Blood,* 19, 501, 1962.
22. **Allen, R. C., Meier, H., and Hoag, W. G.,** Ethylene glycol produced by ethylene oxide sterilization and its effects in an inbred strain of mice, *Nature (London),* 193, 387, 1962.
23. **Reyniers, J. A., Sacksteder, M. R., and Ashburn, L. L.,** Multiple tumors in female germ free inbred albino mice exposed to bedding treated with ethylene oxide, *J. Natl. Cancer Inst.,* 32, 1045, 1964.
24. **Porter, G. and Lane-Petter, W.,** The provision of sterile bedding and nesting materials with their effects on breeding mice, *J. Anim. Tech. Assoc.,* 16, 5, 1965.
25. **Weihe, W. H.,** Temperature and humidity dimatograms fo rats and mice, *Lab. Anim. Care,* 15, 18, 1965.
26. **Lang, C. M. and Vessell, E. S.,** Environmental and genetic factors affecting laboratory animals, impact on biomedical research, *Fed. Proc.,* 35, 1123, 1976.

27. A Guide to Infectious Diseases of Mice and Rats, Institute of Laboratory Animal Resources, Committee on Laboratory Animal Disease, National Research Council, National Academy of Sciences, Washington, D.C., 1971.
28. **Allen, R. C., Wetmore, P. W., and Hoag, W. G.,** Factors effecting the incidence of infantile diarrhea in mice, *Bacteriol. Proc.*, 62, 99, 1962.
29. **Beverly, J. K. A.,** Congenital transmission of toxoplasmosis through successive generations of mice, *Nature (London)*, 183, 1348, 1959.
30. **Briody, B. A.,** Response of mice to ectromelia and vaccinia viruses, *Bacteriol. Rev.*, 23, 61, 1959.
31. **Flynn, R. J.,** Ectoparasites of mice, *Proc. Anim. Care Panel*, 6, 75, 1955.
32. **Gledhill, A. W. and Dick, G. W. A.,** The nature of mouse hepatitis virus infection in weaning mice, *J. Pathol. Bact.*, 69, 311, 1955.
33. **Gledhill, A. W. and Rees, R. J. W.,** A spontaneous entercoccal disease of mice and its enhancement by cortisone, *Br. J. Exp. Pathol.*, 33, 183, 1952.
34. **Griesemer, R. A.,** Bartonellosis, *Natl. Cancer Inst. J.*, 20, 949, 1958.
35. **Habermann, R. T. and Williams, F. P., Jr.,** Salmonellosis in laboratory animals, *Natl. Cancer Inst. J.*, 20, 933, 1958.
36. **Habermann, R. T and Williams, F. P., Jr.,** The identification and control of helminths in laboratory animals, *Natl. Cancer Inst. J.*, 20, 979, 1958.
37. **Levine, N. D.,** Protozoan diseases of laboratory animals, *Proc. Anim. Care Panel*, 7, 98, 1957.
38. **Maurer, F. D.,** Lymphocytic choriomengitis, *Natl. Cancer Inst. J.*, 20, 867, 1958.
39. **Maurer, F. D.,** Mouse poliolyelitis or Theirler's mouse encephalomyelitis, *Natl. Cancer Inst. J.*, 20, 871, 1958.
40. **Nelson, J. B.,** Studies on endemic pneumonia of the albino rat. IV. Development of a rat colony free from respiratory infections, *J. Exp. Med.*, 94, 377, 1951.
41. **Pappenheimer, A. M.,** Epidemic diarrheal diseases of suckling mice, *Natl. Cancer Inst. J.*, 20, 861, 1958.
42. **Pappenheimer, A. M.,** Pathology of infection with the JHM virus, *Natl. Cancer Inst. J.*, 20, 879, 1958.
43. **Pappenheimer, A. M.,** Myocarditis and pulmonary arteritis associated with the presence of ricketsia-like bodies in polymorphonuclear leukocyte, *Natl. Cancer Inst. J.*, 20, 921, 1958.
44. **Saunders, L. Z.,** Tyzzer's disease, *Natl. Cancer Inst. J.*, 20, 893, 1958.
45. **Rowe, W. P., Hartley, J. W., Estes, J. D., and Huebner, R. J.,** Studies of mouse polyoma virus infection. I. Procedures for quantitation and detection of virus, *J. Exp. Med.*, 109, 379, 1959.
46. **Schwartz, J.,** The deep mycoses in laboratory animals, *Proc. Anim. Care Panel*, 5, 37, 1954.
47. **Traub, E,** Epidemiology of lymphocytic choriomeningitis in a mouse stock observed for four years, *J. Exp. Med.*, 69, 801, 1939.
48. **Tyzzer, E. E.,** A comparative study of Grahamellae, haemobartonellae and eperythrozoa in small animals, *Proc. Am. Philos. Soc.*, 85, 359, 1942.

THE GERMFREE SYSTEM FOR AGING AND IMMUNITY*

Julian R. Pleasants

INTRODUCTION

We begin with a paradox. Historically, microbial infections provided our first and most dramatic indication that immune potential declines with age. They could do this because they exploited an immune change which was not grossly visible and produced a gross change in the condition of the aging human patient or experimental animal. Thus, we should be properly grateful to the microbial pathogens for this discovery which may lead to the prolongation of life through immunologic manipulation just as it did initially through the use of antibiotics.

However, the microbial pathogens involved in spontaneous infections of the aged have proved a highly variable, unreproducible measure of immune potential and function, because their presence and numbers in the environment are highly variable. Thus, they may be absent when we want an immune change amplified to an infectious process, or present when we do not want such amplification to occur. Furthermore, the infectious process, once it takes hold, overlays and obscures the state of the immune system at the time the infection began. Of greatest importance may be the fact that experimental reduction of immune potential for research purposes, e.g., by neonatal thymectomy, radiation, cytotoxic drugs or sera, nutritional imbalances, or genetic deficiency, can result in infectious processes destroying the experimental model before aging begins.

Besides their potential for creating severe and often lethal infections, the microbes associated with an animal have a profound influence on the major variable under study, the immune system. Since the microbiota represents a continuous influence during natural aging, we may wish to maintain it as the normal background "noise" of an experiment investigating aging and immunity. Yet, the same type of problem arises as with lethal infections. The microbiota of a conventional (CV) animal is the most variable, least characterized, and least predictable part of the animal. Those members of the microbiota which stimulate or depress the immune system are not characterized qualitatively or quantitatively, and cannot be relied upon to be active when needed or absent when undesired. Even if we wish to maintain the influence of the microbiota during aging, there would be great advantages to having a known, limited microbiota, either constant over time or changing in some predictable way.

We tend to think of the rat or mouse as a model for man which has the same relation to its microbiota that man has to his microbiota. But this is far from true. Rodents and rabbits can be considered semiruminants. They have specialized the cecum for prolonged retention of food residues where an abundant microflora can utilize them. Since the products of such activity would not become readily available to the host during their passage through the colon, the animal consumes part of its feces, (20 to 80% of rat feces)[1] making these bacteria and their products available to the full processes of digestion and absorption. Because of this consumption of large numbers of microbes, and because the rodent stomach has a nonglandular compartment where acidity is low, bacterial numbers and activity are also higher in the upper gut than they would be in man.[2] The rodent's exposure to microbes and microbial products is proportiontely much greater than man's exposure. Even though a germfree (GF) animal

* A glossary of abbreviations follows the text.

will accept and maintain a human-type microflora (a special advantage of using such an animal),[3,4] the influence of this microflora will be proportionately greater in the rodent than in man. In some respects, the GF rodent comes closer to the conventional human analogue than any of the microbially-associated rodents.

In any case, if we want to assess the effect of the microbiota on the processes of aging in general and of immune aging in particular, we need an animal free of microbial influence for comparison. Minimally, it should be free of viable microbes. Ideally, it would be spared contact with dead microbes and with microbial products. With this much control accomplished, it would then be feasible to exclude, from the diet and environment, even nonmicrobial antigens and mitogens.

As the complexity of the immune response has become increasingly evident, it has become necessary to dissect that response into constituent parts, i.e., to employ cell, tissue and organ cultures, transplants, and biochemical measures of immunity. But the integrated immune response carried out by the animal itself remains our ultimate assurance that what we study analytically is not an artifact but a reflection of what occurs in vivo. This is especially true in studies of immune changes with aging, for here the immune system interacts not only within itself but also with other changing systems of the aging animal. Therefore, research tools which might simplify the animal itself and the forces acting upon its immune system, can retain the advantages of an integrated system while avoiding or controlling the complexity and variability introduced into the animal by its most complex, variable and ill-defined constituent, its associated microbiota.

This kind of control is the function of the germfree system and of the animal models it makes possible: the germfree (GF) animal colony free of any demonstrable microbial associates, the germfree antigen-free colony fed ultrafiltered chemically defined diet (GF-CD), the gnotobiotic (GN) animal colony bearing only *known* microbial associates, and the biotoristic (BOR) colony, a term used here to describe a colony limited by germfree technique to the microbiota brought into the isolator system by the original members of the colony, whether that microbiota be conventional (CV), specific-pathogen-free (SPF), or some combination of these with known added species.

The Essence of the Germfree System: Absolute Barriers

The essence of the germfree system, whatever animal model occupies it, is the provision of absolute barriers against the entry of unwanted microbial invaders.[5-8] In addition to the physical barriers of plastic, metal, rubber, and glass which enclose the animals, the system requires the operational barriers of air filtration, food and water sterilization, manipulation by gloves forming an integral part of the barrier system, and the entry and exit of supplies through a sterilizable double door entry port (Figure 1). Details of the system, its operation, and testing, have been supplied in many publications.[9,10] I have recently reviewed these details in the article "Gnotobiotics" in the *CRC Handbook of Laboratory Animal Science.*[11] It is the purpose of the present article to review the needs for GF, GN, or BOR animals in studies of aging and immunity, and to provide information on the availability and suitability of animals to meet those needs. The needs may be summed up in the need for *control* of the microbial variable in order to enhance the precision, sensitivity, and consistency of studies dealing with aging and immunity.

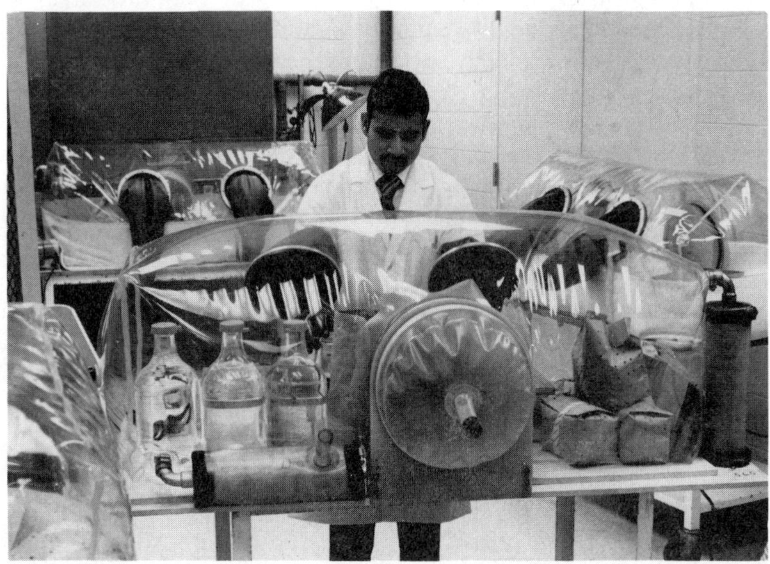

FIGURE 1. A typical flexible film plastic isolator, showing the rubber gloves attached to the plastic wall, the 30 cm diameter entry port for supplies (facing the viewer), the inlet and outlet air filters made of glass wool surrounded by a plastic shroud, and supplies of water, diet, and bedding stored inside the isolator.

THE CONTROL OF INFECTIONS

Prevention of Deaths From Infection to Provide Adequate Numbers Reaching Old Age

Preventing Entry of Outside Pathogens

The adventitious nature of infectious disease in the open animal colony; the fact that it measures not only possible immune decline, but also the size of the infecting dose, and the possibility of prior exposure to the pathogen, make the incidence and severity of spontaneous infection a singularly unpredictable, unreproducible, highly variable measure of immune potential. Some highly virulent pathogens, e.g., Sendai virus,[12] hepatitis virus,[13] and Salmonella,[14] introduced from the outside during an aging experiment can decimate colonies of susceptible strains with little relation to the general state of their immune potential. Against the entry of such virulent pathogens, strict sanitation, and the fact that most animals in animal facilities now originate as SPF animals, have formed the major barriers. In the absence of absolute barriers, however, the entry of such pathogens remains a statistical risk, and the cost of such a risk must be weighed against the costs of maintaining absolute barriers during an aging study.

Preventing the Activation of Indigenous Pathogens During Aging

More relevant to most aging studies than pathogens introduced from outside, is the much greater risk of infections from the buildup of pathogens in an apparently nonpathogenic microbiota as the colony ages. Starting, perhaps, in an individual at the low end of the spectrum of immune potential, a pathogen carried throughout the experiment but never previously expressing itself by disease, may build up by transfer to produce a high exposure rate for others and to achieve a possibly increased virulence.

Under these conditions even individuals less compromised than the initial victim may be lost. A major reason for the development of SPF colonies was the elimination of just such indigenous pathogens, e.g., pneumonia virus of rats,[15] in order to make possible any kind of long-term studies.

Quantitatively at least, the greatest contribution of GF animal research to all basic research, and to long-term studies in particular, has been to provide not only the initial stock of SPF animals, but also the continuing standby source for restocking those parts of a commercial SPF colony which become accidentally contaminated with pathogens. This latter fact is eloquent witness to the superior effectiveness of the GF system in excluding pathogens and to the difficulty of excluding pathogens even in an elaborate system of partial barriers set up primarily to exclude pathogens. If exclusion is difficult in well-engineered commercial SPF animal production facilities, how much more difficult will it be for the experimenter who purchases SPF animals to start an aging colony but must maintain them in animal quarters having less effective barriers than those used for SPF production colonies?

The buildup of infectious agents in aging colonies can become a threat not only to the colony itself, but to neighboring aging colonies which might otherwise resist the pathogen(s) involved, and even a threat to neighboring breeding colonies. This was the experience of an aging experiment that utilized as controls for an aging GF colony, the pioneer SPF colony established at Lobund Laboratory in 1953.[16] A pneumococcal infection (presumably of caretaker origin) built up in the aging rat colony and invaded the nearby breeding colony.[17] Pathogen buildup in aging colonies can thus become a threat to any neighboring animals, to younger members of aging colonies, or to aging colonies subject to other variables. It could even be a threat to caretaker personnel analogous to the deliberate introduction of pathogens (see below). Even when the development of spontaneous infections is desired as a measure of natural aging, it becomes necessary to consider using the GF system to *contain* pathogens as well as to protect the aging colony itself.

Protection For and From Experimentally Introduced Pathogens

Exposure to pathogens, if desired at some point in the research as a test of integrated immune function, can be made in a controlled way within the GF system. If the pathogen is added to a GF or GN animal, response to infection by that pathogen can be monitored without the risk that it will activate some indigenous pathogen to confound the results or that it will be eliminated by the resident microbiota. The pathogenesis of the infection may, however, be different under mono- or poly-associated conditions (see section entitled "Immune Functions Altered by the Microbiota"). Possibly, a more important role of the GF system in research involving experimentally introduced pathogens is the protection of research personnel and neighboring animals from the pathogens in the aging colony. With the addition of one set of operations, the bagging of wastes, the treatment of the bag with antiseptic in the entry-exit port, and the sterile disposal of the bagged wastes, the GF system becomes an effective barrier against the *exit* of pathogens.

Safety standards for protection of personnel and of other animals in contiguous areas of a building are becoming stricter and will probably continue to do so for some time. The great expense of providing separate enclosed rooms for the study of pathogens will make far more attractive the use of the GF system to provide protection both *for* and *from* pathogens. Within the same animal room, isolators make it possible to maintain animals in any state of infectivity and any state of immune deficiency. The cost of isolator maintenance (to be discussed below) will soon seem small in comparison to the space requirements for such studies set by present and future safety standards.

Special Need for Control of Infections When Aging is Superimposed on an Experimentally Induced Immune Deficiency

The GF system's control of infections becomes essential when the object of research is to prolong into old age an experimentally induced severe immune deficiency. GF systems (or incomplete barrier systems as long as they remain effective) have made possible long-term survival of neonatally thymectomized mice,[18] nude mice,[19] mice which have received whole body irradiation followed by allogeneic bone marrow transplants,[20,21] and mice given high doses of cytotoxic drugs or antilymphocyte serum.[22] Under CV or even SPF conditions, mice subjected to such treatment may succumb early to infections with specific opportunistic pathogens or to less specific reactions known as wasting disease, graft-vs.-host reactions, and secondary diseases. Human infants with severe combined immunodeficiency disease have been maintained for periods of years in GF isolators,[23] whereas comparable children under conventional conditions have succumbed to infection during infancy.

Delay of Other Life-Threatening Lesions Associated With the Presence of a Microflora

Experience with GF rats at Lobund Laboratory has shown not only protection against overt infections, but also protection from some other life-shortening conditions which could interfere with aging studies. With the use of present colony diet L485, the kidney and vascular lesions common in CV aging Wistar Lob (WI) rats were delayed under GF conditions.[24-26] The role of the microflora in the origin or progression of these lesions is unknown. It may not be related to pathogenicity at all in the usual sense of the word but is included here because it could be related to subclinical infection. At any rate, the delay in progression of such lesions provides an added bonus for the use of GF animals. In the case of rats, this gain more than offsets the threat to life which is peculiar to GF rodents and rabbits, enlargement[27] and occasional volvulus[28] of the cecum. This hazard is now extremely rare in GF rats on present colony diet L485.[25,26] The hazards of cecal enlargement to aging mice are largely affected by diet and by strain of mouse. This will be discussed below in detail.

GF rats and mice have not shown the decline in circulating thyroid hormones which is found in CV controls at 12 to 24 months of age.[29] When the goal of aging and immunity research is to follow the immune system for as long as possible, and to correlate it with the intrinsic decline of other systems, the GF animal offers an unusual opportunity to prolong the health of other body systems. It can do this without resort to the other frequently used treatments such as early underfeeding[30,31] which could affect many other systems besides the immune system. Comparison and possible combination of these two treatments could offer new insights into the mechanisms of aging and immune decline. Other characteristics of GF rodents, to be discussed below, may affect the aging process. The user of GF animals must be aware of these characteristics in order to interpret his results.

Inadequacy of Partial Barrier Systems in Aging Studies to Prevent Two-Way Transfer of Microbes

Incomplete and small-scale barrier systems may decrease the incidence of pathogen transfer but as long as they cannot totally exclude transfer, they become the potential source of a high degree of variability in the condition of the experimental animals. A filter cap colony of C3H mice, derived from a GF colony 2½ years earlier and provided sterile diet, water, and bedding in cages sterilized at each bedding change, were remarkable for their freedom from parasites such as pinworms and protozoa, which were carried by animals in other rooms of the same buiding. Even fecal streptococci were not visibly evident in fecal and cecal smears. Nevertheless, over a further 12-

month period, trichomonads appeared in 52% of cages, pinworms in 53%, and fecal streptococci in all.[32] If these had been lethal pathogens or had seriously affected some immune parameter being studied, the sporadic character of their occurrence would have made the results so variable as to compromise the meaning and statistical significance of the results obtained. Thus, partially effective barriers create their own special hazards. Against the hazards of sporadic entry of adventitious, indigenous, and opportunistic pathogens, the GF and GN animals are fully protected, and BOR animals are protected against the entry of pathogens after isolation has been established.

THE CONTROL OF MICROBIAL INFLUENCE ON THE IMMUNE SYSTEM

Regardless of whether they cause overt infection, the microbial associates of an animal constitute a major influence on the level of functioning of the immune system. Evidence to this effect, from both GF and nonGF research, will be presented below to substantiate what we intuitively assume. Unless we would further assume, *a priori,* that the immune *potential* of an animal is intrinsically determined, in no way affected by its level of functioning, and in no way capable of disuse atrophy or overuse exhaustion, or optimal use maintenance, we must consider the possibility and probability that the timing and level of immune activation during life will affect the level of immune potential available for meeting challenges in later life. In determining whether this is true and, if so, in what respects, the GF animal must play an essential role.

Intuitively we assume that microbes *stimulate* the overall function of the immune system. We expect an increase of some immune indexes during infections, e.g., circulating immune globulin, circulating WBC. Even husbandry conditions which merely increased an already existing exposure to microbes without causing overt disease, the "dirty colony" conditions described by Makinodan et al.,[33] stimulated a higher peak of primary plaque-forming cell response to sheep red blood cells than occurred in mice with "clean" water and bedding. However, the rate of decline from this peak was also faster in the "dirty" colony, suggesting the possibility of an "exhausting" effect produced by chronic microbial stimulation. The exhausting effect could also occur in comparisons of aged GF animals with those carrying microbial associates, though it has not yet been adequately tested in any kind of system. In other words, the very stimulatory effect which is revealed by higher levels of immune functioning in young animals exposed to microbes might reveal itself in older microbially associated animals by decreased levels of immune function (compared to GF). Therefore, an aging experiment which tested immune function only at the end of the experiment might miss or misinterpret the actual course of events and the role played by the microbiota.

Another danger of misinterpretation arises from the fact that some members of the microbiota can have a *depressing* effect on immune function. Sendai virus infection of CV mice created a deficit in 55 of 63 immune indexes which lasted up to 8 months after apparent recovery from the acute phase of infection.[34] Unless detected, the effect of such an infection can invalidate studies in aging and immunity.

A further complication of interpreting data from aging and immunity studies arises from the fact that some activities of the immune system, e.g., autoimmune reactions, increase with age in SPF or CV animals, at the very time that other functions are decreasing.[35] This reciprocity could be interpreted as a decline in immune *control* mechanisms, allowing some functions to become hyperactive. Another possibility however is that immune decline has permitted increased exposure of body cells to infections by intracellular parasites, e.g., viruses, and thereby increased the risk of stimulating antibodies against cellular components.[35] The GF animal protected from such infections, and the GF antigen-free (GF-CD) animal would provide a useful model for determining the cause of those autoimmune phenomena which are associated with aging.

In determining the usefulness of the GF animal for aging and immunity studies, the reader is referred to the chapter on "Immunological Responsiveness and Aging Phenomena in Germfree Mice," in *Immunology and Aging*.[36]

The review article summarizes the immune responses of germfree mice in general. Most of these data were obtained in mice of the young adult stage by many different investigators. The article describes two aging experiments in which GF and CV animals were compared primarily in terms of long-term survival and in the incidence of specific lesions.[37-39] The authors then give details and data from an aging experiment they themselves conducted in which indexes of immune function at various ages, as well as survival data, were used to compare GF and SPF colonies.[40,41] In addition to briefly summarizing their findings and their summaries, I shall summarize data from a recent report on aging in GF and CV SJL/J mice,[42] data from continuing reports on senescence in GF rats at Lobund Laboratory,[25,26,43,44] and data from our laboratory, both published[45-47] and unpublished,[48] which demonstrate the role of diet in affecting the immune response of GF animals over time. It is not surprising that diet should affect immune functioning in GF animals or that reduction of dietary antigens should diminish *ongoing* immune activity. What is surprising is that, in the absence of microbes, some diets can stimulate total γ-globulin or total circulating WBC beyond the levels found in CV animals fed normal diets.[49]

In the following summary of immunological differences between GF and SPF or CV animals, it is necessary to realize that GF rats are free of all demonstrable microbial associates,[24] but that the mice we continue by force of inertia to call germfree, all carry a leukemogenic virus which produces leukemia spontaneously in AKR mice but produces leukemia in other strains only after they have been subjected to repeated low doses of X-irradiation.[50] All 18 strains of mice tested so far carry the C type particles and the leukemogenic potential, and transmit them *vertically* so that the derivation of GF mice by caesarian section does not eliminate them. In its latent form, the virus presumably has little effect on the immune system, since GF-antigen free mice show very low levels of γ-globulin and ongoing immune function.[47] However, until we can free the GF mouse from its viral associate, we cannot say absolutely what its effect on the immune system or on aging is. For this reason the GF rat would be preferable for aging and immunity studies, but because the mouse seems to be a better model for human responses than is the rat, most studies of immune function in GF animals, as in other animals, have employed the mouse. The GF piglet is an extraordinarily useful animal for studying basic immunology, because the piglet is born with no circulating γ-globulins, and it is possible to formulate diets free of specific antigens in order to study true primary response.[51] Nevertheless, the GF pig is not likely to be used for aging studies because of its size and longevity and will not be considered here. Even the guinea pig is too long-lived to be a likely candidate for aging studies.

Immune Functions Altered by the Microbiota

I. Morphological Development of Lymphoid Organs
   A. GF mice have smaller spleens, lymph nodes, and Peyer's patches.[52-54]
   B. Thymus weight shows no consistent pattern of differences,[40,52,55] but the GF thymus shows less mitotic activity and DNA uptake.[56-58]
   C. GF lymphoid organs show few germinal centers,[52] few pyroninophilic blast and plasma cells,[54] and fewer lymphocytes in general.[54]

II. Background Levels of Immune Function
   A. Total and differential WBC counts are fairly similar in young adult Lo-

bund Carworth Farms Webster (CFW) mice, being more affected by diet (see below) than by microbial status.[47] In the study of Anderson et al.,[40] the total WBC and lymphocyte counts rose with age in GF but declined with age in SPF barrier-maintained mice.

B. Circulating γ-globulins are reduced in GF mice,[47] rats,[47] and guinea pigs,[49] with rare exceptions due to diet.[49]

III. Immune Responses to Challenge

A. GF mice may show a delay in clearance and in intrafollicular localization of some intravenously injected antigens.[60]

B. GF mice often show delayed intracellular degradation of antigens.[61,62]

C. GF chickens responding to human γ-globulin show a slower rise and lower peak of antibody production, but a slower rate of decline so that the overall response is comparable.[63] GF mice showed a less pronounced difference from CV mice in their response.[64]

D. A general tendency to delayed antibody response by GF mice was observed.[64] Later studies related this to delays in clearance and macrophage processing[65] rather than to any impairment of T- and B-cell cooperation. Also implicated, however, were the smaller populations of lymphocytes available in lymphoid organs at the time of challenge.[59] Slower antigen processing could account for the more prolonged peak seen in the GF chicken.[63]

E. Rejection of organ and tumor grafts is normal in GF mice.[66]

F. In contrast to CV mice, neonatally thymectomized GF mice do not develop wasting disease.[18,55] The GF show impaired response to sheep RBC and delayed rejection of skin grafts, but the GF impairment is less than that of neonatally thymectomized CV mice. The ability of GF mice to survive neonatal thymectomy in good health as long as they are kept GF would make them an excellent model for studying the role of the thymus in aging, as Burnett pointed out in 1970.[67]

G. Graft-vs.-host (GVH) disease in whole-body irradiated, allogeneic bone marrow-reconstituted chimeras is minimal in GF animals or bacterially decontaminated animals as long as they are GF.[20,21,68] It is lethal in virtually 100% of CV or SPF mice. This dramatic difference has made it possible to cure GF mice with leukemia or reticulum cell sarcoma by whole body irradiation and reconstitution with allogeneic bone marrow.[21,68,69] The chimeric mice live out a normal life span as long as they remain GF. Precipitious removal from the isolator, even many months after the chimeric state was started, can result in fulminating GVH disease.

H. In GF mice fed natural ingredient (NI) diet, responses of GF spleen cells to the T-cell mitogens PHA and Con A were about 80% of CV levels at 3 and at 8 months of age. Both groups showed about a 20% decline between 3 and 8 months.[70]

I. GF guinea pigs uniformly died when moved from a GF to a CV environment. The pathogen proved to be a strain of *Clostridium perfringens* which could be controlled by antibiotics.[71] GF rats survived such conventionalization after a period of intense immune response.[72] GF C3H mice showed mortality rates correlated with age[73,74] and sex.

J. An unusual susceptibility of GF animals to accidental contamination with presumably viral monoassociates was observed in early GF studies. A fatal nervous syndrome developed in GF chicks hatched from surface-sterilized eggs produced by a particular commercial CV flock.[75] No such symptoms appeared in chicks hatched from these eggs under CV conditions. Change to another commercial source of eggs eliminated the syndrome in GF chicks. A pneumonia developed in GF guinea pigs caesarian-derived from CV mothers of a particular commercial CV colony.[76] The pneumonia did not develop in the CV guinea pigs of this CV colony, nor in GF guinea pigs caesarian derived from a different CV colony. Experimental infections of GF rats and mice with *Salmonella typhimurium*[77,78] and *Shigella* sp.[79] show different pathogenesis from that observed in CV animals. Distemper virus in GF dogs[80] and panleukopenia virus in GF cats[80] cause milder syndromes than those seen in CV controls. GF animals showed either unusual resistance or unusual susceptibility to a variety of parasites, including amoebas[81] and worms.[82] GF mice were susceptible to a human virus resisted by CV mice.[83]

The Effect of Diet on the Immune Responses of GF Animals

There is an understandable tendency to generalize about the effect of the GF state on immune responses on the assumption that the only difference between GF and CV (or SPF) animals is the presence or absence of a living microbiota. But as a result of the absence of a living microbiota, the rat or mouse fed the usual natural ingredient (NI) diet develops a number of physiological differences from the CV control: a lower resting metabolic rate, smaller heart, lungs, and liver, greatly increased cecal size, lower peristaltic rate, slower turnover of intestinal mucosal cells. These will be discussed later. Although some of these characteristics could affect immune function indirectly, nothing is yet known of this possibility, and we will not deal with it here except to say that these characteristics, usually ascribed to the GF state as such, can themselves be modified by diet. What concerns us here is the fact that dietary ingredients which have little effect on immune function in CV animals can have profound effects on the GF animal, perhaps because of decreased degradation, prolonged retention, increased absorption, etc. in the GF gut.

I. Effect of Natural Ingredient (NI) Diets
   A. Gamma globulin in GF guinea pigs fed casein-based diets was higher than in the usual CV animals.[49]
   B. One NI diet prevented death and severe disease in GF rats monoassociated with *Salmonella typhimurium* while another diet provided little protection.[77] The nonprotective diet caused a doubling of circulating WBC in both GF and CV mice before challenge.[47]
   C. Direct PFC responses to SRBC in GF mice fed the standard Lobund NI diet in autoclaved form are twice as high as in mice fed the same diet sterilized by irradiation.[48]

II. Effect of Chemically Defined Diet
   A. Circulating γ-globulin levels were undetectable by immunoelectrophoresis in GF mice fed a chemically defined (CD), water-soluble, membrane filtered (0.20 μm pore size) diet consisting of purified amino acids, glucose, vitamins, minerals, and lipids.[46,47] However, after a year, low but detectable IgG levels appeared.[47] When the diet was further purified by passage through an ultrafilter with 10,000 mol wt cut-off, the IgG lines did not appear over time.[47]
   B. By radial immunodiffusion assay, GF C3H mice at Lobund Laboratory fed ultrafiltered CD diet as above, had barely detectable IgG levels, but

IgM levels only slightly below normal.[70] In Japanese studies with the same diet fed to the Jcl:(ICR) mouse strain, IgG levels were 1/10 those in GF mice fed NI diet and 1/100 those in SPF mice. IgM levels were 1/5 those of either GF or SPF mice fed natural diet; IgA could not be detected in serum or intestinal wall of GF mice fed either diet.[84]

C. Circulating WBC in GF mice fed NI diet were little reduced from CV levels, but GF-CD levels were half those seen in either GF or CV mice.[47,84]

D. Despite low levels of ongoing immune function, GF-CD mice responded to sheep RBC injection with direct PFC counts as high as, and possibly higher than those in CV mice or GF mice fed NI diet.[48]

E. Although displaying a very low level of ^{3}H thymidine uptake in nonstimulated spleen cells, the GF-CD mice responded to PHA and Con A stimulation with uptakes which were equivalent to those of GF mice fed NI diet and about 80% of the CV uptake.[70]

The Problem of Closed Formula Diets

The effects of diet on immune function and their possible amplification under GF conditions, raise an important consideration about the use of commercial diets. Several of the commercial diets prepared especially for GF animals by supplementation with heat-labile vitamins are closed formula diets, that is, the manufacturer guarantees the diet's content of protein, fat, minerals, and vitamins, but may vary the sources of these according to market availability. Yet the *type* of protein in the diet can have important physiological, nutritional, and immunological consequences for the GF animal. Open formula (published composition) diets such as L485[85] used at Lobund Laboratory (Table 1) may still vary because some qualities of wheat or corn vary from batch to batch, but the large differences for GF animals that might result from changing, for example, casein to fish meal or soy protein, are not going to occur. Maximum definition and standardization depend on the use of a chemically defined diet.

Effects of the Microbiota on Immune Changes During Aging

I. Survival as the Measure

A. The initial studies on GF aging by Gordon et al.[37,38] showed that GF mice outlived CV controls, and GF males outlived females, reversing the common pattern. However, the CV mice died earlier than expected for that strain, mostly from infections, and the GF mice suffered from a high incidence of cecal volvulus and intestinal atonia on the diets then in use. In vitro indexes of immune function were not monitored.

B. The second extensive study of aging in GF (ICR) mice, both with and without the stress of radiation, found little difference in survival between GF and CV mice, even when mice dying of cecal volvulus were omitted from the GF sample.[39] The investigators concluded that the presence of a microbiota alters aging processes and late somatic effects of radiation very little.

C. A comparison of GF and CV SJL/J mice during aging noted that the only difference in survival was caused by cecal volvulus among the GF mice.[42]

D. A study comparing survival of GF athymic and C3H mice did not compare them with CV controls, but survival of *some* athymic nude mice to more than 1000 days indicates the potential usefulness of GF isolation for immunologically compromised experimental animals. This survival revealed that the athymic mice had a much greater risk of developing

Table 1
AUTOCLAVABLE DIET L485 FOR GERMFREE RATS AND MICE

	% of diet
Ground corn meal	58.96
50% Protein soybean oil meal	30.0
17% Protein alfalfa meal	3.5
Corn oil (once refined)	3.0
NaCl (iodized)	1.0
Dicalcium phosphate	1.0
$CaCO_3$	0.5
L-lysine (feed grade)	0.5
DL-methionine (feed grade)	0.5
Butylated hydroxytoluene	0.0125
Vitamin premix[a]	1.0
Trace mineral premix[b]	0.025

[a]The 1.0 g of vitamin premix contains:

Retinyl palmitate IU	2646
Cholecalciferol, IU	101.4
α-Tocopheryl acetate, mg	22.1
Vitamin K_3 (menadione sodium bisulfite), mg	8.8
P-Aminobenzoic acid, mg	5.1
Calcium pantothenate, mg	28.7
Choline chloride, mg	198.4
Folic acid, mg	1.1
Niacin, mg	6.6
Pyridoxine HCl (Vitamin B-6), mg	2.2
Riboflavin, mg	3.1
Thiamin NO_3, mg	6.6
Vitamin B-12 mix (0.1% trituration), mg	0.45

[b]The 0.025 g of trace mineral premix contains:

Element	mg element	Salt used as source
Mn	6.6	Manganous oxide
Fe	2.2	Ferrous carbonate
Cu	0.22	Copper oxide
Co	0.066	Cobalt carbonate
I	0.132	Calcium iodate
Zn	1.5	Zinc oxide, zinc chloride

lymphoreticular neoplasms, but a reduced risk of developing solid tumors.[19]

E. Monitoring of aging GF Wistar rats at Lobund Laboratory is an ongoing operation aimed at determining causes of death.[25,26,43,44] GF rats consistently survive beyond 24 months of age when most of the CV controls have died.[44] At 24 months the GF rats show little evidence of the kidney and artery lesions seen in CV rats at that time. Survival of the GF rats past 30 months of age permits the development of many tumors: nine prostate tumors (unusual in rats), and a very high incidence of hepatomas.[44] Monitoring of a small sample of aged discarded GF breeders in rat colonies at Hannover has revealed an unusually increased incidence and variety of endocrine-related tumors compared to CV animals.[86]

F. Older GF guinea pigs[71] and mice[73,74] are much more susceptible to fatal infection following movement to a CV colony than are younger animals.

II. Immune Indexes in Aging GF Mice

A. The studies of Anderson et al.[40,41] compared survival and a number of immune indexes in GF and CV mice of the Charles River CD-1 line. Their findings are summarized below.

1. The survival of GF mice was less than that of SPF mice maintained in an isolator environment similar to that employed for the GF mice.
2. GF mice had fewer neoplasms (31% vs. 51%) but developed them earlier.
3. In the SPF controls, the total leukocyte count and especially the absolute lymphocyte count in the blood declined dramatically between 42 and 522 days of age. In GF mice, however, both measures increased fourfold.
4. γ-Globulin levels of GF mice were always below those of SPF mice but neither group showed a consistent pattern of age-related changes.
5. Amyloidosis occurred to a significant extent in 56% of 86 GF mice, 9% of 88 SPF mice.[87] This finding agrees with the more limited data of Walburg and Cosgrove,[39] who found amyloidosis in 5 of 15 GF mice and in none of 13 CV mice examined for it. Since amyloidosis has been previously associated with antigenic challenge in the presence of a generally hyporeactive immune system,[35] it may be necessary to determine if dietary antigen may be playing an exaggerated role in the GF animal. Bovine milk proteins represent one of the agents used to induce experimental amyloidosis. These may be unusually stimulating under GF conditions, as noted in GF guinea pigs and mice (above).[47]

B. Immune indexes in aging GF or CV SJL/J mice.[42]

Inbred SJL/J mice have a high incidence of reticulum cell sarcoma and reduced life span. GF and CV mice of this strain were compared at 2-month intervals from 4 to 14 months of age for plaque-forming cell (PFC) responses to sheep red blood cells (SRBC), total and differential blood leukocyte counts, serum proteins, circulating IgM and IgG_1, and histological appearance of lymphoid organs. Differences between GF and CV mice were minor compared to immune differences brought about by the developing sarcomas. Most GF SJL/J mice aged 2 to 8 months showed germinal centers in Peyer's patches, contrary to usual observations in other GF strains. Both GF and CV mice showed severe depression of IgG_1 response with advancing age, and a lesser depression of IgM response. The peak of indirect PFC response shifted from day four to day five with advancing age in both GF and CV mice. A few GF mice, but no CV mice, showed IgM responses at 12 to 14 months which equaled or exceeded the average 4 month responses.[42]

C. Immune changes with age in GF mice fed either irradiated natural ingredient diet L485 or CD diet are currently under investigation at Lobund Laboratory. CV and GF C3H/He mice fed natural diet have been carried to 18 months and GF-CD mice to 8 months. Preliminary results (Table 2) show that mitogen responses to PHA and Con A, by GF-L-485 and GF-CD diet mice, while initially only 80% of CV levels, decline with age at the same rate, reaching about 80% of 3 months levels by 8 months and 50% of 3 month levels by 18 months.[70] Stimulation by LPS pro-

Table 2
PHYTOHEMAGGLUTININ RESPONSE AND THYMUS WEIGHTS IN MALE C3H/HeCr MICE AS AFFECTED BY AGE AND MICROBIAL STATUS

Age (months)	Status	PHA response[a] (counts × 10^{-3})	Thymus weight (mg/100 g body weight)
3	CV	203	105
	GF	171[c]	93
8	CV	167[d]	48[d]
	GF	137[c,d]	48[d]
18	CV	109[d,e]	14[d,e]
	GF[b]	94[d,e]	16[d,e]

Note: All mice were fed autoclaved NI diet L485. Mitogen response is expressed in counts × 10^{-3} for 5 × 10^5 spleen cells and 0.5 μg ^{3}H thymidine per well.

[a] Preliminary data. See Reference 70.
[b] This group was accidentally contaminated during the 18th month with a Gram-positive rod that grew only sparsely in the gut.
[c] Significantly different from comparable CV group.
[d] Significantly different from 3 month value.
[e] Significantly different from 8 month value.

duced the lowest responses in CV mice but there was no clear pattern of decline with age in any group. Thymus weights (Table 2) were comparable among the groups at 3 months and declined equally with age to about 50% of 3 month levels at 8 months, and 15% of 3 month levels by 18 months.[70] PFC responses to SRBC had declined by 18 months in CV mice but varied in GF mice from no response to a very high response.

Effect of Partial Barriers on Microbiota Changes During Aging

An interesting sidelight of these investigations is that a line of formerly GF mice maintained under filter caps with sterilized natural food and bedding had circulating γ-globulin levels very close to those of GF mice fed natural diet (20 to 60 mg %)[70] and considerably lower than those found in C3H/He mice kept in the open animal room (200 to 600 mg %). This suggests the possibility that much of the ongoing immune response in CV or SPF mice is a response to certain specific members of the microbiota, rather than a cumulative effect of all of them. It further suggests the possibility of developing defined microbiotas that would normalize the physiological parameters of the animals while greatly reducing the effects of the microbiota on the immune system.

Summary

Effects of the GF state on the immune response show drastic effects on ongoing immune function, but little effect on immune potential (measured by response to challenge) except as a delay probably involving both slower antigen processing and a reduced population of cells ready to be activated. This is reassuring for the usefulness of both CV and GF animals in immunological studies, for it indicates that most CV studies of the past have not been vitiated by unusual immunological effects of microbial associates, and that GF animals can maintain an immune potential comparable to that of CV animals despite a chronically lower level of antigenic-mitogenic stimulation and of ongoing immune response. This means that the special advantages of the GF and GN animal for prevention of infection and for precise control of antigenic-mitogenic stimulation can be fully exploited.

When we consider that the processes of cecal detention and coprophagy in the CV rat or mouse expose it to much more of microbes and microbial products than the human analogue is exposed to, we can well ask if the CV or even SPF animal is a fair model of the type of stimulation which the human being receives from its human microflora (see below). Even when given a human type microflora, the rodent will be much more exposed to it and its activity than a human being would. Perhaps we need all three animal models, i.e., GF, GN (human type microflora), and SPF (rodent flora) to gain an idea of the spectrum of possibilities into which the human analogue may somewhere fit.

CONTROL OF NUTRITION UNDER GF CONDITIONS

Underfeeding early in life or throughout life is now under investigation as a major means for prolonging life[30,31,88] and slowing the rate of immune decline.[89-91] Underfeeding of certain kinds of nutrients can differentially affect the functioning of the cell-mediated or humoral components of the immune system.[92] Immune aging might also be affected by physiological changes. Both underfeeding and GF status affect the resting metabolic rate of rats and mice. Within the GF state, the metabolic rate can be varied from below CV to above CV by changing from NI to CD diet.[93]

It is therefore important to be able to accurately assess an animal's intake of important nutrients. The microbiota of an animal can have a number of significant effects on ingested nutrients, destroying them, sequestering them, altering their digestion and/or absorption. These effects are difficult to estimate unless the GF animal is used. Furthermore, the microbiota undergoes some variation with age and may have different effects in later life. Underfeeding or overfeeding and changes in nutrient proportion or digestibility may themselves alter the microbiota,[94] since these regimens may alter the amount of residues available in the lower gut for microbial action.

The use of GF animals could help explain the mechanism(s) by which underfeeding delays aging and immune decline. Both GF status and underfeeding delay the early activation of the immune system. These observations raise several important questions. Does underfeeding limit the ability of the young animal to respond to challenge, and thereby delay activation? Does underfeeding change the microbiota to a less immunogenic type? Would effects of GF status and underfeeding be additive, both on the delay in early activation and on the rate of immune decline? Does underfeeding produce its effects by changing the basal metabolic rate? Does underfeeding merely reduce the exposure to some harmful trace contaminant of diets, one that may also be affected by the microbiota? Is underfeeding merely a chronic stressor? The GF and especially the GF-CD animal could provide models to test these hypotheses.

The effects of the microbiota can be much more pronounced in rodent models than in man because the rodent has specialized the cecum for prolonged retention of food residues and their fermentation by bacteria. The bacterial products, whether nutritional and/or immunogenic, are made more available to the rodent by way of coprophagy. Usually about 20%, but as much as 80% of feces may be recycled this way.[1] Since the human being lacks both of these adaptations to maximize the contributions of the microbiota, the CV rodent may actually be a poorer model for estimating human effects of different diets than is the GF rodent, although each would have its limitations.

Effects of Microflora on Nutrients Available for Absorption

Studies made in antibiotic-treated or GF animals have established a number of ways in which the microbiota can affect the actual intake of nutrients available for metabolism.

Microbes provide nutrients — Classical cases are vitamin K, vitamin B-12, folic acid and biotin.[95,96] Actual intakes of these and other B vitamins by the host cannot be calculated from the dietary content.

Microbes compete with the host for nutrients — GF studies showed 50% more lysine available to the GF than to the CV rodent from the same diet.[97] When amino acids are being manipulated for differential effects on immune function, this phenomenon needs to be kept in mind.[92]

Microbes affect the absorption of nutrients — Passive absorption is generally better in GF than CV rats.[98] Some histological changes in the gut wall during aging appear to be mediated by the microbiota.[53] If these affect absorption they could account, in part, for the reduced absorption of nutrients by the aged.

Microbes affect the nutritional quality of diets during storage — For example, the chemically defined, water-soluble diet is an excellent culture medium, especially for yeasts. If the CD diet is left in feeding bottles for CV animals more than 1 day, growth of yeasts may affect diet composition. By producing gas, yeasts may also drive the diet out of the bottles before it can be consumed. Some semisynthetic diets fed in moist or agar gel form must be replenished daily under CV conditions.

Side Effect of GF System in Controlling Airborne Particulates

The GF barrier system, as an added bonus, provides control of airborne particulate materials.

Trace minerals — The discoverer of the essentiality of selenium,[99] finds the GF *system* essential for studies of trace mineral requirements.

Airborne toxicants and carcinogens — When these are themselves particles or are adsorbed on particles, or are adsorbable onto glass wool filter materials, they can be removed by the GF system.

The existence of both these possibilities creates the need for isolator controls in studies that might be affected by trace nutrients or toxicants even when control of the microflora is not being considered. Investigators using the barrier system for this purpose should be aware of possible changes in the microflora or in husbandry requirements [see section entitled "Use of the Absolute Barrier System to Control Undefined Microbiotas (SPF or CV)"].

SPECIAL CONSIDERATIONS FOR THE USE OF THE GF SYSTEM IN AGING AND IMMUNITY STUDIES

The Germfree System

As noted in the introduction, the general technology for the use of the GF system has been summarized in an earlier article[11] with references provided for the full details of each use. Basic to all of these uses is the GF *system,* a set of absolute barriers against microbial entry or exit. The GF animal is valuable in itself for studies of aging and immunity, as the preceding discussion has revealed. Any study, however, whether GF or not, in which absolute barriers prove useful, will be indebted to the GF animal for inspiring and testing the design of such systems.

The GF Animal as a Test of the GF System

Suprisingly, this is the function of GF animals which first inspired Professor James

A. Reyniers to develop them.[5] His first interest was in micrurgy, in what it could reveal about the bacteria which underwent transitions from smooth to rough or mucoid colony types. If he could set up his micrurgical apparatus behind absolute barriers, he could carry on complex micrurgical operations without having to worry about microbes getting in from outside. The GF animal, as a combination vacuum cleaner and living culture medium, would provide the most dependable test of the impermeability of the barrier system. However, the challenge of the GF animal in its own right, with its problems and its possibilities, soon overshadowed its role as an adjunct to micrurgy, and became the raison d'être of Lobund Laboratory, the only laboratory continuously devoted, since 1930, to developing, characterizing, and using the GF animal as a research tool. Yet for Professor P. C. Trexler, who joined Professor Reyniers in 1932 and is the developer of the plastic flexible film isolator,[7] the major use of the GF animal may yet be as a test for the integrity of newly developed barrier systems. Regardless of whether the barriers are designed to keep microbes in or out, the GF animal is still the most sensitive indicator of absolute barriers, since it is easier to test a small enclosed space than a large heterogenous "outdoors" for breaks in the integrity of the barrier system. This will make possible continued development of the GF system in the direction of greater simplicity, economy, and convenience. Thus, the GF system will have come full circle to Professor Reyniers' original intention.

The Spectrum of Uses for the GF System

The GF system, developed for and tested by GF animals, opens up possibilities in two directions: (1) increasing the control and definition of an animal's environment, to make the environment not only GF but also free of antigens, mitogens, toxicants, carcinogens, with the possibility of adding any of these to the system in a defined way. These various defined animal models will be discussed in detail below in terms of their use for aging and immunity studies, (2) increasing the stability and reproducibility of animal models not totally defined in terms of their microbiota, but chosen for their usefulness in the past with the hope of maintaining that usefulness in the future. This is a hope only partially attainable by the SPF animal because it is protected by only partial barriers. For most users of SPF animals, the whole elaborate system of SPF barriers is too expensive and space-consuming to maintain after they receive the animals from the supplier. Yet in aging studies, the chance of major change in the SPF microbiota during the course of the experiment is greatly increased by the length of exposure.

Use of the Absolute Barrier System to Control Undefined Microbiotas (SPF or CV)

Problems with Partial Barriers

The very simplicity of some SPF microbiotas, the possibility that some components may have a completely adventitious origin, e.g., from human caretakers, invites the establishment of later adventitious species better suited to the niches in the host's internal environment. Against this latter hazard, a new strategy is being developed in terms of the "colonization-resistant" microflora, a combination of bacteria from CV animal species, not necessarily well characterized, which resists the establishment of transient microbial species.[100] This is a strategy being investigated not only for its application to animal models but for its applicability to human patients after antibiotic decontamination during a period of iatrogenic immune deficiency.

Among the various kinds of partial barriers, well-designed and well-managed laminar flow systems have shown their ability to maintain animals GF for periods of weeks.[101] They have proved especially useful for antibiotic decontamination experiments in which there must be frequent replacement of cages to keep reducing the residual load of microbes. Their success in protecting immunologically compromised human patients from dangerous infections has shown their potential.[102] The laminar airflow protects each cage not only from outside contaminants but also from cross-contamination with microbes from other cages in the same apparatus.[101] In very long-term studies, individual cages might develop different microfloras as a result of accidental additions or deletions, unless the care and feeding of the animals provides sufficient opportunity for cross-contamination.

In contrast to the partial physical barriers available in the usual animal facility and the partial microbial barriers maintained by a colonization-resistant microflora, the GF system offers absolute barriers. Breaks in the barriers do occur, but only as a result of accident. The "holes" are not normally there. For investigators who have so generally accepted the value of the SPF animal while lacking the facilities to keep animals SPF for very long, the GF system ought to seem like the system of choice for long-term studies even with SPF animals. Yet the cost of maintaining a GF system, in terms of floor space, equipment, and caretaker time, has been a major obstacle. The GF system is obviously essential for the GF or GN animal. It is obviously not essential for CV or SPF animals. But a major theoretical obstacle to its use for undefined microfloras has been the concept of the "locked flora".

The Problem of the Microflora Locked Behind Absolute Barriers

Early Studies with GF Animals at Lobund Laboratory

Control animals for the GF animals in early experiments were brought from the CV colony into a metal isolator like that housing GF animals. From that point on, they had no further contact with outside microbes. All supplies and air were sterilized as for GF animals. Under these conditions, the CV animals lost weight and developed diarrheal syndromes.[103] Some died within weeks of their entry into the system. Their gut flora contained only a few very predominant species by that time. The symptoms could be prevented by use of a "visitor", a CV rat fresh from the CV colony. If a new visitor was introduced into the animal's cage each week, the permanent resident no longer displayed the "locked flora" effect. These results led to the concept that the microbiota of a small group of isolated animals would simplify over time, that it took the constant intercommunication of microbes within a large colony of animals to maintain the full complement of what we call the normal flora.[104] Such simplification would not in theory be always harmful, but in the cases observed, the residual flora was in fact pathogenic, and it seemed possible that such would be the usual direction of evolution of a locked flora.

Increased Husbandry Requirements for Locked Flora Animals

Within the next several years, the locked flora effect turned out to be a misnomer for inadequate husbandry. GF animals need less frequent bedding changes than CV animals because their wastes do not produce NH_3, H_2S or other noxious odors. In the early days of GF research, with GF space at a premium, the GF animals were often overcrowded.[105] Crowding stress could not reveal itself by infection and death in the GF animals, but it did reveal itself later when adrenals were found enlarged and thymuses atrophied by comparison with open animal room stock of the same age.[105] When CV animals brought into GF isolators were maintained like the GF, that is, in crowded, and infrequently cleaned cages, they developed the pathogenic "locked flora" effect. When CV animals brought into GF isolators were given more room and were given more frequent bedding changes than either GF or open animal room animals (to make up for reduced air movement within the isolator) they showed none of the gross "locked flora" symptoms.[106]

The "locked flora" concept was thus very useful in calling attention to the added burden of husbandry required by microbially associated animals which are kept in a GF system. However, the concept has remained in the minds of investigators as a nagging worry about the advisability of keeping CV or SPF animals in the GF system for long periods of time. The possibility of microflora simplification seems a real one, comparable to the possibility of genetic drift in small populations. Even if the microflora did not simplify to harmful combinations, it might simplify to different combinations in different isolators, leading to increased variability within the total population under study. Such variability caused by random losses of microbial species would be the analogue of the variability caused by random gains in CV, SPF, or filter cap colonies.

Data on Microflora Simplification Over Time

Several studies have been addressed specifically to the question of flora simplification over time. Pesti and Gordon[106] compared the cecal microfloras of 4- and 24-month-old ICR mice kept either in an open colony room or in a germfree system. The 4-month-old mice had been taken from the open colony room to isolators at 1 month of age, the 24-month-old mice at 6 months of age. A simplification of the microflora did occur, since aged isolator animals showed no counts of *E. coli,* staphylococci, enterococci, anaerobic streptococci, or clostridia, whereas these were present in aged open colony mice. Only bacteroides and aerobic lactobacilli could be cultured from the aged isolator group. These were the predominant organisms in the aged open colony group also, but in addition clostridia had risen to high levels. Since the lost elements of the microflora in isolator animals seemed more likely to include potential pathogens than the stable elements, the simplification in this experiment would appear to be in a nonpathogenic direction. Davis et al.[107] found no simplification in the microflora of beagle dogs kept in a locked environment for 2 years. The predominant genera, by several logs, were the fastidious anaerobes. The microflora remained highly diversified over the 2-year period of observation, and the major groups of microbes were qualitatively and quantitatively similar in dogs housed in the isolator or kept in the open animal room. This was also true in the third aging study with mice (see below).

Microbiota Control in the Control Animals of Previous GF Aging Experiments

The control animals for the 3 GF aging experiments noted earlier differed in their mode of housing. In the first study, the CV controls were kept in an open animal room. These mice did not live as long as the GF mice or as long as the same strain usually lives under CV conditions[37,38] (according to the literature).

The second study compared GF mice with mice maintained in a barrier facility similar to an SPF facility, and with mice kept under open animal room conditions. There was no significant difference in survival among the three groups.[39]

The third study compared GF mice with mice from a conventional colony originally caesarian-derived.[40,41] At the beginning of the aging experiment these mice were placed in isolators and maintained by GF procedures although it is not clear if the barriers maintained were absolute. In this experiment the isolator-housed CV mice outlived the GF group. The authors reported that the CV mice harbored the usual murine viruses and bacteria throughout the experiment despite their unusual housing and diet.

The Concept of the Biotoristic Animal

Microflora simplification thus appears possible but does not occur consistently and has not proved harmful since the early days of inadequate husbandry for isolator-reared CV animals. For CV or SPF animal stocks which have proved their value as experimental models, the GF system offers the possibility of stabilizing the animal-microbe ecosystem against additions from the outside. Only future experience can test the ability of such an ecosystem to maintain its variety and complexity over time. This kind of animal model, free of the disadvantages of the GF animal (see below), and free of the risk that unwanted microbes may be added to its microbiota in an open animal room, could well be the major animal model for future studies of aging and immunity. I have therefore coined a term for it to distinguish it from GN and GF animals in which the operative defining concept is one of *known* microbial associates (or none). When the operative concept to be expressed is one of *limiting* or setting boundaries to a microbiota (whether its composition is known or unknown), the suffix *(h)oristic* can be taken from the Greek noun *horos* (boundary) and the Greek verb *horizein* (to set bounds, confine). Our word "horizon" originally denoted a boundary. Thus, an animal or environment with an absolute barrier set against entry of microbes, and its biota therefore limited to what is already there, can be called biotoristic. What is essential to it is maintenance in an absolute barrier system, since only such maintenance can set absolute limits to the existing microbiota. With continued improvement of the GF system in the direction of economy and of large-scale operation to simplify husbandry, the biotoristic animal should become a much more widely used model system for aging studies and particularly studies in aging and immunity.

The GF Animal

Obtaining the GF Animal

The GF system will limit the animal to whatever microbiota it had when it entered the system. Generally, a new mammalian species or strain enters the system directly from the uterus.[108] The shell of an oviparous animal is sterilized before or during its passage into the system.[109] Whatever microbe was present and viable in utero or in ovo is still there. Antibacterial decontamination has proved effective for the elimination of bacteria and fungi from CV mice[101,110] and probably could be applied to other species, but the process does not eliminate viruses, and the chance of a virus occurring in a CV animal has proved greater than the chance of a virus occurring in utero. Nevertheless the use of antibiotic decontamination and laminar flow maintenance has made possible long-term survival of allogeneic mouse radiation chimeras.[21] Such decontamination might be the method of choice for obtaining a GF species if it should prove possible to eliminate in an adult female animal a virus which could not be eliminated in utero. But this possibility is purely speculative.

At the moment, the method of choice for obtaining GF mammals is caesarian section (hysterotomy) performed with a combined incision through the floor of the isolator and the abdominal wall of a pregnant CV or SPF female.[108] Alternatively, a hysterectomy can be performed, the uterus being lifted out whole with its openings clamped shut and passed through a germicidal trap into the isolators.[108] Inside the isolator the young are cleaned, washed with antiseptic, stimulated to breathe, and either hand-fed[111,112] or foster-suckled by mothers of an existing GF strain.

Many GF rat and mouse strains already exist in commercial colonies and at the National Institutes of Health (NIH), Lobund Laboratory, or other laboratories. These can be used directly or as foster mothers for new strains. Newborn GF guinea pigs require no foster nursing.[113] Although GF guinea pigs[113] and rabbits[114] can reproduce, they are not reared in reproducing colonies for reasons of economy, with the disadvantage to be noted below. Syrian hamsters have not yet been obtained GF. GF Mongolian gerbils can be obtained using GF mice as foster mothers, but they have not yet reproduced GF, although GN gerbils reproduce at Lobund Laboratory.

Establishing the GF or GN Pedigree

The GF mammal in the GF system is only as GF as it was in utero. A number of microbes, bacterial, viral, parasitic, are capable of passing the placental barrier. Others may even be present in egg or sperm. Nevertheless, the GF Lobund Wistar rat is indeed GF by a whole battery of microscopic, cultural, and serological tests.[24] This fact does not guarantee that every other rat colony originating by hysterotomy or hysterectomy is GF. Each new operation on a pregnant animal carries with its the risk that the young already have a microbial associate in utero or acquire one during the operation from contact with maternal blood or tissue. Every time a new species or strain is introduced into the GF system, its GF status must be established by the full battery of tests. Transplacental transmission of *Bacillus piliformis* has been shown in mice and rats.[115] One GF rat colony was found to harbor salivary gland virus.[116] A study of *Mycoplasma pulmonis* transmission across the rat placenta reported its sporadic occurrence.[117] The first dogs caesarian-delivered into the GF system at Lobund were characterized as germfree but not worm-free.[118] First generation GF guinea pigs[76] and chickens[75] have occasionally been reported to show symptoms of viral infection although no virus could be demonstrated. When the pregnant females or the eggs were obtained from a different colony, no such symptoms appeared. As noted earlier, all so-called GF mice carry a leukemogenic virus.[50] All of 18 mouse strains tested for it carried it.

For the above reasons, GF animals for experimental aging studies should come from reproducing colonies with a pedigree of tests. Only in such colonies is there time for extensive and repeated testing since the last caesarian operation. Ideally, they would come from what Professor P. C. Trexler designated an α-colony,[119] one that not only has a full pedigree of negative tests, but has never had a known break in its barrier system. In practice, however, once a pedigree has been established by extensive testing, we rely thereafter on relatively simple biweekly testing for the presence of microbial contaminants that can grow on common aerobic and anaerobic media.[9,120] Even if there has been a break in the system, e.g., a tear in a glove or envelope which was patched as soon as discovered, followed by transfer of the animals to another GF isolator, the failure of any of the ubiquitous microbes to get through the break makes it highly unlikely that rare or exotic microbes would have passed through the break.

The Genetic Pedigree

The need for establishing the microbial pedigree of a GF colony after each new caesarian-derived entry tends to limit the number of such entries. But this can affect the genetic pedigree of the animal colony itself, especially if it came from an out-bred colony.[121] Maintaining heterozygosity and genetic continuity with some CV or SPF colony calls for more frequent entries into GF, and therefore further need for extensive testing. However, commercial breeders of SPF animals keep large colonies of GF animals for restocking any SPF units which have acquired pathogens. These GF colonies have become large enough to maintain their own heterozygosity, and they retain genetic continuity with the SPF colonies by the entry of GF animals into the SPF colonies, not by bringing caesarian-derived animals into the GF colonies. For small operations, the use of inbred strains avoids much of this problem, although inbred lines can drift apart. The original GF rats and mice at Lobund Laboratory all originated from single litters, caesarian-derived from outbred matings. Yet they have maintained steady reproduction through 45 rat generations and 50 mouse generations. Genetic drift, inherent in isolated lines, is indicated by the fact that prostate tumors arising spontaneously in the Lobund Wistar line can be passed only in them, and not in other Wistar lines.[122] Hydronephrosis has appeared in some segments of two GF rat colonies and was eliminated by selection of breeders from among unaffected rats. These problems are not unique to GF colonies except insofar as they remain small.[121]

Special Characteristics of GF Rodents that May Affect Aging Studies

The reduced level of ongoing immune function in GF animals was expected and hoped for when they developed as animal models. This difference from microbially-associated animals has been outlined in previous sections. However, several other anatomical and functional differences have been noted consistently in GF rodents and rabbits. Insofar as they can affect the results of aging experiments or the interpretation of such results in the investigator who uses GF animals must be aware of these differences, and of the measure of control over them which can be achieved by dietary means or by association with known microbes.

The Enlarged Cecum

Since the first GF guinea pigs were reported in 1895,[123] cecal enlargement has been a hallmark of the GF status in GF rodents and rabbits.[27,124] Other species, chicken,[125] dog,[126] and pig,[127] have shown a change in cecal *contents* analogous to that seen in rodents and rabbits. These changes include greater fluidity,[123-127] reduced chloride concentration,[128] and increased concentration of mucoproteins or their derivatives.[129] Only in rodents and rabbits is this consistently accompanied by cecal enlargement.[124] The enlargement raises the weight of the full cecum to 5 to 20 times its size in CV or SPF controls fed the same diet. For a particular species or strain, the ratio of GF/CV cecal weights is stable, but the actual sizes are much influenced by the type of diet fed and its mode of sterilization. Diet had already been shown to vary cecal size in CV rodents over a fourfold range.[130] The same range will usually be found in the GF animals, the GF/CV ratio remaining the same. Within the GF system, however, cecal enlargement is exacerbated by stress. Subordinate guinea pig males had ceca three times as large as that of the dominant male.[113] Stressed GF mice have shown fivefold enhancement of cecal enlargement.[131] This fact needs to be considered if stress is going to be superimposed on an aging study. It seems possible that underfeeding, especially of animals housed in groups, might be a stress in this sense, but it has not yet been tested.

Effects of Cecal Enlargement or of Cecal Contents

Poor Reproduction

Development of reproducing colonies of GF animals has generally depended on developing empirically for each species a diet which reduced GF cecal size while maintaining nutritional adequacy. The first GF rabbit reproduction was obtained only after cecal ligation was used.[114] An improved diet made this operation unnecessary.[114] Poor reproduction in GF AKR mice appears related to their rapid development of severe cecal distention.[132]

Cecal Volvulus

In terms of the use of GF rats and mice in aging studies, this was in the past the most relevant hazard of GF life.[37-42] In a case of cecal volvulus, the enlarged cecum turns several times in the same direction. This can cause a constriction of various parts of the intestine. If the mesenteric vasculature is also twisted and constricted, the animal dies quickly of shock. If only the movement of chyme is blocked, the intestinal tract may fill up above the point of blockage and the animal dies several days later. Besides obvious cases of constriction of the gut and/or mesentery, very large cecal size was associated in the first GF mouse aging study with an atonia of the gut and failure of the chyme to pass through. This developed without any obvious point of constriction occurring.[37,38] Among the 80 mice studied in that investigation, 9 died with clear-cut cecal volvulus and 36 others with intestinal atonia. The diet used was L-462, a diet containing 4% lactose (as part of the 10% whole milk powder). This ingredient can cause some cecal distention even in CV mice.[130]

In the second aging experiment, 26% of the GF mice died from cecal volvulus, most of these deaths occurring in the first half of the normal life span.[39] Their diet was a closed formula commercial ration, and there is therefore no way of knowing if it contained ingredients such as lactose which would have some cecum-distending effect. In the third GF aging experiment, the GF mice were fed an autoclaved commercial natural ingredient diet, again a closed formula ration but different from the one used in the second study. The authors noted that GF mice died "on occasion" from volvulus of the cecum,[40,41] but did not give the incidence, so that it was presumably much less than in the two previous studies, although enough to affect the shape of the survival curves.

In the SJL/J aging study, the difference between GF and CV survival curves was entirely due to deaths from volvulus. Cecal size rose abruptly at 8 months, reaching 50% of body weight in some individuals.[133] In the study comparing survival of GF C3H and nude mice, volvulus occurred in 1/132 C3H mice and 9 of 114 athymic mice. These mice were fed a closed formula commercial diet.[19]

In contrast to the above, aging GF Lobund Wistar rats fed autoclaved diet L485 have shown no incidence of volvulus among 132 rats which died at an average age of 36 months.[44] It should be noted that in the GF rat, the cecal size as a percent of body weight declines with age, primarily because the adult cecal size remains steady while the body weight continues to increase even into old age. In the GF mouse[133] and guinea pig,[113] however, relative cecal size increases with age, and a greater risk of cecal volvulus might be expected. Among the GF breeding colonies of Swiss-Webster, CFW,C3H mice at Lobund Laboratory fed autoclaved diet L485, no incidence of cecal volvulus has been noted in recent years. GF C3H male mice have been fed irradiated diet L485 for 18 months without any incidence of cecal volvulus.[134] Among GF breeding colonies at the National Cancer Institute, volvulus has been observed in GF mice of the C57BL/6N, GR/N and DBA/2N strains, but not in AKR/N, C3H/HeN, BALB/CAnN, nude athymic, or NIH Swiss strains.[28] The risk of volvulus in new GF strains cannot be predicted. For all GF rat strains used at Lobund Laboratory, and for the three strains of mice just mentioned, the risk appears very low when the diet is L485.

The same cannot at the present time be said about aging GF mice fed chemically defined antigen-free diet. During the course of diet development, GF C3H female mice were maintained on CD diet up to 2½ years, when they died of multiple types of tumors,[134] but there has been a marked incidence of cecal volvulus in GF male C3H mice set aside specifically for aging studies. Out of 72 such mice, 11 (15%), died of cecal volvulus by the age of 8 months, and 5 others (7%), died of intestinal blockage by large fur balls which had moved out of the stomach.[134] Paradoxically, cecal size in 8-month-old GF-CD mice (5.4% of body weight) was less than in the 8-month-old GF mice fed L485 (8.6% of body weight) which showed no cecal volvulus.[134] Since the incidence of cecal volvulus and trichobezoars in the GF-CD breeding colony is much lower than reported above, and these mice are exposed to filter paper nesting material used by pregnant and nursing females, the effect of such fibrous material is being tested on a group of aging GF-CD mice. This material is not chemically defined, and is possibly antigenic, but if it prevents volvulus, it may enable us to determine the mechanisms involved. It is possible that GF-CD animals require a form of fiber for normal physiological functioning, but at the moment, no chemically defined, totally nonantigenic fiber is known, and something like filter paper may be the lesser of two evils. On the other hand, since death from cecal volvulus appears to be a risk largely in the first half of life,[39] those which survive the first half of life on CD diet may experience little risk thereafter and be acceptable models for the effect of minimal antigenic stimulation on immune potential during aging.

Effects of Cecal Enlargement and/or Cecal Contents on Basal Metabolism (O_2 Consumption)

In GF rats fed NI diet the MR is 20% less than in comparable CV rats, the heart and lungs are reduced in size, and blood flow to the liver is reduced 30%.[135] In GF mice, the MR and heart weight are 10 to 15% less than in CV mice fed NI diet.[93] These effects can be attributed to the characteristics of the GF cecum, because cecectomy of weanling GF rats brings these parameters into the CV range.[136] Materials have been detected in high levels in GF rodent cecal contents which make the intestinal vasculature refractory to stimulation by catecholamines so that much higher levels are required to produce the same degree of constriction.[137] In GF C3H mice fed CD diet, however, MR and heart size are actually greater than observed in either GF or CD mice fed NI diet L485.[93] As noted above, cecal enlargement in 8-month-old GF-CD mice is about 60% of what it is in GF-NI mice but this difference is obviously not equivalent to cecectomy.

The investigator doing aging studies with GF rats or mice must be aware of this difference in MR between GF and CV rats and mice fed NI diets, and the fact that the GF-CD mice have a MR above that of CV-NI mice. These differences might be exploited to help determine the role of MR changes in the delay of aging by underfeeding.

The GF rat and mouse fed NI diet show no decline in levels of circulating thyroid hormones in the age range 18 to 24 months, when the CV levels have declined to ⅔ of their 3 to 4 month levels.[29] The role of the cecum or of MR changes in this difference is presently unknown. This difference might also be exploited to elucidate the role of the thyroid in aging and immunity.

Preventing the Effects of Cecal Enlargment

Diet

It has already been demonstrated that diet has a profound effect on cecal enlargement and on its sequelae.

Cecetomy

When a diet must be chosen which is likely to cause considerable cecal enlargement or a new diet must be used whose cecal effects are unknown, then a simple and dependable procedure for cecectomy has been developed for GF rats which prevents cecal enlargement without the occurrence of any compensating colonic hypertrophy.[138] This brings MR into the CV range.[136] It would, of course, prevent cecal volvulus.

Defined Microfloras to Eliminate Cecal Enlargment and its Sequelae

Much research has gone into discovering such defined microfloras. Since the resulting animal is no longer GF, it will be discussed below under GN animals.

Quantitative Differences in Other Aspects of Anatomy or Function Between GF and CV Animals

In general, there is a slower rate of peristalsis in the GF rodent than in the CV rodent, although the amount of difference depends on the type of diet, whether semisynthetic or NI.[139,140] The feces of the GF rodent are generally softer, more fluid, less well formed than those of CV rodents but this is not a diarrhea resulting from rapid passage of chyme. Rather it represents the inability of the colon to extract sufficient water from GF cecal contents even during prolonged passage to the anus. The rate of sloughing of the GF intestinal mucosal epithelium is about ½ the CV rate.[141] There is generally more efficient passive absorption of substances by the GF gut[98] despite the fact that in some cases there is less total mucosal surface in the GF animals.[124]

In view of the immunogenicity of intestinal contents, shown by GF studies[47] and by use of specific antigens in CV animals,[142] the above characteristics of the GF gut could be significant in some types of study of aging and immunity.

Housing for GF Animals in Aging Studies

Isolators

A variety of isolator systems are available for GF animals, from room size plastic envelopes with cages on a ferris wheel assembly, to cookie jars with filter top lids used in short-term experiments.[143] They are fabricated of steel,[6,8] aluminum,[144] rigid,[145] or flexible plastic.[7] Depending on the material and the design, they can be sterilized with steam under pressure,[6] peracetic acid,[7] ethylene oxide,[39] formaldehyde vapors, and presumably by radiation. For the technical details, other publications can be consulted. The most common form of such a GF system is the flexible plastic isolator consisting of a 2 ft × 2 ft × 4 ft envelope of 0.002 in. thick vinyl film (Figure 1). A pair of arm length rubber gloves are sealed to the plastic wall opposite a 12 in. diameter cylindrical entry port made of rigid plastic, approximately 6 in. in length.

Caging Arrangements

Within this system it is possible to place 6 to 8 shoe box type plastic mouse cages 11 in. × 7 in. × 5 in., or 4 shoe box type plastic rat cages. The number will be determined by the amount of supplies stored in the isolator and the space needed for working with the animals. Frames have been devised for stacking the cages two-high in the same size isolator and nearly doubling the number of cages possible. The center must still be left open for manipulating the entry port.

Major concern in all cage arrangements within the isolator must be the provision of adequate airflow to all cages, similarity of environment for all cage positions (or rotation to make up for dissimilarity), and the ease and safety of manipulation within the isolator. Over the span of an aging experiment, arrangements of materials which carry only a small risk per day of causing a tear in glove or plastic will multiply that risk to unacceptable levels. Cages must obviously be capable of passing through the largest opening in the wall of the isolator and must be able to withstand the sterilization procedure chosen. The investigator must go over each piece of equipment and remove any burrs or sharp points which could puncture rubber or plastic. When gloves are attached to an isolator by heavy compression rings, even a blunt object which bumps the rubber glove against an edge of the compression ring can cause puncture. A rubber band cut from an inner tube and glued to the compression ring to cover its edge has been found useful in preventing such punctures.

Housing Plan for Aging and Immunity Experiments — Group vs. Individual Housing

Even though GF animals cannot die of infections from overcrowding, their immune system will be affected by any deviation from good husbandry standards (see below). A major dilemma for the planner of any aging and immunity research is group housing vs. individual housing. Group housing constitutes a stress for subordinate animals which can affect their immune responses and cause variability within the group.[146] Isolation stress also affects immune response.[147] Because individual housing had to be developed for GF-CD mice in order to be sure that each mouse received its full measured supplement of defined lipids each day, the caging designed for them may be useful for other studies of aging and immunity, especially those in which underfeeding is carried out. In the latter case, group housing could lead to great individual variation in the amount eaten, to an over rapid intake of food, and to the stress of competition for a limited food supply.

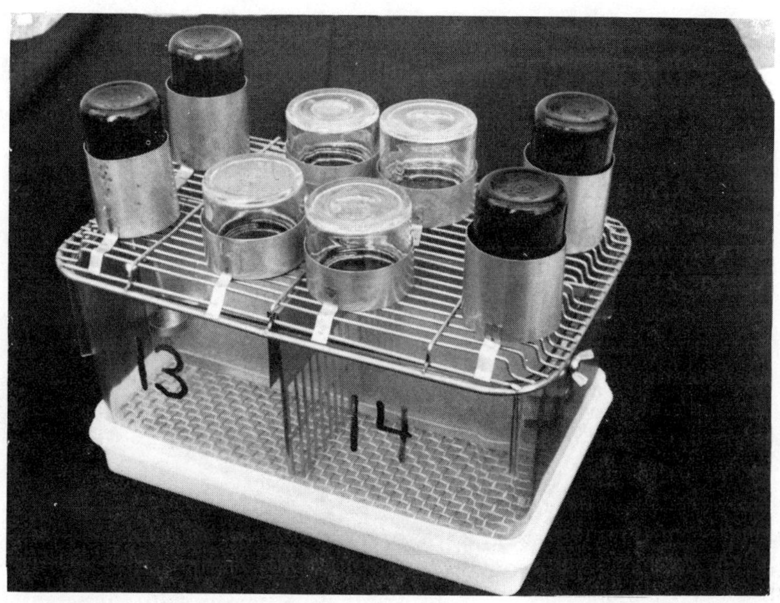

FIGURE 2. A holding cage for aging animals designed to provide individual housing with a minimum of isolation stress. Any two animals are separated only by a wire partition so that visual and tactile contact remains possible. The brown bottles are used to hold chemically defined, water-soluble diet. Holes 1.7 mm in diameter have been drilled in the plastic tops of both diet and water bottles. The small stainless steel cup welded to the solid metal divider is used for the daily measured supply of defined lipids.

To provide individual housing with minimal isolation stress for GF-CD mice a plastic shoe box cage is divided into four compartments of a size to meet minimal space requirements for one animal. The longitudinal divider is of stainless steel sheet metal. The cross-divider is made of welded wire, so that any two mice have visual and tactile contact with each other, yet neither can attack and dominate the other. This cage has been used for aging C3H male mice, both GF and CV, on both CD and NI diet (Figure 2).

Control of Noxious Agents in the Environment

Peracetic Acid

For its rapid sterilizing effect on surfaces, and convenience of use, peracetic acid is the sterilant routinely used for introducing supplies into a plastic isolator through its entry port.[7] Since peracetic acid sterilizes only surfaces and is rapidly inactivated by organic matter, materials which contain microbes where peracetic acid cannot reach them (e.g., food pellets) must be presterilized in a supply cylinder[7] or in a sealed container which has been sterilized by irradiation or ethylene oxide (which can penetrate many materials). When the entry port is opened to the inside of the isolator, vapors of peracetic acid spread to the inside of the isolator. GF rats and mice have shown no obvious effect of this periodic exposure but GF puppies showed obvious respiratory distress[148] and GF snails died from even trace amounts of peracetic acid vapor in the air.[149] Peracetic acid has been shown to be a weak cocarcinogen but a stronger promoter.[150] Periodic exposure to it over a lifetime could conceivably affect the health and pathologic experience of aging rats and mice. For this reason, three systems have been devised for removing peracetic acid fumes from entry ports. One airs out the port by diverting isolator air into the port and out another opening into a hood or neutralizing bath.[148] Another system uses a spray of sterile sodium carbonate to neutralize and inactivate the peracetic acid, since it is nonvolatile and nonstable above pH 6.5.[151] A third uses a special transfer isolator for making entries into the animal isolator.[152]

Ethylene oxide sterilization of bedding, in a retrospective study, was associated with increased neoplasms in GF mice,[153] but other experimenters have found no association. Some anticorrosion additives in central system steam supplies may be carcinogenic (e.g., morpholine). Direct steam generation in the laboratory can avoid this problem.

Husbandry of GF Animals

No changing of cages or bottles is required. A pleasant surprise is the discovery that GF animals do not require the removal, cleaning, sterilization, and replacement of cages and water bottles, thus saving one of the major burdens of conventional animal care. Bedding is merely changed when it appears wet. Adequate airflow and appropriate animal numbers per cage will minimize the number of times such changes need be made.

There is a need for protective gloves inside the isolator. A major consideration in GF aging studies is to minimize the risk of a break in the gloves or other parts of the barrier. Even if it slows down the daily care of the animals, the wearing of protective gloves over the isolator glove hands inside the isolator will help eliminate the greatest single threat to the integrity of the GF system.

Diets for GF Animals

The nutrition of GF animals has been thoroughly reviewed.[95,96] The important roles of diet in the GF rodent, not only for nutrition but for gut physiology and immune stimulation, have already been pointed out. Much experience with GF animals has already gone into determining the effects of various diets on physiology and immunology. These can serve as models for formulation of diets. At the present time it is not possible to predict precisely how a new, untried, and unusual diet will affect overall nutrition, cecal size, or immune function. It is not even possible to predict how the same diet will affect the GF animal after different modes of diet sterilization. NI diet fed to GF guinea pigs caused much more cecal distention after irradiation than after autoclaving.[154] A semisynthetic diet reacted oppositely to the two kinds of sterilization. Another NI diet caused much less cecal distention in GF guinea pigs when autoclaved as a wet mush than as a dry pellet.[113]

The most satisfactory NI diet for GF rats and mice at Lobund Laboratory has been diet L485 (Table 1).[85] It supports consistent reproduction and maintains rats to an advanced age without nephrosis or arterial lesions or cecal volvulus. A satisfactory semisynthetic diet (Table 3) has also been well tested.[155]

If it is necessary to feed aging GF animals a type of diet developed for other aging studies but never tested in GF animals, the following requirements of a GF animal diet must be kept in mind.

Essential Requirements for an Aging Colony Diet

The sterilized diet must meet nutritional requirements without any help from the microflora in producing nutrients or aiding digestion. In practice this means it must contain generous levels of all the known B vitamins. Studies with GF-CD animals have shown no requirement for still unknown nutrients produced by microbes or found only in natural foods.[156] Protein requirements are reduced by GF status.[157] Calcium is absorbed so well by GF rodents that some reduction might be needed to prevent calcification.[158,159] In GF rabbits, the *form* in which iron was presented determined its nutritional adequacy. Iron in its natural form in soybean meal was much more effective

Table 3
AUTOCLAVABLE PURIFIED DIET L474E12 FOR GERMFREE RATS AND MICE

	% of diet
Casein, vitamin free	24.0
Corn oil	3.0
LADEK 55[a]	2.0
Cellophane spangles	5.0
i-Inositol	0.1
DL-methionine	0.3
Salts L27[b]	1.0
$CaCO_3$	1.7
K_2HPO_4	1.0
Na_2HPO_4	1.0
B mix 75[c]	0.5
Rice starch	60.4

[a]The 2 g of LADEK 55 contains:

Vitamin A concentrate, natural ester	1600 IU
Vitamin D_3 (cholecalciferol)	100 IU
Vitamin E, mixed tocopherols	37.5 mg
DL-α-tocopheryl acetate	10.0 mg
Vitamin K_3 (menadione)	10.0 mg
Corn oil to 2 g	

[b]The 1.0 g of salts L27 contains (all in mg):

NaCl, iodized	515
$MgSO_4$	400
$Fe(C_6H_5O_7)_2$	60
$MnCO_3$	20
CuO	2.5
ZnO	2.5
$CoCl_2 \cdot 6H_2O$	0.05
NaF	0.01
MoO_3	0.005
KBr	0.01
Na_2SeO_3	0.01

[c]The 0.5 g of B mix 75 contains (all in mg):

Thiamine	6.0
Riboflavin	3.0
Niacinamide	5.0
Niacin	5.0
Calcium pantothenate	30.0
Choline chloride	200.0
Pyridoxine · HCl	2.0
Pyridoxamine · 2HCl	0.4
Biotin	0.1
Folic acid	1.0
p-Aminobenzoic acid	5.0
0.1% Trituration vitamin B-12 in mannitol	25.0
Rice starch carrier	217.5

than a larger amount of iron in the form of iron salts. CV rabbits obtained sufficient iron from either form.[114]

The diet must retain its nutritional adequacy *after* sterilization and storage in the isolator. In diets designed to be autoclaved, this usually means increasing thiamine to about ten times its natural content, and other B vitamins to about four times their natural content.[95] Such fortified diets are on the market as autoclavable or sterilizable diets. Although autoclaving may make part of the protein content unavailable, the generally high levels of protein in laboratory animal diets (25% protein for L485)[85] compensate for such losses.

Irradiation of diet has been extensively studied in England, where it is the rule rather than the exception. Most nutrients except oxidizable vitamins like E and A will survive irradiation better than autoclaving.[160,161] Irradiation of diets in plastic bags or in cans offers great convenience for the investigator. Bags of irradiated diet may be sprayed into the entry port with peracetic acid, without the trouble of connecting the isolator to a supply cylinder or supply isolator. Diets containing sugars may be irradiated with little change, whereas they turn into caramel when autoclaved.

On the other hand, autoclaving, especially in the presence of added water, may improve digestibility of NI diets (see below for cecal effects). Added water also improves vitamin B retention during autoclaving,[162] but may increase the time required for bringing the diet up to sterilizing temperature, and in one case increased the risk of spore survival during autoclaving. Autoclaving has been the commonest method of diet sterilization in the U.S. but the autoclaving of diet in supply cylinders can produce dietary deficiencies when the time of sterilization is extended much beyond the 20 min at 15 lb steam pressure which is commonly used. The narrow margin between the time required for sterility and the time which produces deficiency means that the procedure must be carefully controlled and monitored, especially in terms of removing air from the cylinder as quickly and completely as possible, so that maximum temperature is reached rapidly in all parts of the load. Central steam sources may contain contaminants such as antirust agents which could be carcinogenic.

Filtration of nutrients dissolved in water or in oils is completely nondestructive and the ideal method of sterilization. It of course limits the nutrients to those which are water-soluble or oil-soluble. Nutrients in solution such as sugars and amino acids, or B vitamins and minerals, can interact readily. Therefore losses of nutrients can occur rapidly during storage.[163] Prevention of such losses may be reduced by frequent entry of fresh diet,[156] by refrigeration of diet in the isolator,[84] and by separation of the diet into two solutions until just before feeding.[156]

The diet must cause minimal cecal enlargement and a low incidence of volvulus. As indicated above, the effect of a diet on cecal size can only be determined empirically. Also, as noted earlier, CD diet causes less cecal enlargement than NI diets but a much higher incidence of volvulus. In general, diets containing dried milk products increase cecal distention of GF rodents. GF guinea pigs get more cecal distention from drinking their own GF mother's milk than they do from being fed a solid (mush-type) NI diet.[113] A semisynthetic diet of casein, rice starch, cellophane spangles, corn oil, vitamins, and minerals, causes less cecal distention in rats than NI diet, but it is not known how it would affect volvulus in much older animals.

Desirable Characteristics of a Diet for Study of Aging and Immunity

Defined and controlled nutrient intake. Ideally, it should be possible to vary any nutrient independently of any other. In NI diets it is not possible to vary protein, e.g., without changing other variables. Semisynthetic diets offer this possibility. Satisfactory semisynthetic diets have been developed and used extensively for GF animals.[155] If we wish to vary amino acids independently, or individual vitamins and minerals, the chemically defined water-soluble diet offers the possibility of varying 50 different nutrients independently (Tables 4 and 5).

Defined and controlled immunogenicity and mutagenicity. NI diets provide a broad spectrum of immunogens and mitogens. Sterilization may widen the spectrum. CV mice fed autoclaved L485 diet produced twice as many plaque-forming cells against

Table 4
CHEMICALLY DEFINED WATER-SOLUBLE DIET
L489 E11

To 156 mℓ Ultrapure H_2O at 70°C, Add the Following (All L-Form)

Leucine	1.54 g	Asparagine	0.84 g
Phenylalanine	0.60	Arginine HCl	0.66
Isoleucine	0.88	Threonine	0.60
Methionine	0.86	Lysine HCl	1.44
Tryptophan	0.30	Histidine HCl · H_2O	0.60
Valine	1.00		

Cool to 45° and Add (All L-Form Amino Acids)

Glycine	0.24 g	Alanine	0.48
Proline	1.20	Na Glutamate	2.76
Serine	1.08	Tyrosine-Ethyl · HCl	0.50

When All Dissolved, Add

Ferrous gluconate	0.04 g	NaCl + KI (0.55 mg)	0.07 g
Salts 35D[a]	0.086	B-mix 111E4[b]	0.072
Ca glycerophosphate	4.24	Choline Cl	0.25
Mg glycerophosphate	1.16	K acetate	1.5
$CaCl_2 \cdot 2H_2O$	0.15		

In 118 mℓ Ultrapure H_2O at 80°C, dissolve

α-D-dextrose, anhydrous 77.4 g
Cool, combine both solutions.
Filter through Amicon Diaflo PM-10 membrane with 10,000 mol wt cut-off.

[a]0.086 g salt mix 35D contains, in mg

Mn $(acetate)_2 \cdot 4H_2O$	45	$(NH_4)_6Mo_7O_{24} \cdot 4H_2O$	0.3
$ZnSO_4 \cdot H_2O$	33	$NiCl_2 \cdot 3H_2O$	0.3
Cu $(acetate)_2 \cdot H_2O$	3	Co $(acetate)_2 \cdot 4H_2O$	0.09
Cr $(acetate)_3 \cdot H_2O$	2	Na_3VO_4	0.18
NaF	1.7	Na_2SeO_3	0.018
$SnSO_4 \cdot 2H_2O$	0.3		

[b]0.072 g B mix 111E4 contains, in mg

Thiamine HCl	1.00	Riboflavin	1.5
Pyridoxine HCl	1.25	Niacinamide	7.5
Biotin	0.20	i-Inositol	50.0
Folic acid	0.30	Ca pantothenate	10.0
Vitamin B-12 (pure)	0.12		

Table 5
LADEK 69E6

Lipid Supplement. Each Mouse Receives Daily in a Stainless Dish 0.25 mℓ (0.225 g) of LADEK 69E6 Containing

Purified soy triglycerides[a]	0.22	g
Vitamin A (retinyl) palmitate	4.3	μg (7.8 IU)
Vitamin D_3 (cholecalciferol)	0.0192	μg (0.77 IU)
DL-α-Tocopherol	2.2	mg
DL-α-Tocopheryl acetate	4.4	mg
Vitamin K_1 (phylloquinone)	48.0	μg

[a] Soybean oil saponified, esterified with methanol, distilled, and transesterified with glycerol. It contains: 11.8% tripalmitin, 1.5% tristearin, 23.8% triolein, 54.8% trilinolein, and 8% trilinolenin.

sheep red blood cells as mice fed irradiated L485.[48] NI diets vary over time in their immunogenic effects even when they are open formula diets. Closed formula diets would be very unpredictable in their effects, since the highly immunogenic proteins and carbohydrates can be varied by the manufacturer without notice. Chemically defined, water-soluble diets offer the most completely nonantigenic diet possible for the following reasons: the nutrients consist of the very same nutrients which circulate naturally in the blood; they could not be considered as foreign. The nutrients have been highly purified chemically and by treatment with activated charcoal. Because they are low-molecular weight and water-soluble, they can be ultrafiltered to remove impurities above a given molecular size, e.g., 10,000 mol wt, 1,000 mol wt. For practical reasons, the diet used at Lobund and in Japan has been filtered through a 10,000 mol wt filter, because most effective antigens and mitogens exceed that size. Sterilization by ultrafiltration does not alter the diet nutritionally and it removes rather than creates antigens.

Because of the potential importance of the GF-CD animal model in studies of aging and immunity, it will be discussed further in the following section.

The GF Animal Fed Chemically Defined Antigen-Free Diet (GF-CD Animal)

The advantages of the GF-CD animal model for aging and immunity studies have been noted. Experience with this model will be brought together here because of its potential importance.

Hand Rearing vs. Colony Rearing

It had originally been hoped that a rat or mouse could be reared *from birth* on CD diet, thus bypassing even the potential immunogens of maternal milk. Although GF rats could be hand-fed the diet to weaning after one day of maternal nursing, they could not be carried from birth. Their condition at weaning was also unsatisfactory. Efforts therefore centered on rearing GF-CD animals in a reproducing colony. GF-CD rat colonies twice initiated reproduction, but nursing mothers were lost by contamination in one case, trichobezoars in another. Because of the cost of maintaining GF-CD rats, all further development has been done with GF-CD mice.

Qualitative Adequacy of GF-CD Diet

A GF-CD CFW mouse colony demonstrated the qualitative adequacy of this diet by breeding through five generations.[156] If any nutrient had been completely missing, reproduction could not have continued so long. Quantitative deficiency, however, was indicated by low weaning weights and a high perinatal mortality. Post-weaning growth was normal. Present diets (see below) have improved weaning weights and perinatal survival.

Requirements for Lactation: Nesting Material

Although the animals were normally maintained in stainless wire cages without bedding, it was found essential to provide nesting material for nursing mothers. No defined form of nesting material has yet been found. Whatman® ashless filter paper, cut into strips, provides the required nesting material with minimal nutrient addition, but its antigenicity seems probable. It was found necessary to continue this nesting material for 10 to 14 days after weaning. Without it, mice fed this type of diet develop a temporary seborrhea which retards growth and sometimes causes death. Limiting the intake of defined oil during this immediate post-weaning period further helps to prevent the seborrhea.

Colony Performance on Present Diets

A colony of GF-CD C3H/HeCr mice is now maintained, this inbred line having been chosen to minimize the antigenicity of animal-to-animal contact. On present diet formulations, these mice have normal weaning weights and a low normal post-weaning growth rate. One individual has lived as long as 2½ years on this type of diet. As described earlier, these mice have extremely low circulating γ-globulins, as did the Jcl:(ICR) mice reared on a similar diet in Japan.[84] Nevertheless, the nutritional adequacy of the diet has been shown by their ability to respond to challenges. While the mice both at Lobund and in Japan have shown a decline in reproductive ability over successive generations, very recent changes in the proportions of amino acids and lipids, and in the form of housing for nursing mothers, have dramatically improved perinatal survival in later generations and litters.

Physiological Characteristics of GF-CD Mice

The use of CD diet has eliminated three physiological anomalies of the GF-NI mouse compared to the CV-NI mouse. The GF-CD mouse has a MR and heart size comparable to the CV mouse and not to the GF-NI mouse.[93] Furthermore, it does not show the slight delay in reaching adult thyroid hormone levels which occurs in GF-NI mice.[29] Its cecum is smaller than that of GF-NI mice, although still three to five times the CV size.[134]

Aging of GF-CD Mice

An aging experiment with GF-CD C3H mice was set up to answer a basic question of immunity and aging: Will the absence of antigenic stimulation throughout life postpone immune decline, accelerate immune decline, or have no effect on it? GF-CD male mice housed as shown in Figure 2 have been carried through 14 months. Except for the difference in circulating γ-globulins, these mice, when tested at 8 months, showed immune responses to challenge similar to those of GF-NI mice.[70] This indicates the nutritional adequacy of the diet for immune response. The low γ-globulin level indicates its low immunogenicity.

These mice showd an unexpectedly early incidence of volvulus (*15%*) by 8 months of age.[134] This occurred despite the fact that relative cecal size was less than in GF-NI mice and did not increase between 3 and 8 months as it did in GF-NI mice. An experiment is under way to determine if fiber in the form of filter paper bedding is necessary to prevent volvulus and trichobezoars in GF-CD mice. If so, fiber may be a potential antigen that GF-CD mice will have to live with. Other dietary variables will also be tested for their effect on volvulus. From the 8th to the 14th months, no further volvulus occurred. In the aging GF mouse study of Walburg and Cosgrove[39] volvulus tended to occur in the first half of life. Once past 8 months of age, the GF-CD mice may not be further threatened by it.

Although the CD diet continues under study to improve its adequacy for reproduction, its ability to maintain normal growth and immune potential makes the GF-CD mouse a highly desirable animal model for assessing the role of antigens and mitogens in general, or of specific antigens and mitogens, in aged-related immune decline.

Cost of CD Diet

At 1979 prices, diet ingredient costs are approximately $0.25 per mouse per day and $0.75 per rat per day. Diet preparation, filtration, and daily feeding at least double the time required for animal maintenance. Cages have been modified in the Lobund machine shop for a total cage cost of $35.00 for space for four aging mice or two breeding mice (Figure 2).

The Gnotobiote Associated With Known Microbial Species

The GF animal is the simplest gnotobiote, since its biota consists of one living species, the animal itself. The GF rat qualifies for the designation GF[24] but the mouse which is still called GF is strictly speaking only gnotobiotic (GN), carrying a latent leukemogenic virus.[50] Other GF species would require more exhaustive testing over time in a reproducing colony to determine if they are strictly GF.

The GN Mouse

I have discussed the GN mouse under the heading of the GF animal (above) for the following reasons: it is referred to as GF in the literature; the virus in its latent fom may be without any effect on the animal; and we have no simple way to refer to it that will tell us it contains the latent leukemogenic virus and nothing else. When, however, an investigator carries these mice through long-term studies, he must be aware of the fact that the mice do carry a leukemogenic virus. This virus might become activated in advanced age, have long-term cumulative effects on the immune system even without causing leukemia, and/or cause other kinds of neoplasm in GF mice. When leukemia does occur, the investigator will be faced with the problem of determining whether it was caused by the leukemogenic virus or would have occurred anyway. Out of 90 aged GF Wistar rats, 2 developed leukemia, although no virus or virus-like particle has ever been detected in this rat colony.[44] In the second aging study with GF mice, leukemia had a higher incidence in GF than in CV mice.[39] In the third aging study, leukemia was less prevalent in the GF than in CV mice but thymic lymphosarcoma had a much higher incidence in the GF than the CV mice.[40,41] Although neoplasms in general were less frequent in the GF mice, there was a tendency for neoplasms to occur earlier in GF.[40,41] It is possible that the leukemogenic virus could express itself in more than one way.

Changes in the Expression of Pathogenic Potential By A Microbial Monoassociate in the Absence of Other Microbes

A number of examples were given previously. The concept may be relevant both to the expression of the leukemogenic virus of mice and to microbial associates deliberately added to GF animals for aging studies. The investigator needs to be aware of such possibilities.

Use of Microbial Associates to Eliminate the Unusual Anatomic and Functional Characteristics of the GF Animal

GN rats and mice have been maintained through long periods in studies designed to develop a defined microflora which would normalize the anomalies of the GF rodent without producing pathogenic effects.[164-167] The prime index of GF status in the rodent has been cecal enlargment. No single microbial associate or combination of a few defined species has succeeded in reducing cecal size all the way to what it is in CV or SPF animals. However, large groups of bacterial species, particularly anaerobes, isolated from cecal contents of CV rodents have brought cecal size to CV levels.[165] One group of defined microbes, the "hexaflora" of Schaedler has been extensively studied, although it does not completely reduce cecal size to CV levels.[166] It offers the advantages of clear definition, stability of the species over time in the same relative proportions, and ease of detection, isolation, and enumeration of the species involved. Minor variations on this hexaflora have been studied, with various deletions, additions and substitutions. These animals maintain good health and generally CV- or SPF-like characteristics.[164]

Use of Microbially Associated Gnotobiotes in Aging Studies

These associated GF animals have not been systematically studied for aging. In a small sample kept at Lobund, C3H mice with a modified hexaflora showed mammary tumors earlier than expected (GF C3H mice as such do not carry the Bittner virus). However, the results are only suggestive at this time.

Human Type Microflora in GN Animals

GF animals can accept and maintain at high levels microbial species predominant in man, thus producing an animal model closer to the human analogue.[3,4] Such a microflora would soon be displaced by the murine microflora in animals maintained in SPF or CV colonies. Animals with such floras have not yet been used in aging studies but may provide a unique model for some types of study.

Increased Husbandry Demands for GN Mice Compared to Either GF or CV Mice

As discussed previously under the locked flora concept, when animals with a CV or SPF microbiota are confined in an isolator, they require more frequent cleaning of bedding, cages, and water bottles than GF animals do. Usually they require more of such cleaning than open colony room animals do, because the open animal room has more mass air movement to remove humidity and noxious odors than does a GF isolator.

In addition to the increased frequency of cleaning, there is much more labor involved in each cleaning operation for animals with a broad spectrum of microbial associates. Changing water bottles and cages for GN animals is an involved process requiring large-scale exits and entries through the port and increased risk of contamination in the process. In practice, however, it has proved possible to maintain "hexaflora"-type associated animals without changing of cages and water bottles; hexaflora mice, rats, and gerbils at Lobund Laboratory have shown no flora simplification or signs of ill health. Selection of associated bacteria which produce little or no ammonia from animal wastes would simplify husbandry even further.

If a defined microflora is to be added to GF animals for an aging experiment, and there is no previous experience with it as there is for the "hexaflora" and its modifications, the investigator must be prepared for the posibility of flora simplification, shifts in relative proportions of species, and an increased burden of husbandry.

Possible Differences in Dietary Requirements for GN Animals

Well-tested diets like L485 have proved adequate for GF, CV, SPF, and GN animals, but new and exotic microbial species added to GF animals could affect diet adequacy or other effects of diet. Some monoassociates actually increase cecal distention rather than reduce it.[131]

Summary

With the present possibilities for minimizing the risk of cecal volvulus through use of diets like L485 the demand for developing defined normalizing microfloras may be lessened. If confirmed, the recent discovery that CD diet increased the low MR of GF mice to at least CV levels[93] may offer a way of normalizing this anomaly under GF conditions. It will be necessary to determine if this CD diet effect is the result of a compensating anomaly. Nevertheless, for studies of immunity and aging where a general stimulation of the animal is desired, there are available well-studied combinations of representatives of the major types of intestinal bacteria and yeasts.

Isolator Controls for Animals Maintained in the GF System

The GF isolator system affects not only the transfer of microbes but also the transfer of air and airborne particles and some odors, the transmission of sound and light, and the type of contact with the caretaker. It requires the use of sterilized diet, bedding and water, and may involve exposure to the fumes of peracetic acid. When the investigator using GF animals wants to set up control groups whose environmental exposure differs from the GF only in the variable of having a microbiota, then isolator controls are essential. Such controls would appear to require as demanding a husbandry as the biotoristic animals described above. This is not the case, however, if the investigator is willing to take some risks of pathogen entry. A major burden of husbandry in biotoristic animals results from the need to change cages and water bottles as well as bedding. Systems have been developed for maintaining defined flora colonies under filter caps by carrying out all cage changes, feeding, and watering in a laminar flow hood.[168] For biotoristic isolator maintenance, cage changes could be made in a laminar flow hood with an entry port built into the side for attachment to an isolator entry port. The hood can be stocked with sterilized supplies for transfer into the control isolator. For an even simpler system, an entry port wall made of canvas is being developed which forces sterile air out of the sides of the entry port.[169] Wrapped and sterilized cages, bottles, diet, and bedding can be passed into the isolator without absolute security but with greatly reduced risk of the entry of airborne pathogens. Actual maintenance of control animals in laminar flow hoods could be a feasible compromise, since animals with an existing microflora would resist establishment of rare accidental microbes. However, the airflow patterns would not be identical to those in isolators, and some cages might acquire an accidental contaminant while other cages would not. The originator of the flexible film isolator, P. C. Trexler, is continuing development of simplified absolute barrier or low-risk isolators for easy maintenance of large colonies and long-term experiments.

Summary

The development of the GF animal as an experimental tool has provided investigators of aging and immunity with:

1. An absolute barrier system which can be used to protect aging animals from adventitious entry of microbes which could affect their survival or immune responses. It also serves to *contain* microbes when necessary. Within the barrier system microbes can circulate freely to maintain homogeneity of microbial exposure within the animal group.
2. A background of information on diets and husbandry to meet the special requirements of GF animals, and some GN animals. Diets tested include natural ingredient, semisynthetic, and chemically defined, antigen-free diets.
3. A background of data on physiological characteristics of some GF and some GN animals. These could interact with survival and immune responses in aging studies.
4. A background of information and some generalizations about immune responses in a variety of GF animal species.
5. Pilot studies on aging of GF mice and rats which indicate their suitability for aging studies.

GLOSSARY OF ABBREVIATIONS

BOR — Biotoristic — A coined term derived from the Greek *biota,* and *horizein,* to set bounds or limits. It refers to animals having an undefined microbiota but maintained within absolute barriers to prevent influx (and sometimes efflux) of microbes.

Although no additions to the confined microbiota can occur, losses of species may occur over time (locked flora effect).

B-cell — Bone marrow-derived lymphocyte.

CD — Chemically defined. Applied to diets made up entirely of ingredients capable of chemical definition, e.g., amino acids, simple sugars, and lipids, vitamins and minerals.

Con A — Concanavalin A.

CV — Conventional — This applies to animals maintained in open colony rooms by traditional animal rearing practices. It includes animals which have never known any break in the transmission of the ancestral microbiota, as well as animals once GF, GN, or SPF, which have later been exposed to animals with the ancestral microbiota. The composition of the microbiota will vary with the history of the colony. Such animals may be maintained in isolators as controls for GF or GN animal experiments, but if the isolator is not maintained as an absolute barrier, the animals would still be designated as CV rather than BOR.

GF — Germfree — As applied to an enclosed environment GF indicates that the environment is enclosed by absolute barriers, both physical and operational, which prevent the entry of any living microbe. As applied to animal or plant species, GF means that the organism has been demonstrated by microscopic, cultural, and serological tests to be free of viable microbial associates. The validity of application of the term depends on the comprehensiveness of the tests and the reliability of the barriers maintained since the tests. As applied in practice to mice, GF has been and is still frequently used to refer to mice otherwise GF which carry a latent form of leukemogenic virus. No strictly GF mice are now known to exist, since the virus is transmitted vertically in all strains tested. This use of the term GF is unsatisfactory, and must always be qualified for accuracy.

GN — Gnotobiotic — From the Greek *gnotos* (known) and *biota*. This term applies to animals or plants with defined microbial associates. Such application requires that they be maintained within an absolute barrier system and subjected to tests to identify all microbial species with which they are associated. In practice, GN usually refers to animals formerly GF which have received inocula of identified microbial species.

GVH — Graft versus host.

IgA — Immune globulin of the A class.

IgG — Immune globulin of the G class.

IgM — Immune globulin of the M class.

LPS — Lipopolysaccharide.

Mol wt — Molecular weight.

MR — Metabolic rate as determined by oxygen consumption of fasting, quiet animals.

NI — Natural ingredient — Term applied to diets containing ingredients derived from natural feedstuffs by simple processing.

PFC — Plaque-forming cells.

PHA — Phytohemagglutinin.

RBC — Red blood cells.

SPF — Specific-pathogen-free — In theory, this term could be applied to any animal proven by exhaustive test to be free of specific pathogens. In practice, SPF animals are descended from GF or GN animals which have been maintained behind stringent but not absolute barriers and have been subjected to repeated tests for the pathogen(s) specified and found negative.

SRBC — Sheep red blood cells.

T-cell — Thymus-derived lymphocyte.

WBC — White blood cells.

REFERENCES

1. **Barnes, R. H., Fiala, G., and Kwong, E.**, Decreased growth rate resulting from prevention of coprophagy, *Fed. Proc.*, 22, 125, 1963.
2. **Bauchop, T.**, Stomach microbiology of primates, *Ann. Rev. Microbiol.*, 25, 429, 1971.
3. **Dymsza, H. A., Stoewsand, G. S., Enright, J. J., Trexler, P. C., and Gall, L. C.**, Human indigenous flora in gnotobiotic rats, *Nature (London)*, 208, 1236, 1965.
4. **Gibbons, R. J., Socransky, S. S., and Kapsimalis, B.**, Establishment of human indigenous bacteria in germ-free mice, *J. Bacteriol.*, 88, 1316, 1964.
5. **Reyniers, J. A., Ed.**, *Micrurgical and Germfree Methods*, Charles C Thomas, Springfield, Ill., 1943.
6. **Reyniers, J. A.**, Design and operation of appratus for rearing germfree animals, *Ann. N.Y. Acad. Sci.*, 78, 47, 1959.
7. **Trexler, P. C. and Reynolds, L. I.**, Flexible film apparatus for the rearing and use of germfree animals, *Appl. Microbiol.*, 5, 406, 1957.
8. **Gustafsson, B. E.**, Lightweight stainless steel systems for rearing germfree animals, *Ann. N.Y.Acad. Sci.*, 78, 17, 1959.
9. **Wostmann, B. S., Ed.**,Gnotobiotes: Standards and Guidelines for the Breeding, Care and Management of Laboratory Animals, National Research Council, National Academy of Sciences, Washington, D.C., 1970.
10. **Coates, M. E., Gordon, H. A., and Wostmann, B. S., Eds.**, *The Germfree Animal in Research*, Academic Press, London, 1968.
11. **Pleasants, J. R.**, Gnotobiotics, in *Handbook of Laboratory Animal Science*, Vol. 1, Melby, E. C., Jr. and Altman, N. H., Eds., CRC Press, Boca Raton, Fla., 1974, 117.
12. **Zurcher, C., Burek, J.D., Van Nunen, M. C. J., and Meihuizen, S. P.**, A naturally occurring epizootic caused by Sendai virus in breeding and aging rodent colonies. I. Infection in the mouse, *Lab. Anim. Sci.*, 27, 955, 1977.
13. **Rowe, W. P., Hartley, J. W., and Capps, W. I.**, Mouse hepatitis virus infection as a highly contagious, prevalent, enteric infection of mice, *Proc. Soc. Exp. Biol. Med.*, 112, 161,1963.
14. **Gleiser, C. E.**, Diseases of laboratory animals-bacterial, in *CRC Handbook of Laboratory Animal Medicine*, Vol.2, Melby, E. C., Jr. and Altman, N. H., Eds., CRC Press, Boca Raton, Fla., 1974, 271.
15. **Nelson, J. B.**, Studies on endemic pneumonia of the albino rat: IV. Development of a rat colony free from respiratory infections, *J. Exp. Med.*, 94, 377, 1951.
16. **Reyniers, J. A.**, The control of contamination in colonies of laboratory animals by the use of germfree techniques, *Proc. Anim. Care Panel*, 7, 9, 1957.
17. **Wagner, M.**, personal communication, 1979.
18. **Wilson, R., Sjodin, K., and Bealmer, P. M.**, The absence of wasting in thymectomized germfree (axenic) mice, *Proc. Soc. Exp. Biol. Med.*, 117, 237, 1964.
19. **Holland, J. M., Mitchell, T. J., Gipson, L. C., and Whitaker, M. S.**, Survival and cause of death in aging germfree athymic nude and normal inbred C3Hf/He mice, *J. Natl. Cancer Inst.*, 61, 1357, 1978.
20. **Jones, J. M., Wilson, R., and Bealmer, P. M.**, Mortality and gross pathology of secondary disease in germfree mouse radiation chimeras, *Radiat. Res.*, 45, 577, 1971.
21. **Pollard, M., Chang, C. F., and Srivastava, K. K.**, The role of microflora in development of graft-versus-host disease, *Transplant. Proc.*, 8, 533, 1976.
22. **Pollard, M. and Sharon, N.**, Prevention and treatment of spontaneous leukemia in germfree AKR mice, *Proc. Soc. Exp. Biol. Med.*, 137, 1494, 1971.
23. **Wilson, R. and Mastromarino, A.**, Gnotobiotic human infants, *Am. J. Clin. Nutr.*, 30, 896, 1977.
24. **Pollard, M.**, Senescence in germfree rats, *Gerontologia*, 17, 333, 1971.
25. **Pollard, M.**, Spontaneous diseases in germfree animals, in Research Animals in Medicine, Harrison, L. T., Ed., Department of Health, Education and Welfare, Publ. No. 72-333, National Institutes of Health, Bethesda, Md., 1974, 1005.
26. **Pollard, M. and Kajima, M.**, Lesions in aged germfree Wistar rats, *Am. J. Pathol.*, 61, 25, 1970.
27. **Gordon, H. A.**, Morphological and physiological characterization of germ-free life, *Ann. N.Y. Acad. Sci.*, 78, 208, 1959.
28. **Djurickovic, S. M., Ediger, R. D., and Hong, C. C.**, Volvulus at the ileocecal junction in germfree mice, *Lab. Anim.*, 12, 219, 1978.
29. **Wostmann, B. S. and Bruckner-Kardoss, E.**, Thyroid hormones in older germfree rats and mice, *Fed. Proc. Abstr.*, 38, 1030, 1979.
30. **Ross, M. H. and Bras, G.**, Lasting influence of early caloric restriction on prevalence of neoplasms in the rat, *J. Natl. Cancer Inst.*, 47, 1095, 1971.

31. **Fernandes, G., Good, R. A., and Yunis, E. J.,** Attempts to correct age-related immunoeficiency and autoimmunity by cellular and dietary manipulation in inbred mice, in *Immunology and Aging,* Makinodan, T. and Yunis, E., Eds., Plenum Press, New York, 1977, 111.
32. **Pleasants, J. R. and Wostmann, B. S.,** unpublished data, 1979.
33. **Makinodan, T., Chino, F., Lever, W. E., and Brewen, B. S.,** The immune systems of mice reared in clean and in dirty conventional laboratory farms. II. Primary antibody-forming activity of young and old mice with long life spans, *J. Gerontol.,* 26, 508, 1971.
34. **Kay, M. M. B.,** Long term subclinical effects of parainfluenza (Sendai) infection on immune cells of aging mice, *Proc. Soc. Exp. Biol. Med.,* 158, 326, 1978.
35. **Kay, M. M. B.,** Autoimmune disease: the consequence of deficient T-cell function?, *J. Am. Geriatr. Soc.,* 24, 253, 1976.
36. **Anderson, R. E., Doughty, W. E., and Troup, G. M.,** Immunological responsiveness and aging phenomena in germfree mice, in *Immunology and Aging,* Makinodan, T. and Yunis, E. J., Eds., Plenum Press, New York, 1977, 151.
37. **Gordon, H. A., Bruckner-Kardoss, E., and Wostmann, B. S.,** Aging in germ-free mice: life tables and lesions observed at natural death, *J. Gerontol.,* 21, 382, 1966.
38. **Gordon, H. A., Bruckner-Kardoss, E., and Wostmann, B. S.,** Aging studies in colonies of germ-free and conventional animals, in *Age With a Future,* Proc. 6th Int. Congr. Gerontology, Munksgaard, Copenhagen, 1964, 220.
39. **Walburg, H. E., Jr. and Cosgrove, G. E.,** Aging in irradiated and unirradiated germfree ICR mice, *Exp. Gerontol.,* 2, 143, 1967.
40. **Anderson, R. E., Scaletti, J. V., and Howarth J. L.,** Radiation-induced life shortening in germfree mice, *Exp. Gerontol.,* 7, 289, 1972.
41. **Anderson, R. E., Doughty, W. E., Stone, R. S., and Howarth, J.,** Spontaneous and radiation-treated neoplasms in germfree mice, *Arch. Pathol.,* 94, 250, 1972.
42. **Seibert, K., Pollard, M., and Nordin, A.,** Some aspects of humoral immunity in germ-free and conventional SJL/J mice in relation to age and pathology, *Cancer Res.,* 34, 1707, 1974.
43. **Pollard, M. and Teah, B. A.,** Spontaneous tumors in germfree rats, *J. Natl. Cancer Inst.,* 31, 155, 1963.
44. **Pollard, M. and Luckert, P. H.,** Spontaneous tumors in aged germfree Wistar rats, *Lab. Anim. Sci.,* 29, 74, 1979.
45. **Wostmann, B. S., Pleasants, J. R., and Reddy, B. S.,** Water-soluble nonantigenic diets, in *Husbandry of Laboratory Animals,* Conalty, M. L., Ed., Academic Press, London, 1967, 187.
46. **Wostmann, B. S., Pleasants, J. R., Bealmear, P., and Kincade, P. W.,** Serum proteins and lymphoid tissues in germ-free mice fed a chemically defined, water soluble, low molecular weight diet, *Immunology,* 19, 443, 1973.
47. **Wostmann, B. S., Pleasants, J. R., and Bealmear, P.,** Dietary stimulation of immune mechanisms, *Fed. Proc.,* 30, 1779, 1971.
48. **Webb, P. M., Wostmann B. S., and Pleasants, J. R.,** unpublished data, 1979.
49. **Olson, G. S. and Wostmann, B. S.,** Electrophoretic and immunoelectrophoretic studies of the serum of germfree and conventional guinea pigs, *Proc. Soc. Exp. Biol. Med.,* 116, 914, 1964.
50. **Kajima, M. and Pollard, M.,** Wide distribution of leukemia virus in strains of laboratory mice, *Nature (London),* 218, 188, 1968.
51. **Kim, Y. B., Bradley, S., and Watson, D.,** Ontogeny of the immune response. IV. The role of antigen elimination in the true primary immune response in germfree, colostrum-deprived piglets, *J. Immunol.,* 99, 320, 1967.
52. **Dukor, P., Miller, J. F. A. P., and Sacquet, E.,** The immunological responsiveness of germ-free mice thymectomized at birth. II. Lymphoid tissues and histopathology, *Clin. Exp. Immunol.,* 3, 191, 1968.
53. **Gordon, H. A. and Pesti, L.,** The gnotobiotic animal as a tool in the study of host microbial relatioships, *Bacteriol. Rev.,* 35, 390, 1971.
54. **Olson, G. B. and Wostmann, B. S.,** Lymphocytopoiesis, plasmacytopoiesis and cellular proliferation in nonantigenically stimulated germfree mice, *J. Immunol.,* 97, 267, 1966.
55. **McIntire, K. R., Sell, S., and Miller, J. F. A. P.,** Pathogenesis of the postneonatal thymectomy wasting syndrome, *Nature (London),* 204, 151,1964.
56. **Bealmear, M. and Wilson, R.,** Histological comparison of the thymus of germfree (axenic) and conventional CFW mice, *Anat. Rec.,* 154, 261, 1966.
57. **Burns,W., Bauer, H., and Einheber, A.,** Quantitative morphology of the thymus in normal and irradiated germ-free mice, *Fed. Proc.,* 23, 547, 1964.
58. **Webb, P. M., Chanana, A. D., Cronkite, E. P., Joel, D. D., and Saissure, J.,** Comparative uptake of ^{125}I-iododeoxyuridine and ^{3}H-thymidine, and DNA renewal studies in germ-free and conventional mice, *Cell Tissue Kinet,* 13, 227, 1980.

59. **Pollard, M. and Sharon, N.**, Responses of the Peyer's patches in germ-free mice to antigenic stimulation, *Infect. Immun.*, 2, 96, 1970.
60. **Miller, J. J., III, Johnson, D. O., and Ada, G. L.**, Differences in localization of Salmonella flagella in lymph node follicles of germ-free and conventional rats, *Nature (London)*, 217, 1059, 1968.
61. **Bauer, H., Horowitz, R. E., Watkins, K. C., and Popper, H.**, Immunologic competence and phagocytosis in germ-free animals with and without stress, *JAMA*, 187, 715, 1964.
62. **Horowitz, R. E., Bauer, H., Paronetto, F., Abrams, G. D., Watkins, K. C., and Popper, H.**, The response of the lymphatic tissue to bacterial antigen. Studies in germ-free mice, *Am. J. Pathol.*, 44, 747, 1964.
63. **Wostmann, B. S. and Olson, G. B.**, Precipitating antibody production in germ-free chickens, *J. Immunol.*, 92, 41, 1964.
64. **Bauer, H., Paronetto, F., Burns, W. A., and Einheber, A.**, The enhancing effect of the microbial flora on macrophage functions and the immune response. A study in germ-free mice, *J. Exp. Med.*, 123, 1013, 1966.
65. **Bosma, M. J., Makinodan, T., and Walburg, H. E., Jr.**, Development of immunologic competence in germ-free and conventional mice, *J. Immunol.*, 99, 420, 1967.
66. **Miller, J. F. A. P., Dukor, P., Grant, G., Sinclair, N. R. St. C., and Sacquet, E.**, The immunological responsiveness of germ-free mice thymectomized at birth. I. Antibody production and skin homograft rejection, *Clin. Exp. Immunol.*, 2, 531, 1967.
67. **Burnett, M.**, *Immunological Surveillance*, Pergamon Press, New York, 1970, 217.
68. **Pollard, M. and Truitt, R. L.**, Allogeneic bone marrow chimerism in germ-free mice. I. Prevention of spontaneous leukemia in AKR mice, *Proc. Soc. Exp. Biol. Med.*, 144, 659, 1973.
69. **Pollard, M. and Truitt, R. L.**, Allogeneic bone marrow chimerism in germfree mice. II. Prevention of reticulum cell sarcomas in SJL/J mice, *Proc. Soc. Exp. Biol. Med.*, 145, 488, 1974.
70. **Webb, P. M., Schmitz, H. E., Pleasants, J. R., and Wostmann, B. S.**, Mitogen responses of germfree mice fed chemically defined or natural diet, *Fed. Proc. Abstr.*, 38, 764, 1979.
71. **Madden, D. L., Horton, R. E., and McCullough, N. B.**, Spontaneous infection in ex-germfree guinea pigs due to *Clostridium perfringens*, *Lab. Anim. Care*, 20, 454, 1970.
72. **Gordon, H. A. and Wostmann, B. S.**, Responses of the animal host to changes in the bacterial environment: transition of the albino rat from germfree to the conventional state, in *Recent Progress in Microbiology*, Tunevall, G., Ed., Almquist and Wiksell, Stockholm, 1959, 336.
73. **Outzen, H. C.**, Ageing and resistance to infection in germfree C3Hf mice, in *Germ-free Biology: Experimental and Clinical Aspects*, Mirand, E. and Back, N., Eds., Plenum Press, New York, 1969, 207.
74. **Outzen, H. C. and Pilgrim, H. I.**, Differential mortality of male and female germfree C3H mice introduced into a conventional colony, *Proc. Soc. Exp. Biol. Med.*, 124, 52, 1967.
75. **Gordon, H. A., Wagner, M., Luckey, T. D., and Reyniers, J. A.**, An encephalomeningeal syndrome selectively affecting newly hatched germfree and monocontaminated chickens, *J. Infect. Dis.*, 105, 31, 1959.
76. **Phillips, B. P. and Wolfe, P. A.**, Pneumonic disease in germfree animals, *J. Infect. Dis.*, 108, 12, 1961.
77. **Knight, P. L., Jr. and Wostmann, B. S.**, Influence of *Salmonella typhimurium* on ileum and spleen morphology of germfree rats, *Indiana Acad. Sci.*, 72, 78, 1964.
78. **Margard, W. L. and Peters, A. C.**, A study of gnotobiotic mice monocontaminated with *Salmonella typhimurium*, *Lab. Anim. Care*, 14, 200, 1964.
79. **Maier, B. R. and Hentges, D. J.**, Experimental *Shigella* infections in laboratory animals. I. Antagonism by human normal flora components in gnotobiotic mice, *Infect. Immun.*, 6, 168, 1972.
80. **Griesemer, R. A.**, Virus disease research utilizing germfree animals, in *Advances in Germfree Research and Gnotobiology*, Miyakawa, M. and Luckey, T. D., Eds., CRC Press, Boca Raton, Fla., 1968, 287.
81. **Phillips, B. P.**, Studies on the amoeba-bacteria relationship in amebiasis, *Am. J. Trop. Med. Hyg.*, 13, 391, 1964.
82. **Newton, W. L., Weinstein, P. P., and Jones, M. F.**, A comparison of the development of some rat and mouse helminths in germfree and conventional guinea pigs, *Ann. N.Y. Acad. Sci.*, 78, 290, 1959.
83. **Schaffer, J., Beamer, P. R., Trexler, P. C., Breidenbach, G., and Walcher, D. N.**, Response of germ-free animals to experimental virus monocontamination. I. Observation on Coxsackie B virus, *Proc. Soc. Exp. Biol. Med.*, 112, 561, 1963.
84. **Hashimoto, K., Handa, H., Umehara, K., and Sasaki, S.**, Germfree mice reared on an "antigen-free" diet, *Lab. Anim. Sci.*, 28, 38, 1978.
85. **Kellogg, T. F. and Wostmann, B. S.**, Stock diet for colony production of germfree rats and mice, *Lab. Anim. Care*, 19, 812, 1969.

86. **Pitterman, W. and Deerberg, F.,** Spontaneous Tumors and Lesions of the Lung, Kidney, and Gingiva in Aged Germfree Rats, in 5th Int. Symp. on Gnotobiology, Abstr., Stockholm, Sweden, June 9 to 12, 1975, 27.
87. **Anderson, R. E.,** Disseminated amyloidosis in germ-free mice, *Am. J. Pathol.,* 65, 43, 1971.
88. **Young, V. R.,** Diet as a modulator of aging and longevity, *Fed. Proc.,* 38, 1994, 1979.
89. **Weindruch, R. H., Kristie, J. A., Cheney, K. W., and Walford, R. L.,** Influence of controlled dietary restriction on immunologic function and aging, *Fed. Proc.,* 38, 2007, 1979.
90. **Good, R. A., Jose, D., Cooper, W. C., Fernandes, G., Kramer, T., and Yunis, E.,** Influence of nutrition on antibody production and cellular immune responses in man, rats, mice and guinea pigs, in *Malnutrition and the Immune Response,* Susskind, R. M., Ed., Raven Press, New York, 1977, 169.
91. **Fernandes, G., Yunis, E. J., and Good, R. A.,** Influence of diet on survival of mice, *Proc. Natl. Acad. Sci. U.S.A.,* 73, 270, 1976.
92. **Jose, D. G. and Good, R. A.,** Quantitative effects of nutritional essential amino acid deficiency upon immune responses to tumors in mice, *J. Exp. Med.,* 137, 1, 1973.
93. **Wostmann, B. S., Bruckner-Kardoss, E., and Pleasants, J. R.,** unpublished data, 1979.
94. **Thompson, G. E.,** Control of intestinal flora in animals and humans: implications for toxicology and health, *J. Environ. Pathol. Toxicol.,* 1, 113, 1977.
95. **Wostmann, B. S.,** Nutrition and metabolism of the germfree animal, *World Rev. Nutr. Diet,* 22, 40, 1975.
96. **Coates, M. E.,** Gnotobiotic animals in nutrition research, *Proc. Nutr. Soc.,* 32, 53, 1973.
97. **Stoewsand, G. S., Dymsza, H. A., Ament, D., and Trexler, P. C.,** Lysine requirement of the growing gnotobiotic mouse, *Life Sci.,* 7, 689, 1968.
98. **Heneghan, J. B.,** Influence of microbial flora on xylose absorption in rats and mice, *Am. J. Physiol.,* 205, 417, 1963.
99. **Schwarz, K.,** Control of environmental conditions in trace element research: an experimental approach to unrecognized trace element requirements, in *Trace Element Metabolism in Animals,* Mills, C. F., Ed., E. and S. Livingston, London, 1970, 25.
100. **Van der Waaij, D. and Berghuis, J. M.,** Determination of the colonization resistance of the digestive tract of individual mice, *J. Hyg.,* 72, 379, 1974.
101. **Van der Waaij, D. and Andreas, A. H.,** Prevention of airborne contamination and cross-contamination in germfree mice by laminar flow, *J. Hyg.,* 69, 83, 1971.
102. **Vossen, J. M. and van der Waay, D.,** Reverse isolation in bone marrow transplantation: ultraclean room compared with laminar flow technique. II. Microbiological and clinical results, *Rev. Eur. Etud. Clin. Biol.,* 17, 564, 1972.
103. **Luckey, T. D.,** Gnotobiology and aerospace systems, in *Advances in Germfree Research and Gnotobiology,* Miyakawa, M. and Luckey, T. D., Eds., CRC Press, Boca Raton, Fla., 1968, 317.
104. **Luckey, T. D.,** Potential microbic shock in manned aerospace systems, *Aerospace Med.,* 37, 1223, 1966.
105. **Gordon, H. A. and Wostmann, B. S.,** Morphological studies on the germfree albino rat, *Anat. Rec.,* 137, 65, 1960.
106. **Pesti, L. and Gordon, H. A.,** Effects of age and isolation on the intestinal flora of mice, *Gerontologia,* 19, 153, 1973.
107. **Davis, C. P., Cleven, D., Balish, E., and Yale, C. E.,** Bacterial association in the gastrointestinal tract of beagle dogs, *Appl. Env. Microbiol.,* 34, 194, 1977.
108. **Sacquet, E.,** General technique of maintaining germfree animals, in *The Germfree Animal in Research,* Coates, M. E., Gordon, H. A., and Wostmann, B. S., Eds., Academic Press, London, 1968, 1.
109. **Coates, M. E.,** Chickens and quail: production and rearing, in *The Germfree Animal in Research,* Coates, M. E., Gordon, H. A., and Wostmann, B. S., Eds., Academic Press, London, 1968, 79.
110. **Srivastava, K. K., Pollard, M., and Wagner, M,.** Bacterial decontamination and antileukemic therapy of AKR mice, *Infect. Immun.,* 14, 1179, 1976.
111. **Pleasants, J. R., Wostmann, B. S., and Zimmerman, D. R.,** Improved hand rearing methods for small rodents, *Lab. Anim. Care,* 14, 37, 1964.
112. **Pleasants, J. R.,** Small laboratory mammals: production and rearing, in *The Germfree Animal in Research,* Coates, M. E., Gordon, H. A., and Wostmann, B. S., Eds., Academic Press, London, 1968, 47.
113. **Pleasants, J. R., Reddy, B. S., Zimmerman, D. R., Bruckner-Kardoss, E., and Wostmann, B. S.,** Growth, reproduction, and morphology of naturally born, normally suckled germfree guinea pigs, *Z. Versuchstierkd.,* 9, 195, 1967.
114. **Reddy, B. S., Pleasants, J. R., Zimmerman, D. R., and Wostmann, B. S.,** Iron and copper utilization in germfree rabbits as affected by diet and germfree status, *J. Nutr.,* 87, 189, 1965.

115. **Fries, A. S.,** Studies on Tyzzer's disease: transplacental transmission of *Bacillus piliformis* in rats, *Lab. Anim.,* 13, 43, 1979.
116. **Ashe, W. K.,** Properties of the rat submaxillary gland virus haemagglutinin and antihaemagglutinin and their incidence in apparently healthy gnotobiotic and coventional rats, *J. Gen. Virol.,* 4, 1, 1969.
117. **Ganaway, J. R., Allen, A. M., Moore, T. D., and Bohner, H. J.,** Natural infection of germfree rats with *Mycoplasma pulmonis, J. Infect. Dis.,* 127, 529, 1973.
118. **Phillips, B. B.,** Parasitological survey of Lobund germfree animals, *Lobund Reports No. 3,* University of Notre Dame Press, Notre Dame, Ind., 1960, 172.
119. **Trexler, P. C.,** A rationale for the development of gnotobiotics, *Lab. Anim.,* 12, 257, 1978.
120. **Wagner, M.,** Determination of germfree status, *Ann. N. Y. Acad. Sci.,* 78, 89, 1959.
121. **Dinsley, M.,** Gnotobiotic animals II, in *The UFAW Handbook on the Care and Management of Laboratory Animals,* 4th ed., T.-W.-Fiennes, R. N., Ed., Williams & Wilkins, Baltimore, 1972, 12.
122. **Pollard, M.,** Animal model: transplantable adenocarcinoma of the rat prostate gland, *Am. J. Pathol.,* 86, 277, 1977.
123. **Nuttall, G. H. F. and Thierfelder, H.,** Thierisches Leben ohne Bakterien im Verdauungskanal, *Z. Physiol. Chem., Hoppe-Seyler's,* 21, 109, 1895.
124. **Gordon, H. A.,** Is the germfree animal normal? A review of its anomalies in young and old age, in *The Germfree Animal in Research,* Coates, M. E., Gordon, H. A., and Wostmann, B. S., Eds., Academic Press, London, 1968, 127.
125. **Reyniers, J. A., Wagner, M., Luckey, T. D., and Gordon, H. A.,** Survey of germfree animals: the white Wyandotte bantam and white Leghorn chicken, *Lobund Reports No. 3,* University of Notre Dame Press, Notre Dame, Ind., 1960, 7.
126. **Heneghan, J. B., Gordon, H. A., and Wostmann, B. S.,** personal communication, 1979.
127. **Miniats, O. P. and Valli, V. E.,** The gastrointestinal tract of gnotobiotic pigs, in *Germfree Research: Biological Effect of Gnotobiotic Environments,* Henegan, J. B., Ed., Academic Press, New York, 1974, 575.
128. **Asano, T.,** Inorganic ions in cecal content of gnotobiotic rats, *Proc. Soc. Exp. Biol. Med.* 124, 424, 1967.
129. **Lindstedt, G., Lindstedt, S., and Gustafsson, B. E.,** Mucus in intestinal contents of germfree rats, *J. Exp. Med.,* 121, 201, 1965.
130. **Reussner, G., Jr., Andros, J., and Thiessen, R., Jr.,** Studies on the utilization of various starches and sugars in the rat, *J. Nutr.,* 80, 291, 1963.
131. **Luckey, T. D.,** Stress, Diet, and Microflora Interaction in Cecum Enlargement of Gnotobiotic Mice, in Proc. 5th Int. Symp. on Gnotobiology, Stockholm, Sweden, June 9 to 12, 1975, 69.
132. **Teah, B. A.,** personal communication, 1979.
133. **Seibert, K. A.,** Study of germfree and conventional SJL/J mice in relation to pathology, humoral immunity, and immunosuppression, Ph.D. thesis, University of Notre Dame, Notre Dame, Ind., 1973.
134. **Pleasants, J. R.,** unpublished data, 1979.
135. **Gordon, H. A., Wostmann, B. S., and Bruckner-Kardoss, E.,** Effects of microbial flora on cardiac output and other elements of blood circulation, *Proc. Soc. Exp. Biol. Med.,* 114, 301, 1963.
136. **Wostmann, B. S., Bruckner-Kardoss, E., and Knight, P. L., Jr.,** Cecal enlargement, cardiac output and oxygen consumption in germfree rats, *Proc. Soc. Exp. Biol. Med.,* 128, 137, 1968.
137. **Baez, S. and Gordon, H. A.,** Tone and reactivity of vascular smooth muscle in germfree rat mesentery, *J. Exp. Med.,* 134, 846, 1971.
138. **Bruckner-Kardoss, E. and Wostmann, B. S.,** Cecectomy of germfree rats, *Lab. Anim. Care,* 17, 542, 1967.
139. **Gustafsson, B.E. and Norman, A.,** Influence of the diet on the turnover of bile acids in germ-free and conventional rats, *Br. J. Nutr.,* 23, 429, 1969.
140. **Sacquet, E., Garnier, H., and Raibaud, P.,** Étude de la vitesse du transit gastrointestinal des spores d'une souche thermophile stricte de *Bacillus subtilis* chez le rat holoxènique, le rat axènique, le rat axèniuqe caecectomisé, *C. R. Acad. Sci. Paris,* 164, 532, 1970.
141. **Abrams, G. D., Bauer, H., and Sprinz, H.,** Influence of the normal flora on mucosal morphology and cellular renewal in the ileum. A comparison of germfree and conventional mice, *Lab. Invest.,* 12, 355, 1963.
142. **Hemmings, W. A., Ed.,** *Antigen Absorption From the Gut,* MTP Press, Lancaster, England, 1978.
143. **Luckey, T. D.,** Nutrition and biochemistry of germfree chicks, *Ann. N.Y. Acad. Sci.,* 78, 127, 1959.
144. **Pilgrim, H. I. and Thompson, D. B.,** An inexpensive autoclavable germfree mouse isolator, *Lab. Anim. Care,* 13, 602, 1963.
145. **Phillips, A. W., and Balish, E.,** Growth and invasiveness of *Candida albicans* in the germfree and conventional mouse after oral challenge, *Appl. Microbiol.,* 14, 737, 1966.
146. **Vessey, S. H.,** Effects of grouping on levels of circulating antibodies in mice, *Proc. Soc. Exp. Biol. Med.,* 115, 252, 1964.

147. **Baer, H.**, Long-term isolation stress and its effects on drug response in rodents, *Lab. Anim. Sci.*, 21, 341, 1971.
148. **Heneghan, J. B. and Gates, D. F.**, Effects of peracetic acid used in gnotobiotics on experimental animals, *Lab. Anim. Care*, 16, 96, 1966.
149. **Vieira, E. C., Nicoli, J., and Rogana, S. M. G.**, Some Problems in Rearing Germfree Aquatic Animals in Isolators, in Proc. 6th Int. Symp. on Gnotobiology, Ulm, Federal Republic of Germany, June 6 to 10, 1978, 100.
150. **Bock, F. G., Myers, H. K., and Fox, H. W.**, Co-carcinogenic activity of peroxycompounds, *J. Natl. Cancer Inst.*, 55, 1359, 1975.
151. **Trexler, P. C.**, Rapid removal of peracetic acid fumes from isolators, *Lab. Anim.*, 14, 47, 1980.
152. **Trexler, P. C.**, Transfer isolator to protect personnel from exposure to peracetic acid, *Lab. Anim.*, 13, 163, 1979.
153. **Reyniers, J. A., Sacksteder, M. R., and Ashburn, L. I.**, Multiple tumors in female germfree inbred albino mice exposed to bedding treated with ethylene oxide, *J. Natl. Cancer Inst.*, 32, 1045, 1964.
154. **Horton, R. E. and Hickey, J. L. S.**, Irradiated diets for rearing germfree guinea pigs, *Proc. Anim. Care Panel*, 11, 93, 1961.
155. **Wostmann, B. S. and Kellogg, T. F.**, Purified starch-casein diet for nutritional research with germfree rats, *Lab. Anim. Care*, 17, 589, 1967.
156. **Pleasants, J. R., Reddy, B. S., and Wostmann, B. S.**, Qualitative adequacy of a chemically defined liquid diet for reproducing germfree mice, *J. Nutr.*, 100, 498, 1970.
157. **Gustafsson, B. E.**, Introduction of specific microorganisms into germfree animals, in *Nutrition and Infection*, Ciba Study Group No. 31, Little, Brown, Boston, 1967, 16.
158. **Reddy, B. S.**, Calcium and magnesium absorption: role of intestinal microflora, *Fed. Proc.*, 30, 1815, 1971.
159. **Smith, J. C., Jr., McDaniel, E. G., and Doft, F. S.**, Urinary calculi in germfree rats: alleviated by varying the dietary minerals, in *Germfree Research: Biological Effect of Gnotobiotic Environments*, Heneghan, J. B., Ed., Academic Press, New York, 1973, 285.
160. **Ley, F. J., Bleby, J., Coates, M. E., and Paterson, J. S.**, Sterilization of laboratory animal diet using gamma irradiation, *Lab. Anim.*, 3, 221, 1969.
161. **Coates, M. E., Ford, J. E., Gregory, M. E., and Thompson, S. J.**, Effects of gamma-irradiation on the vitamin content of diets for laboratory animals, *Lab. Anim.*, 3, 39, 1969.
162. **Zimmerman, D. R. and Wostmann, B. S.**, Vitamin stability in diets sterilized for germfree animals, *J. Nutr.*, 79, 318, 1963.
163. **Greenstein, J. P., Birnbaum, S. M., Winitz, M., and Otey, M. C.**, Quantitative nutritional studies with water-soluble, chemically defined diets. I. Growth, reproduction and lactation in rats, *Arch. Biochem.*, 72, 396, 1957.
164. **Celesk, R. A., Asano, T., and Wagner, M.**, The size, pH and redox potential of the cecum in mice associated with various microbial floras, *Proc. Soc. Exp. Biol. Med.*, 151, 260, 1976.
165. **Syed, S. A., Abrams, G. D. and Freter, R.**, Efficiency of various intestinal bacteria in assuming normal functions of enteric flora after association with germ-free mice, *Infec. Immun.*, 2, 376, 1970.
166. **Schaedler, R. W., Dubos, R., and Costello, R.**, Association of germfree mice with bacteria isolated from normal mice, *J. Exp. Med.*, 122, 77, 1965.
167. **Sacquet, E., Lachkar, M., Mathis, C., and Raibaud, P.**, Cecal reduction in "Gnotoxenic" rats, in *Germfree Research: Biological Effect of Gnotobiotic Environments*, Heneghan, J. B., Ed., Academic Press, 1973, 545.
168. **Sedlacek, R. S. and Mason, K. A.**, A simple and inexpensive method for maintaining a defined flora mouse colony, *Lab. Anim. Sci.*, 27, 667, 1977.
169. **Trexler, P. C.**, personal communication, 1979.

Index

INDEX

A

G

H

I

J

K

L

M

N

P

W

X